Praise from Veterinarians, Authors & Book Reviewers

"The future is upon us and this **ground-breaking book** is a vital cornerstone. In dealing with cancer, our worst illness, this Survival Guide is educational, logical, expansive, embracing, honest – and so needed."

> Dr. Marty Goldstein, DVM
> Holistic veterinarian and Host, *Ask Martha Stewart's Vet* on Sirius Radio

"The message of this book jumps off the written page and into the heart of every reader, and will become the *at home* **bible for cancer care of dogs.** The authors have given you a sensible and systematic approach that practicing veterinarians will cherish. I found the book inspiring and, clearly, it will become part of my daily approach to cancer therapy for my own patients."

> Dr. Robert B. Cohen, VMD
> Bay Street Animal Hospital, New York

"Picking up *The Dog Cancer Survival Guide* is anything but a downer: it's an 'empowerer.' It will **make you feel like the best medical advocate for your dog.** It covers canine cancer topics to an unprecedented depth and breadth – from emotional coping strategies to prevention – in plain English. Read this book, and you will understand cancer stages, treatment options, and types, and much more. If you have just had the dreaded news, pick up a copy and it will guide the decisions your dog trusts you to make."

> Laure-Anne Viselé
> Dog behavior specialist and technical dog writer, CanisBonus.com

"I wish that I had had *The Dog Cancer Survival Guide* when my dearly beloved Flat-coated Retriever, Odin, contracted cancer. It would have provided me alternative courses of action, as well as some well needed "reality checks" which were not available from conversations with my veterinarian. It should be on **every dog owner's book shelf**--just in case..."

> Dr. Stanley Coren, PhD, FRSC
> author of many books, including *Born to Bark*

"A comprehensive guide that **distills both alternative and allopathic cancer treatments in dogs**… With the overwhelming amount of conflicting information about cancer prevention and treatment, this book provides a pet owner with an easy to follow approach to one of the most serious diseases in animals."

> Dr. Barbara Royal, DVM
> The Royal Treatment Veterinary Center, Oprah Winfrey's Chicago veterinarian

"Dr. Dressler and Dr. Ettinger have succeeded at the incredible task of writing a book that really helps pet parents who are struggling with the many decisions faced when their beloved animal has been diagnosed with cancer. Presenting and explaining **both complementary and conventional medical options for the treatment of cancer in 'one book' is a giant step** in the direction of 'one medicine' offering integrative medical choices to pet parents for the betterment of their animal's health."

> Dr. Bob Goldstein, VMD
> Veterinary Director for Healing Center for Animals, Westport CT

"*The Dog Cancer Survival Guide* is a great resource for pet parents whose dogs have been diagnosed with cancer. This **easy-to-read book** provides important information about canine cancers and discusses both conventional and holistic treatment options. Besides being informative, the book helps guide people as they navigate throu gh a difficult and emotional path."

> Dr. Ruth MacPete, DVM
> Practicing veterinarian, writer and media personality

"As a holistic dog care author, I knew exactly which experts to consult when my sweet Maltese Jiggy developed a large liver tumor. But even with advice from a top cancer specialist and help from a half dozen veterinary friends, I still had numerous questions. Exactly how should I adjust Jiggy's diet? What supplements should I add? What else could I do to help him? I found the answers I sought and more in Dr. Dressler's book. I was particularly impressed by the thoroughness of the information. The book is easy to read, but **wonderfully complete**. If your dog has cancer, I urge you to get two things: a second opinion ... and this book."

> Jan Rasmusen
> National award-winning author, *Scared Poopless: The Straight Scoop on Dog Care*

"*The Dog Cancer Survival Guide* is **indispensable reading** for any dog owner dealing with cancer… this book guides, supports and educates you!"

> Pennie Clark Ianniciello
> Costco Book Buyer

"*The Dog Cancer Survival Guide* is like a **crash course in canine cancer for the layperson**. It takes a bit of the mystery out of the dreaded disease by teaching some of the what, why, and how regarding cancer and cancer treatment. After reading it, you will be better equipped to help your best friend live life to the fullest, regardless of the prognosis."

> Therese Kopiwoda
> Pet Blogger and Founder of PetsitUSA.com

Praise from Readers

True Tails from Readers of *The Dog Cancer Survival Guide, First Edition*

Caesar Smashed the Statistics Because of This Book

"Caesar was diagnosed with a Mast Cell Tumor Grade/Stage III when he was just over a year old. We had a clean removal of the tumor from his inner rear thigh, and began chemo very shortly after. It was a very scary time, but we were fortunate to have a great vet who made some fantastic recommendations to a local pet store. The pet store owner made a recommendation to a lady who specifically deals with Boxers, and she recommended *The Dog Cancer Survival Guide*. We have recommended the guide to our vet and anyone we know who is going through this horrible process. Caesar has six month checkups and he is now approaching four years old. He has smashed most of the statistics out there and I directly attribute that to Dr. Dressler's book, our support group and the diet he is now on."

–MATT CANTINE, WHITE HOUSE, TENNESSEE

The Only Comprehensive Research ... With a Personal Touch

"Dr. Dressler's book was the only comprehensive research I was able to find on this subject. I found it to be thorough when dealing with all aspects of cancer in dogs with a personal touch that made me feel that he was addressing me personally."

– MIKE BERTULEIT, BOWLING GREEN, KENTUCKY

Our Reference

"We learned a significant amount from the book, and we continue to use it as a reference. Our standard poodle has had a tremendous boost out of chemo (there has been only one round of the 19 week protocol), and we are now at over nineteen months since the end of chemo and we are approaching two years since diagnosis. Apocaps is central to her regimen still, and we use and have used many other recommendations from the book as well. She has lived, and more importantly she has thrived, well beyond the statistical norm, and we credit the book and Apocaps for much of that success. Dr. Dressler is honest and realistic about prognosis, and yet he offers hope and evidence-based advice, and the learned and professional integration of conventional and alternative approaches is something that we did not find anywhere else.""

– BOB ANDERSEN, BROADWAY, VIRGINIA

Eighteen Months (and Counting) Without Spending $10,000

"The radiation oncologist that we saw after the tumor was removed suggested five weeks of radiation, for five days a week, all for the "small price" of $10,000! They only did the treatments between 8am and noon, making it virtually impossible for anyone who holds a job, but you could leave your dog there for the day for an additional charge of $35per day!! I was beside myself, but I also just wanted it all to go away, so initially, I was willing to pay. However, the more I thought about what that would be like for Yoda, I couldn't bring myself to do that. I thought, if his days are indeed numbered, I don't want to burn his little leg so that he can't run and chase bunnies and squirrels and deer. It was about the quality of his life. I had to find an alternative, and I couldn't be happier with the outcome. The radiation oncologist and his vet told me that if I didn't have the treatment done, his tumor would grow back in three to six months. Well it has been one year and six months and the growth hasn't come back! Certainly, he is aging and isn't as agile and playful as he was when he was a puppy, but his 10th birthday is April 30th and I couldn't be more happy! Ever since I adopted him (three days prior to his first birthday!) he has had a steak for his birthday. This year I may make it a filet mignon! THANK YOU for your book, because it gave me the support, strength and encouragement I needed to turn this entire situation from doom-and-gloom to complete possibility for something different."

– LORI, BETHESDA, MARYLAND

Took Me by the Hand ... and Became My "Bible"

"I read **The Dog Cancer Survival Guide The Dog Cancer Survival Guide** fervently. It has become my "bible" in taking care of my dog. This book has helped not only my dog feel better, but me, too!!! Any dog lover who is facing cancer in a beloved dog truly needs to read and devour the information in **The Dog Cancer Survival Guide**. This amazing book "took me by the hand" and has given me avenues that I never would have known about otherwise. I cannot recommend this amazing book enough or sing it's praises loud enough!!! Thank you, Thank you, Thank you, Dr. Dressler!!"

– CYNTHIA MCKINNON, SANFORD, FLORIDA

Helped Me Make Better Decisions: Worth Every Penny

"This book was extremely helpful to me. Even if it had not helped extend Apollo's life - which I am convinced it did as we were given maybe 6 months and we got 18 months - it explains things that you didn't hear at your appointment or were too overwhelmed to absorb. It helped me understand how canine cancer works and what to expect. This also prepared me for Apollo's appointments because I was able to ask educated questions and feel that I was a part of his healthcare team and not just his advocate. This book helped me make better decisions for Apollo so that we could preserve his quality of life for as long as possible. There are a lot of sad truths in this book that as a dog owner suffering from cancer, you don't really want to read ... but they are helpful. This book was worth every penny and I would (and have) recommended it to anyone who has a dog diagnosed with cancer."

– SANDY MILLER, PALO, IOWA

Even the Vet Thinks "We Beat This"

"My dog is a beagle named Gordon. We rescued him in 2000; we don't know how old he was at the time. In September of 2009 he suddenly got very sick. "Critically ill" my vet said. He ended up having a splenectomy. Lab results of the biopsy: hemangiosarcoma. Median life expectancy: 3-6 months. I asked the vet every question I could hoping there was a sliver of hope. Could the lab results be wrong? Could the splenectomy have removed all the cancer cells? Has a dog ever beat it? Our family agreed we didn't want to put him through any chemo or radiation. Well, a few weeks later I had Dr. Dressler's book in my hand and was following his Full Spectrum cancer care. I was cautiously optimistic. It's been 18 months since his surgery and he's doing great. The vet has even said that he "thinks we beat this." I've made some adjustments accordingly, but I still make Gordon's food and use the supplements according to Dr. Dressler's recommendation. I credit Dr. Dressler and his research and his book every bit as much as my vet and his surgery for saving Gordon's life."

– KIM GAU, STOW, OHIO

No Regrets

"When I heard the diagnosis that my dog had cancer I had no idea where to start, what to do. After taking some time to contemplate what was in front of us, I realized I needed more than just "medical" language, more than just a clinical approach. I needed a game plan for us and for our dog. I know her and love her and needed to make the right choices. The bottom line for me was "no regrets". I needed to make sure I understood the range of alternatives available, that I was making choices that were "right" given all the circumstances and that I would have peace whatever the outcome. The Dog Cancer Survival Guide gave me a starting place, empowered me to ask questions, push for alternatives, challenge the status quo and change the landscape. Whatever happens now, there will be no regrets on my part."

-VALERIE SACHS, PEPPER PIKE, OH

An Answer to Our Prayers

"When we first found out that our ten year-old Labrador had cancer, we had a sonogram done of his entire body. It showed that the cancer, which had started in his anal gland, had spread to several of his lymph glands, some of which were grossly enlarged. The vet, on seeing the sonogram results, told us our dog had 6 to 8 weeks to live. We immediately started using the strategies in Dr. Dressler's book, including the high-protein, low-carb diet, the cancer-busting supplements, the immunity-strengthening methods, and the self-esteem building activities. We first used alternated using Luteolin and EGCG, as well as Doxycycline, Modified Citrus Pectin, K-9 Immunity and Transfer Factor, Multivitamins, and Fish Oil. Then, when Apocaps came on the market, we used only Apocaps, along with the K-9 Immunity and Transfer Factor, Multivitamins, and Fish Oil. We used all of Dr. Dressler's immune boosting strategies, including having our dog in a completely dark room for nine hours of sleep each night. We gave our dog some type of exercise every day, whether it was a short walk, chasing a Frisbee in the yard, or playing ball in the house. We also played fetch and tug-of-war games with him. We also gave him hugs and plenty of petting every day. You could tell that he was happy...his tail was always wagging. Our dog lived not only 8 weeks, but 18 MONTHS longer, largely, we believe, due to Dr. Dressler's suggestions. He amazed every veterinarian we knew! We were so thankful to have the blessing of this extra time with him. In addition, his quality of life during all these extra months was very good. He was not constantly nauseous and fatigued, as he would have been if we had pursued chemotherapy. He was his normal, happy, energetic self. And when we realized the end was finally near, Dr. Dressler's advice on how to make the final decision and how to deal with the stress and sadness of losing our beloved friend really helped us. I can't tell you how thankful we are for this book! It was truly an answer to our prayers."

— HEATHER G., SAN ANTONIO, TEXAS

Like Having a Second (or Third) Opinion

"Having *The Dog Cancer Survival Guide* is truly like having a second opinion (in my case a third, along with my general practice vet and the canine oncologist overseeing Sparkle's treatment). It was so reassuring to me to have good questions to ask, and to see that what my vets are recommending agree with Dr. Dressler."

— SUSAN MCKAY, WINNIPEG, MANITOBA

If She Didn't Look at His Chart, "She'd Never Know Buddy Was Sick"

"I was devastated when I learned Buddy's cancer had returned. The same ache in my stomach, the tearing of my heart came back. He had seemed to recover nicely from the melanoma. I had great vets. His affected toe had been amputated. His previous x-rays were clear. How could this have happened again? I immediately started searching the internet. The news was so grim that I felt nothing but despair. How could I watch my pet, my friend, suffer through this? I clicked on Dr. Dressler's site and scanned the info on his book. I realized that I had to play an active role in Buddy's" treatment. I immediately ordered the book (e-mail copy.) I downloaded the 300+ pages as soon as i got home from school and began reading. While the news was still alarming I began to feel a little hope. Notes and read up on the research cited. I jotted down questions and was ready form my initial appointment with Buddy's new oncologist. I listened, questioned, and re-hashed what the oncologist explained to me. I quizzed her about her background, research practices and philosophy of medicine. I was amazed she actually agreed about the medication (doxycycline) to give to Buddy. I began Buddy on the Apocaps and massage therapy. We began daily walks and a dietary change from Beneful to an almost grain-free dog food. I spent more time telling him how grateful I was to him and much more time on my knees praying for a miracle. I began to "beef up" Buddy's weight and chart his progress. I held my breath and expected the worse. It hasn't happened yet. Buddy's blood count is great, his weight is up and his attitude is wonderful. While the doctor says is too soon to tell, she has suggested that he is getting better. She has actually said on more than one occasion that if she didn't have Buddy's chart in front of her she would never suspect he was at all sick. I keep waiting for the miracle of Buddy being healed. In the meantime, I know there are options to sitting back and letting the worse happen. I am more optimistic and grateful for Dr. Dressler's book. It has brought me closer to God, given me hope for the future, peace of mind, and avenues to follow to help Buddy and the rest of my family cope with this "trying" situation."

– DEBBIE GRANGER, CHESTERFIELD, MISSOURI

Grateful for Real Information Backed by Real Research

"We were very grateful to find such a resource as this book. There is so much misinformation on the net and so many self-proclaimed or new age experts today, it was a blessing to find real information backed by real research. Thank you!"

– STEVEN MCAFEE, FORT WAYNE, INDIANA

Nothing Is Sugar Coated

"DO NOT GIVE UP! Read the book, cry, laugh, and love with your pet. Use the book to formulate a realistic game plan in regards to attacking the disease to the best of your abilities. When you love a pet as evidently you do (given you found this book and Dr. D), you'll find trying will make a world of difference to you and will reflect on your pet as well. It was well worth the time, effort and money spent and I would pay tenfold for this information. Dr. Dressler presented everything in a REAL light. Nothing was sugar coated but at the same time the recommendations all had supporting information as to the "why" this can work, and how the research has come about."

– JULIAN TREVINO, ROSEVILLE, MICHIGAN

You Won't Be Disappointed

"Buy this book; you won't be disappointed. It will help you prepare yourself for all the challenges that come along with your dog having cancer. So many of the things he recommends seem so logical and are things you need to do to help yourself before you can help your dog. You find yourself saying "Wow, this makes so much sense" but yet it was something you hadn't actually thought of yourself."

– CHRISTINE DARG, WINNIPEG, MANITOBA

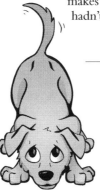

Special quantity discounts available for bulk purchases by veterinary and animal related organizations.

For details, please contact Maui Media at 1-800-675-3290 or via our website: www.MauiMedia.com

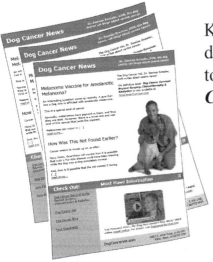
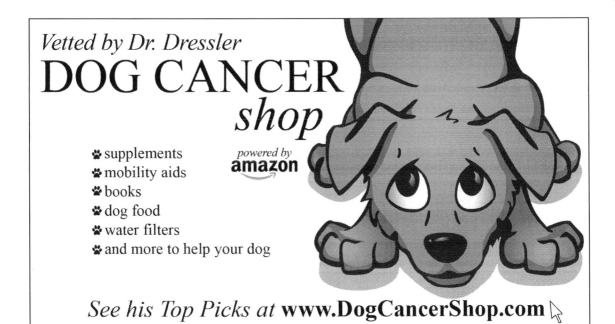

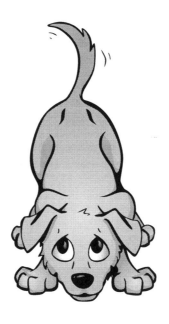

The Dog Cancer Survival Guide

Full Spectrum Treatments to
Optimize Your Dog's Life Quality & Longevity

Dr. Demian Dressler, DVM

with Dr. Susan Ettinger, DVM, Dip. ACVIM
Diplomate American College of Veterinary Internal Medicine (Oncology)

Maui Media, LLC
Maui, Hawaii

Published by
Maui Media LLC
www.MauiMedia.com

The Dog Cancer Survival Guide
Full Spectrum Treatments to Optimize Your Dog's Life Quality & Longevity
By Dr. Demian Dressler, DVM
with Dr. Susan Ettinger, DVM, Dip. ACVIM
Edited by Molly Jacobson

ISBN 978-0-9752631-5-0

www.DogCancerSurvival.com

Library of Congress Control Number: 2011929069

Back cover photo credit: Michelle Brady

Second Edition

Contents

Introduction

Glenda watched as I examined Max,[1] her nine-year-old Golden Retriever.[2] The surgical stitches from his bone biopsy looked fine: no swelling, no irritation, and a nice, clean mark. He would barely have a scar. Unfortunately, a scar was the least of his problems. I scratched his rump, and his big flag of a tail wagged in response. I turned to Glenda. "How has he been doing since his bone biopsy?"

"You were right about using cream cheese to hide his pills – he took them with no complaints … but he's still limping." She paused. "Did you get the report?"

"Yes, the biopsy report came in this morning," I said, rocking my head back and forth to loosen my neck. "The area of bone I showed you on the X-ray does not look good. It's a cancer named osteosarcoma."

Glenda looked like she'd been slapped. *Please don't cry,* I thought.

"What?"

"Osteosarcoma. Max has bone cancer."

"So my dog is going to die of cancer?"

"Well, we have different options. It's a little early to say how things will turn out," I dodged. I wasn't sure she was really ready to hear the survival statistics or contemplate the complex choices ahead of her.

"I thought you said this was an *infection.* You said it looked like an infection on the X-ray. I'm having a hard time believing what you're telling me."

"Infection was one of the possibilities we discussed. The other main possibility was cancer. Sometimes the two can look similar on an X-ray. We did the biopsy so we could be sure of the diagnosis. I'm really sorry. I wish the biopsy had come back negative."

Glenda placed one hand on her forehead, fingers shading her eyes. Her other hand dropped to Max's head as he leaned against her thigh. I waited, ready to offer tissues. After a moment, Glenda

---

[1] Not their real names. Throughout this book I will use real stories from my veterinary practice to illustrate important concepts and ideas. To protect the privacy of my clients and ensure clarity, I combine circumstances and client stories and change names and identifying factors. There are a few exceptions, which I note in the text. Readers of the previous edition of *The Dog Cancer Survival Guide* have also submitted stories about their own dogs, and these stories are clearly marked as "True Tails."

[2] Traditionally, breed names are not capitalized unless there is a proper name (English bulldog, Labrador retriever, etc.). I am breaking this grammatical rule by capitalizing every breed name, because, one, the text flows better that way, and, two, I don't want readers to think I am favoring some breeds over others.

wiped her eyes and cleared her throat.

"What are the options?"

Here we go, I thought, it's not going to get any easier to tell her this, so just start talking.

"The treatment options are surgery, chemotherapy, and radiation."

It was hard to look directly into Glenda's eyes, so I shuffled the papers in Max's file as I continued.

"Surgery, in the case of bone cancer, means amputation. Yes, dogs can walk on three legs, but no, it likely will not cure the cancer in the end.

This cancer has usually spread through the body by the time it is diagnosed. Without treatment, median survival is about two months, and owners usually choose to euthanize the dog because of the decline in life quality.

Chemotherapy added to the surgery extends median survival time to about ten months to a year, give or take.

Radiation can take away the pain for a few months, usually four or five."

I was finished listing treatments, so I stopped talking.

"Is that all? That's it?" Glenda whispered.

"Yes," I confirmed. "Those are the options we have."

"But, I, I mean…" Glenda stammered, "How, how did Max even get this?"

I resumed my standard cancer lecture.

"No one really knows exactly how cancer starts. It's a multi-factorial disease, which means many things can increase the odds of its happening."

"Is it his food?"

"Well, not really."

"I have heard vaccines can do it. What about toxins or something? Should he be wearing sunscreen?"

There was no one way to answer Glenda's questions, but, I didn't know how to explain that to her.

"We don't know the actual cause of cancer. The person who figures that out will get the Nobel Prize." I trailed off. Helping Glenda to understand and deal with Max's cancer diagnosis could take hours, and the next client was waiting.

We both knew I was avoiding her questions.

Glenda sighed and asked for some time to digest the bad news. I agreed, took out Max's sutures, dispensed more pain medication, and showed them out.

The visit had taken over half an hour. *I'm late,* I thought as I hurried Glenda's paperwork to the receptionist. *I've got to get back in the game and treat my next patient.*

The rest of the day was busy. I had few breaks, and those were filled with paperwork, ordering prescriptions and running my hospital. I felt distracted. Max's big brown eyes kept showing up in my thoughts. I saw him wagging his tail at me and comforting Glenda. *Dogs can be so generous. Too bad we're not more like them.*

I didn't know it yet, but Max's generosity was about to inspire a change in my career.

It's not unusual to feel exhausted at the end of a day filled with broken bones, infections, heart disease, diabetes and cancer, but that evening found me particularly drained; Max's predicament was still weighing on my mind.

I had recently noticed that more and more cancer cases were showing up in my practice. I repeated the same lines over and over: "Your dog has cancer ... radiation, surgery, chemotherapy ... crummy statistics ... no other options." Then, short on time, as most vets are, I hurried the poor dog lovers out the door, leaving them to wipe their eyes and wonder what to do.

I'm a healer, I thought, as I walked to my car. *Why couldn't I help more? How could I leave Glenda crying and Max still sick? I want to be able to do more. I'm tired of going home at night, feeling powerless and demoralized.*

Something is very wrong.

If I hadn't been so physically, emotionally, and mentally tired, I may have shrugged off these thoughts. But, something was different that night. Max had gotten to me somehow. So, instead, I contemplated these thoughts, especially the last one.

Something is very wrong.

Could that really be true? And if it were true, was there something I could do about it? Could I make what was wrong right?

I graduated from Cornell University, the top veterinary school in the country[3]. I had been practicing fifty to sixty hours per week since 1997. I had loads of information cemented into my brain, and incredible experience. And yet, I could not cure Max's cancer. I couldn't cure cancer in most of my patients.

---

[3] U.S. News & World Reports.

Glenda's world had turned upside down today, and I couldn't give her what she really needed: good answers, a solid plan, and (maybe just as important), hope and comfort.

My tired mind raced on. *What if there <u>are</u> other options? What else is there? There must be more to know, and there must be better tools. There are so many medical systems I have never used. What if I haven't learned all there is to learn?*

This may not sound like a radical train of thought to you, but for a conventional vet, it's tantamount to heresy. I have been trained to be skeptical of any practice, herb, technique, or medicine that has not been proven to work in a double-blind, placebo-controlled study. Unless it met this "gold standard," I scoffed at the treatment as unlikely to work ... and trying it would be a waste of time, money, or both.

Until that night, I thought this was a scientific mindset. But now, I wondered if I was just closed-minded.

By the time I turned into my driveway, I was questioning everything.

Did Max's diet actually contribute to his cancer? What about vaccines? Do toxins in our environment affect dogs? My first-rate veterinary education had never addressed many of these angles.

My conscience nagged me. *What did I really know?* It had been a few years since I left school. I had had little time to keep up with the latest research.

*When did I last read original cancer literature? Are chemotherapy, radiation, and surgery **really** all that veterinary medicine can offer Max? Is he getting short-changed? What else can I do besides what I have been trained to do? There must be more options!*

Since that night, I have been searching for the answers to these and many more questions. I rediscovered a passion for research, and have been tireless in my search for answers about the causes of dog cancer and, of course, the best treatments. As it turns out, there are more options, and there is more we can do.

Your Survival Guide

"Cancer" is the last word dog lovers want to hear from their veterinarian. Many feel their dogs are part of the family, and those two syllables can release a torrent of fear, confusion, anger, guilt, and grief, just as if a human family member were sick. I've seen clients "numb out" in front of me, burst into disbelieving, hysterical laughter or violent rages, and even threaten suicide.

I can understand where these extreme responses come from, because I am a lifelong dog lover, too. At first, this diagnosis can seem as urgent, hopeless, and final as a tsunami towering on the horizon.

Dog cancer *is* an emergency, and if it is the tsunami you are facing, think of this book as your survival guide. When tsunami warnings sound in my home state of Hawaii, authorities remind us to pack food and water, gather our loved ones, and quickly but calmly move to higher ground.

In that spirit, this book is written to help you calm down, think clearly, and choose wisely from among the tools that have been credibly shown to help canine cancer.

Full Spectrum Cancer Care

Every cancer case is as unique as the dog herself[1], but it's also true that cancer cases are similar to each other. Cancers can be similar in how they begin, develop, spread, and affect surrounding tissues. On the other side of the equation, the body always mobilizes certain systems to try to fight off the cancer.

By taking a bird's eye view of dog cancer and accounting for these common factors, I've developed a standard plan that can be used to target any dog cancer diagnosis, no matter what type it may be. I call my approach Full Spectrum cancer care because it includes everything I've found that has been shown to be helpful for dogs with cancer.

Conventional western medical tools are included, but my Full Spectrum approach also includes the very best options from alternative medicine, botanical nutraceuticals, supplements, strategic immune system boosters, nutrition, emotional management strategies, and even some cutting edge mind-body medicine techniques that deliberately modify brain chemistry.

There's No Expiration Date

You may have heard "there's nothing we can do," or "the only options are chemotherapy and radiation."

You may have heard your dog has one week or two months or six months left.

It doesn't matter what you've heard. No one has a crystal ball, no matter how many letters or credentials line up after his name. These estimates – and, by the way, most of the numbers in this book – are educated guesses, based on general rules of thumb.

As you'll learn later, not even veterinary oncologists (animal cancer specialists) all agree on those rules of thumb. **Your individual dog does not have an expiration date, and there is plenty you can do to help.**

Imagine looking back at this time in your life, five years from now, and having not a single regret. You can help your dog fight cancer, and, just as important – maybe more important – you can honor your dog's life by living each moment to the fullest, starting now.

---

[1] It is clumsy to refer to dogs as he/she, so I alternate their genders throughout this book. I do the same when referring to veterinarians and other professionals.

_____ • _____

Your individual dog does not have an expiration date, and there is plenty you can do to help. Imagine looking back at this time in your life five years from now and having not a single regret.

_____ • _____

We both have jobs here. My job is to lay out a well-researched, practical and comprehensive survival guide, including every available tool credibly shown to help fight cancer and help your dog.

Your job is to take a deep breath (you'll learn later why breathing is so important), read, and take action on what you learn.

Even if you feel miserable right now, reading this book is an act of hope and optimism. This is good news, because, in my experience, the pragmatic dog lover who is willing to learn does the best job of dealing with and fighting dog cancer.

The Dog Cancer Vet

I'm a skeptic by nature, so if an author claims to know something about a subject, I want to know a little bit about him before I give him my trust. No matter who we may be, we all have our own experiences, perspectives, and objectives. Knowing something about the author's background helps me to understand how he arrives at his conclusions, and whether he may have any underlying biases or a hidden agenda.

I recommend you adopt a similar attitude as you learn about your dog's cancer. Take everything you hear and read (even in this book) with a grain of salt. As you'll discover, cancer is not simple, and there are many competing theories, treatments and approaches. What works for one dog may not work for another.

At this time there is no one cure for systemic cancer and, therefore, no absolute right way to treat it. With all of the possibilities out there, you will need to use discernment to weigh all the factors and find the best way to treat your dog's cancer.

In the spirit of full disclosure, I'm going to tell you a little more about my own story, so you can get to know me, and be alert to my particular biases and attitudes.

First things first: I am a dog lover, through and through. When clients tell me their dog is their best friend, I know exactly what they mean. If loving dogs is genetic, I inherited it from my mother, Lucy. She is the founder of the Pacific Primate Sanctuary on Maui, and yet, she still finds room in her home and heart for a pack of five Chihuahuas. My love of dogs gives me a unique understanding of how painful it is to have a dog with cancer, and that has helped me to write this book.

Second (and this is important): I am not an oncologist. I am a general practice vet who works in one of the most isolated places on Earth. Hawaii is about 3,000 miles from California, in the middle of the Pacific. There are very few veterinary specialists; I simply don't have the option to refer advanced cases out of my practice. I deal with every type of animal illness and concern, every day. This makes my experience broad and very wide in scope compared to many of my colleagues on the mainland. I am sometimes forced to take a broad view of illnesses and look for overall patterns to help me treat patients, and this can result in unusual methods and unconventional ideas.

Even though I'm not an oncologist, I've been nicknamed the "dog cancer vet" by readers and clients, because of my special interest in canine cancer, which was sparked by Max. I spend my extra time devoted to researching and writing about it on my blog www.DogCancerBlog.com.

I've studied every aspect of canine cancer treatment. I read oncology textbooks cover to cover. I pore over every paper I can find. I talk to every researcher I can get on the phone and pepper those I can't with emails. I fly to veterinary oncology conferences and follow every lead that presents itself in my search for dog cancer answers.

———— • ————

"The pragmatic dog lover, who is willing to learn does the best job of dealing with and fighting dog cancer."

———— • ————

Until I started this research, I identified myself as a conventional vet. I did not have much respect for "alternative" or "holistic" vets who – in my opinion – were not as scientific as I.

But over time, as I followed leads offered by cutting-edge research, I found myself going, in a sense, "down the rabbit hole." Like Alice entering Wonderland, things no longer appeared black and white. Rules I had lived by seemed to bend. Assumptions I'd been taught were turned upside down. I found myself venturing far from conventional medicine: first into alternative medicine, and then beyond, to places, theories, and therapies I never would have guessed had anything to do with treating cancer.

I started applying what I had learned with dogs in my practice, and saw results I could never have expected. Not everything worked perfectly, or worked exactly as I hoped it would. But it was surprising to me how many therapies, beyond chemotherapy, surgery, and radiation, can help a dog with cancer.

In the first years of my research, I was really burning the midnight oil, while still running my full-time veterinary hospital. I was glad to be helping the dogs in my practice, of course; what bugged me was that this information was scattered all over the place.

Just like many dog lovers who get a cancer diagnosis, I had started with the Internet as my first source of information, and boy, was there a lot of it out there. Some of it, I just couldn't stomach. Online forums and blogs are filled with people sharing their own stories or recommendations – but how much of this can be trusted? When I look at them from a medical perspective (even my expanded one), many posts are definitely suspect.

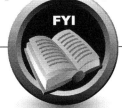

Dogs and Humans: Closer Than We Know

When it comes to cancer, dogs are physiologically very similar to humans: so much so that they are often the preferred test animals in human cancer treatment trials. Because of this, most veterinary cancer treatments actually come from human medicine. (Only two drugs have been FDA-approved specifically for dog cancer, both very recently.) Usually, once a treatment has been approved for human use, vets start evaluating it in dogs, including optimal dosing schedules and possible side effects.

Knowing this, I decided to try using botanicals that are currently being tested for use in humans. We will likely use them in dogs eventually, so why wait ten or twenty years for human approval, when cancer is the number one killer of dogs today?

*You'll see sidebars like this one used throughout this book. These special sections add to or enhance the regular text.

Simple but Powerful

After sifting through personal anecdotes, hyperbole, outright product sales pitches and miscellaneous gobbledygook, what I found really shifted my entire medical perspective on animal health and disease.

Some very simple lifestyle shifts may help fight cancer, for example: changing the diet and using certain supplements.

I also learned how much emotions impact disease development in humans, and was impressed by the possibility that our dogs' emotions could impact canine cancer development. Our own human emotions, by influencing our thought processes, could also ultimately have an impact on the outcome of canine cancer.

I was surprised to find that some cutting-edge human cancer research is not looking for a cure in isolated chemicals. Instead, these research labs are exploring natural botanicals – agents found in plants – which induce apoptosis in cancer cells.

Apoptosis is the completely normal process that causes the natural death of a cell when it has lived to the end of its life. Cancer cells can turn apoptosis off, allowing themselves to grow indefinitely, at the expense of the body. Certain botanicals, called "apoptogens," can turn apoptosis back on in the cancer cell, causing it to die a natural death (or, in the more colorful language of cancer researchers, "commit cell suicide").

I wrote about all of this cutting-edge research,

including information about some powerful apoptogens, in the first edition of this book. I received three main pieces of feedback about that edition:

The emotional management tools really helped dog lovers to calm down, think clearly and choose wisely.

Dogs like the diet I recommend, and it seems to help them feel better.

The apoptogens I recommend are not only effective, but also difficult to procure and clumsy to combine.

This feedback reflected the challenges I was having with my clients on Maui. Finding and preparing the apoptogens I recommend was tiresome and taking too much time out of already busy lives.

The good news was: these apoptogens, when given, were actually helping dogs. Dogs with lethargy and pain were perking up, sometimes within a day of taking the supplements. Even more exciting, some dogs (not all, but a significant number) experienced a shrinking of their tumors.

My natural skepticism had not let me imagine this outcome, and it was humbling to realize how much there was still to learn. As I continued to work with these cutting edge apoptogens, I grew happier with the results and ultimately decided to make them easier to find and administer and finally, invented a supplement. Today, you can find Apocaps online at Amazon.com (both in the U.S. and in Europe), in veterinary practices across the U.S., and at www.DogCancerShop.com.

Backlash

Not everyone has been happy with my work. I give some controversial advice, and I have received backlash from some of my colleagues, who believe their methods and livelihoods are being questioned. The "dog cancer vet" nickname rankles some oncologists, and I've even been threatened professionally. One blog comment I received – anonymous, but claiming to be from an oncologist – called me a "heretic" and warned me I was "playing with fire."

I shared this with a sympathetic colleague, who reminded me of the story of Ignaz Semmelweis. After giving birth in his mid-1800's Vienna hospital, mothers died of puerperal fever at a huge rate of 18%. Once his doctors were required to wash their hands after performing autopsies, the death rate dropped to just 2%. Semmelweis was an early proponent of the theory of germs (it inspired his policy change), which no one had yet proven to the satisfaction of the medical community. Despite his obvious success, he went to his grave discredited as a radical and a heretic. Years later, Louis Pasteur finally "proved" Semmelweis was correct in claiming that germs were responsible for, among other things, puerperal fever.

I take inspiration from Semmelweis, and many other thinkers and inventors, who take a wide-angle view to discover new methods. I'm hoping that by looking at dog cancer in this way, reviewing the basics of how the body works, and looking ahead to future breakthroughs, we can find new angles and maybe – dare I say it? – even hope to cure cancer, someday.

I Meet Dr. Susan Ettinger (Again)

After I invented Apocaps, it was clear the first edition of my book needed updating and revising. My publisher and I started planning the second edition.

During this time, I attended a veterinary oncology conference, where I ran into a friend from vet school, Dr. Susan Ettinger. Dr. Ettinger is a hotshot veterinary oncologist at the prestigious Animal Specialty Center, in Yonkers, New York.

After catching up with each other, Dr. Ettinger realized I was the vet who blogs at www.DogCancerBlog.com and the author of this book. She narrowed her eyes and said, "Who supervised your section on oncology?" When I told her I had, she sniffed.

"You should have an oncologist do it."

"Why don't you?" I asked.

Our partnership makes perfect sense. As a medical oncologist in a large specialty practice, she prescribes chemotherapy every single day of her career … but she's open to new ideas and concepts. I'm interested in treatments beyond the conventional options … but I don't exclude them.

Luckily for all of us (although perhaps not so much for her very patient husband and two young sons), she agreed we would make a good team, and joined me as my co-author.

Dr. Ettinger's contribution is invaluable. While most of the book is still in my voice, her experience and formal oncology training has informed every paragraph. She has expanded and solidified the scope of the section on conventional medicine, so much so that our editor asked her to write entire chapters in her own voice. Her section contains her best recommendations from conventional medicine for twelve common dog cancers.

Dr. Ettinger and I are physically separated by an ocean and a continent and our collaboration stretches one quarter of the way around the planet. It also spans the Full Spectrum of what's available for canine cancer treatments. This book tells you everything we want you to know if your dog has cancer of any kind.

How This Book Is Organized

The Dog Cancer Survival Guide, 2nd Edition, is divided into five parts, plus five appendices and an index.

Section I: My Dog Has Cancer, Now What? This section covers a lot of ground, including how to tinker with your mindset, so you can make good decisions about your dog's cancer.

Section II: What You Should Know about Dog Cancer covers some of the most important things you must know about the root causes of cancer, so you can make good decisions for your dog.

Section III: Full Spectrum Cancer Care takes you through the five most important facets of cancer care: conventional medicine, apoptogens, strategic boosting of the immune system, diet, and modifying your dog's brain chemistry.

Section IV: Making Confident Choices gives you a step-by-step framework from which you can make decisions for your own dog's cancer case. There is also a section on end-of-life care, advice for working with your veterinarian or oncologist, and some advice about how to get and stay organized.

Section V: From the Oncologist is Dr. Ettinger's section of the book. She describes each of the twelve common canine cancers in detail, including lymphoma, mast cell tumors, mammary cancer, osteosarcoma, hemangiosarcoma, transitional cell carcinoma, oral cancers, malignant melanoma, nasal tumors, soft tissue sarcomas, brain tumors, and anal gland tumors. She gives her most up-to-date recommendations for treatments from a conventional perspective and discusses the most common chemotherapy drugs, including their side effects.

Two Authors, One Voice

Writing about cancer is tricky, because so little is known *for sure.* While most of the time Dr. Ettinger and I agree with each other, we do disagree on some occasions. In these cases, it will be noted in the text, or you will see a sidebar explaining the difference in our perspectives.

My strongest recommendation is that you start at the beginning of the book and read all the way through, including Dr. Ettinger's chapter on your dog's cancer. When you do this, you will have learned how to handle your dog's cancer in the most thoughtful, compassionate, and "full spectrum" manner I can imagine.

Sidebar Symbols

There are many sidebars throughout this book which contain information that enhances the main text or goes into great depth on a subject. Here are the symbols we use for each type of sidebar so you'll be able to "tell at a glance" what information is presented.

 These sidebars allow me to present my ideas and get larger points across that may be only briefly discussed in the main text.

 Because most of the book is my voice, it might sound like Dr. Ettinger isn't contributing. She is, of course, but these sidebars give her a chance to step out from "behind the scenes" and give her own thoughts in her own words.

 These sidebars present information that is crucial to your understanding of the topic under discussion or for dog cancer in general.

 If something was stated earlier that needs to be repeated, you'll be reminded in these sidebars.

 These sidebars usually illustrate specific examples of what's being discussed in the main section.

 These sidebars alert you if there are important exceptions to the topic under discussion.

 As you'll find out, I look at cancer as a living system. In these sidebars I have the space to share this "wide angle view" with you.

 You will see these sidebars when I need to remind you to consult with your vet for specific advice about the topic at hand.

 These sidebars are written by readers of the first edition of this book. They are "true tails" of personal experiences with dog cancer. Each True Tail was written to – and for –

you, the reader of this edition, by other dog lovers who have benefitted from this guide and my Full Spectrum approach. We could only include a fraction of those we received; but hopefully these voices will remind you that you are not the first one to deal with dog cancer. There are people who understand what you are going through, and have reached out deliberately to support you at this time.

This Book Does Not Substitute for Your Veterinarian's Guidance

I want to remind you that this book is in no way a substitute for professional, in-person care from your own vet. Dr. Ettinger and I do not recommend you follow any advice for treating cancer without having a vet examine your dog and diagnose your dog.

A lot of what we recommend we would not advise for a healthy dog, or for a dog that is sick with an illness other than cancer. Because of this, I urge you to bring your vet into the conversation we have in these pages. This book is designed to help you work closely with him or her.

Part I:
My Dog Has Cancer ...
Now What?

In this section of the book we'll lay the foundation for Full Spectrum cancer care. We'll talk about your role in your dog's cancer care, answer the three most pressing questions dog lovers have and remind you of your dog's inherent "super powers," in preparation for learning more about dog cancer.

Chapter 1: Your Role

When your dog has cancer, everything changes. An otherwise typical moment – your dog running after a ball – can seem precious and fleeting. Some people stay up at night, watching their dog's breathing, wondering how many more breaths she has. Time flies by … or slows down. Your whole life may seem unstable. You may ride the "emotional rollercoaster," or you may feel stuck in an "emotional rut."

This disorientation and emotional upset is normal, of course, but it can interfere with getting your dog the help she needs right now. Over the years, I have noticed that dog lovers who adopt a certain kind of attitude, role and mindset seem to have the most success dealing with their dog's cancer. I'll describe that role in this chapter, and I encourage you to consider adopting it for yourself and your dog.

Be Your Dog's Guardian

If you are like most dog lovers, you may still have difficulty believing you must deal with dog cancer at all.

Disbelief is a normal reaction; as a fellow dog lover, I truly sympathize. But disbelief doesn't help your dog. Changing your thoughts, from "I can't believe this" into "I can deal with this," is your first priority.

Your first step takes you from being a *Dog Lover* to becoming a *Dog Guardian*.

What's the difference? It's subtle, but important.

For a *Dog Lover,* a dog is a family member, and watching a beloved family member get sick or feel pain is extremely upsetting. A Dog Lover's primary mode of relating is through shared emotional bonding.

A *Dog Guardian* feels the same way about her dog, but her first priority is protecting her dog. This is an important responsibility, because dogs have evolved to become dependent on us, and dogs with cancer are particularly vulnerable. As your dog's guardian, you will now face many confusing decisions, and you will need to stay calm in order to choose wisely.

In the extreme urgency of dealing with a dog cancer diagnosis, you could imagine the role of a guardian as much like the role of a bodyguard. The world's best-trained bodyguards are United States

Secret Service Agents, so let's take a look at how they operate.

If the President of the United States is in physical danger, his Secret Service agents take charge of his person and his actions. Even if the President wants to stay in a dangerous place – to help others or to make sure his family is all right – his guardians will not allow it. Their priority is the President's safety. They are empowered, confident, and mentally and physically prepared to deal with anything, even with the President, himself. They protect him, defend his boundaries, assess situations with wisdom and fight when necessary.

Guardians, whether they guard Presidents or pooches, set their own priorities and take action based only on those priorities.

As your dog's guardian, you acknowledge that you are in charge, that only you know your dog as well as you, and that no one else (not even your vet) can truly know what is best for you and your dog. You are her fiercest advocate for health and happiness. You take advice from well-informed and trusted sources; you also make the final decisions. You are empowered.

So, then, what is your first priority, if you are your dog's guardian? When I had just graduated from veterinary school, my answer was "Finding the right treatment as soon as possible."

Today, after years of research and experience, I know better. Your first priority is to clear your mind and heart of emotional upset.

"Your first priority is not to find the right treatment for your dog. Your first priority is to clear your mind and heart of emotional upset."

First Priority: Deal with Your Emotions

Many readers feel uncomfortable with that last sentence. A cancer diagnosis is extreme, pressing and deadly. Doing anything that isn't directly related to treating the cancer itself can seem like a waste of time. Surprisingly, dealing with disorienting emotions like disbelief, grief, anger, numbness, and shock is directly related to treating the cancer.

I didn't always think that emotions played such a big a role. As an analytical scientist, I generally feel more comfortable talking about treatment options than talking about feelings.

My research changed my mind. There are certain realities that affect all humans, no matter how emotional or analytical we think we are. Let's get a few reality checks.

Reality Check Number One

If you are emotionally aroused (angry, sad, fearful, shocked, or numb), your brain is most likely blocked from learning anything new. Numerous studies have shown this to be true, and both Dr. Ettinger and I have personally experienced this phenomenon in our own practices.

When emotionally upset, our brains tend to narrow their focus to the topic causing the distress. Later, we remember mostly what upset us, and little else.

You may have already experienced this. Think back to the appointment at which your vet gave you the diagnosis of canine cancer. Can you remember the details of what he advised? Or do you just remember hearing the words "cancer" or "six months"? Some people just remember the sweat on the vet's forehead, or the color of his scrubs. Others remember that they're supposed to feed a high protein diet, but not the median survival time for this cancer, the name of the recommended oncologist, or what supplements to get.

> ### My Husband – The Vet – Didn't Know How To Deal, Either
>
>
>
> "When LP was first diagnosed, we were distraught and felt completely hopeless. My husband is an equine vet - yet he couldn't deal with such devastating news any better than I did. We were emotional disasters - yet when I read Dr. Dressler's book, I realized that everyone goes through the exact same things we were. We need to be strong for our dogs, we need to be focused. We don't know where this journey will take us but we are now on a steady course. LP is a happy guy, he's doing well right now and we're taking one day at a time. I am sure this has helped LP."
>
> – Susie, Millwood, Virginia

If you are reading this book while angry, sad, fearful, or numb, you run the risk of missing crucial information. You're likely to fixate on an isolated fact that matches your current mood, while ignoring the context and the relevant advice. When you clear some of those emotions first, you will absorb what you read better: you won't have to read a chapter over and over to understand it, or worse, make mistakes based on a faulty reading.

As Abraham Lincoln once said, "Give me six hours to chop down a tree and I will spend the first four sharpening the axe."

Releasing your emotions – whatever they are – is not a waste of time; in fact, it is an efficient use of your time. The simple exercises outlined in the next chapter don't take long. If you ignore them and just suppress your emotions, you'll be wasting energy and time you probably need right now.

There is another reason you should deal with your emotions:

Reality Check Number Two

During periods of great stress, the human brain is likely to rely on old, usually unconscious, patterns or "rules of thumb" to make decisions, not logic.

The brain helps us live efficiently by building shortcuts for routine tasks. You may remember learning to tie your shoe, and how difficult it was to memorize all those steps in the right order. Today, you can tie your shoe while reading the paper, having a conversation or even when you're half asleep. Your brain has built up rules of thumb so that you can tie your shoe on automatic pilot.

Using rules of thumb can be very effective when the stakes are low, but disastrous when the stakes are high, when we're in a new situation, or when existing rules of thumb are irrelevant.

Unfortunately, if the brain is under what scientists call "disruptive stress," (a cancer diagnosis certainly causes this level of stress for most guardians dealing with dog cancer), the part of the brain that is most active is usually the older (sometimes called "reptilian") brain. This part of the brain is not rational; it's instinctive. It tends to apply any rule of thumb that seems vaguely related, whether it is helpful or not. Depending upon the situation, this could be fatal.

For example, a guardian may have known a human who died of cancer after a long series of terribly painful chemotherapy treatments. This experience could have caused the creation of a rule of thumb about chemotherapy: *all cancer patients suffer during chemotherapy treatments, and then they die anyway.*

If the vet recommends chemotherapy, the guardian's "old" brain may apply this rule of thumb as soon as that word is spoken. The "higher" brain might be blocked, so that information about side effects, remission rates, and median survival times is discarded as irrelevant. As a result, the guardian instinctively decides not to use chemotherapy. For some cancers, for some dogs, and for some guardians, this automatic decision could be the right one. But for some cancers, for some dogs, and for some guardians, this automatic decision might be a grave error that is regretted for years.

Keep this critical fact in mind: when you are under great stress, your brain has an instinctive tendency to make automatic decisions without processing all of the available information and without consulting your brain's center of logic. Managing your stress levels by managing your emotions can help you to avoid automatic, faulty decision-making.

There is one more reason managing emotions is a guardian's first priority.

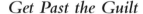

Get Past the Guilt

"Getting past the guilt at the very beginning is absolutely essential. You are no good to your dog while you're wrapped up in yourself."

– *Mignon Owens, Jessup, Maryland*

Reality Check Number Three

Even the most logical of human minds tends to lean toward delusional thinking during times of stress.

A brain under great stress doesn't handle information well, especially if there are gaps in its knowledge or if there is a great deal of complexity. Instead, the brain tends make up "facts" and simplify complicated issues. In certain situations, the otherwise normal human brain actually leans toward what researchers call "delusional thinking."

"I have to understand what caused her cancer," a client told me. "I need closure on this. It's driving me crazy. I can't think about anything else."

We went over her dog Lucky's medical history, but found no single, obvious cause for her hemangiosarcoma. "This is typical," I explained, "We will probably never know the one cause of the cancer. More likely, it was caused by many things, happening over a long period of time."

There was a long pause on the line. She finally said, "It was the vaccine. They gave her a third round of vaccinations when she was three months old, and something inside said not to let them do it. But I did. That's what it was."

"I agree there is some evidence connecting cancer with vaccinations," I said. "But I can't possibly agree, with absolute certainty, that a vaccination given ten years ago definitely caused this cancer today. It's more likely that several things came together to cause this condition."

"That was definitely it. I knew they shouldn't have done it!" she replied.

This is an example of what can happen to a normal brain under great stress. My client simply could not deal with not knowing a specific answer to her burning question. In response, her brain made up a story ("it was the vaccine") that simplified everything. She felt better, momentarily. However, if her next dog actually needs a vaccination, then today's delusional thinking could become tomorrow's dangerous rule of thumb.

A cancer diagnosis represents treacherous

> ### *Permission to Grieve: for One Week!*
>
> **TRUE TAILS**
>
> "When we first found out about Gordon's cancer, all I wanted to do was hold him and cry. But if we ended up losing him, what would our last few weeks together have been like? So, with Dr. Dressler's point in mind, I gave myself permission to grieve but for no longer than one week. When that week was up, I was going to put the sadness aside and love and enjoy my dog every minute I still had him. Once I read Dr. Dressler's book I had hope and faith that something could be done. That alone gave me a brighter outlook. Once I started to implement his recommendations, the outlook got even brighter. I am confident that Gordon could sense all this positive energy and love for him and responded to it."
>
> – *Kim Gau, Stow, Ohio*

territory for the normal brain. Cancer diagnoses are frustratingly devoid of complete, accurate information. For example:

> *Has it spread?* We don't think so – but we can't be sure.
>
> *Will the surgery get it all out?* We hope so, but we won't know until we get the biopsy back. And, even then, we still won't know for sure.
>
> *How long does he have?* We can talk about median survival times, but those aren't directly relevant. Those times are true for a particular group of dogs in a particular study – but not for your particular dog, now.

No matter how much we know about cancer, we know too little, and cancer is an inherently complex illness. The stress generated by these two facts in our human brains is enormous. In this situation, delusional thinking is *very likely* to happen for any one of us. Delusion is a bad place from which to make decisions about cancer care. No matter how sane you may be, during times of unmanaged stress you and I and every other human are *likely* to make delusional decisions. Reducing your stress is critical.

It's All about You

Like it or not, **you** are the "X factor" in treating your dog's cancer. Your mind and heart can be your best advisors or your worst enemies.

There are several exercises that can help you to decrease your emotional burden, reconnect to a clear-thinking mindset, and re-establish a clean, nurturing, compassionate relationship with your dog.

The emotional management exercises in the next chapter can be used at any time, and checking them out now is your first priority. Just as a Secret Service agent is always on the watch for trouble, a dog guardian is vigilant and keeps his mind and heart clear.

Chapter 2: Mission Critical: Emotional Management

This chapter contains several emotional management exercises, which I consider "mission critical" for any guardian while dealing with dog cancer. Sound dramatic? It may be. Let me tell you a story about how upset emotions negatively influenced one dog's cancer outcome.

Jake was still reeling from hearing about his dog Fluke's cancer diagnosis. After a minute, he blurted, "He's dying anyway. Let's just put him down and get it over with."

I jumped in. The diagnosis, while serious, was not an immediate death sentence. In fact, this particular cancer seemed to respond very well to the supplements I sometimes recommend, and had a good track record with chemotherapy, too. Several clients had gained months of good quality life with almost no side effects. Jake had time to consider all of Fluke's options while starting her on some inexpensive dietary and mind-body treatments. Her pain could be managed, and she could actually feel better, while we tried to give her more time.

But, Jake's mind was made up. He was not "going to put Fluke through this," and he "couldn't watch Fluke die a slow, painful death." He wanted it quick, painless, and now.

Jake is a very loving guardian, so I knew he wasn't being heartless. Although he didn't share his personal story with me, I would bet a hefty sum that he once watched a loved one go through a

Desperate Times Call for Goofy Exercises

"Many of these exercises seem goofy or ridiculous, but I figured in desperate times ... so I tried all of them. Imagine my surprise when almost all of them had me noticing a significant change in my dog's attitude. Even the smallest thing can help. Don't we always say "attitude is everything?" In doing **Pledge of Thanks** on a regular basis throughout any given day I was amazed to find out just how much I underappreciated my best buddy. I now have an even more responsive and enthusiastic best friend. I truly believe a happy dog is a healthier one. Lucky for me it works for people too – my outlook has improved drastically."

– Holly Rydman,
Olympia, Washington

painful, prolonged death process, and thought he was saving his dog from a fate worse than euthanasia. Jake had a rule of thumb running his brain, and that rule of thumb spoke up and made the decision for him. There was no talking him out of it, no matter how much evidence I had.

Catching yourself in moments like this is critical to taking good care of your dog. If you've ever flown on a commercial airliner, you remember that you are advised in the pre-flight announcements that in an emergency, you must put on your own oxygen mask before you start helping others – even your own children. The reason for this is simple: if you are gasping for air and about to pass out, you can't help those who really need you.

Guardians get to choose their emotional states. It may seem a little wacky to say this – but consider it for a moment. There is probably a part of your life in which you set aside everything else to focus on the task at hand. Maybe it is when you go to work, or when you play a sport, or when you spend time with your kids. Most people can literally choose to feel something different, if they must.

The clearer your mind and heart are, the easier you learn. The more you learn about cancer and

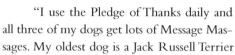

Is It Time for My Massage?

"I use the Pledge of Thanks daily and all three of my dogs get lots of Message Massages. My oldest dog is a Jack Russell Terrier named Gorilla and last year was a rough one for him. He went through an agonizing vestibular incident, lost most of his sight and toward the end of the year had a series of seizures that left us suspecting that a brain tumor was the cause of his fading cognition and failing health. Massage has always been a part of my dog's lives because it is my profession. I have a school in Seattle called the Northwest School of Animal Massage and Gorilla is the school mascot! ... last year, those massages became as important to me as they were to Gorilla. The time I spent cradling his frail body and lovingly stroking his coat lifted both of our spirits and empowered me as his guardian to be able to provide him comfort. When he didn't want to eat, massaging him would revive his appetite and then help him keep his food down. When he was restless and couldn't sleep through the nights, I would lie on the floor with him massaging his crown and his belly until he was snoring peacefully. And when his vestibular incident left him with a dramatic head tilt and sore muscles that nearly immobilized him, the massage helped restore his posture and his independence. Using many of the suggestions from Dr. Dressler's book and website and with the help of a TCM Veterinarian who provides acupuncture and herbal supplements, Gorilla has regained a lot of his former vigor and is entering his fourteenth year in better weight, with more energy and a renewed enthusiasm for his daily activities. I know we still have some tough days ahead with an inevitable heartbreak at its end, but in the meantime, I am thankful for every glorious moment I have with my amazing dog. Oops... gotta go...someone is looking at me as if to say, 'Is it time for my massage?'"

- Lola Michelin, Shoreline, Washington

how to treat it, the wiser the decisions you will make about your dog's treatment. The calmer you are, the more likely your dog will be calm, too.

Your dog is completely dependent upon you, and, as you probably already know, she can pick up on your emotions easily. As you'll find out, a dog who is depressed or stressed is not able to heal as easily as a content and calm dog. Managing your emotions is a mission critical step to take in treating your dog's cancer.

The following exercises address most of the major emotions that guardians experience. Even if you feel the urge to skip this next section, my strong recommendation is that you read through all of the exercises and complete as many as apply to you right now. Later, if you need to, you may want to come back and use one of these exercises, exactly as you would an oxygen mask on an airplane. Three Deep Breaths is especially helpful and, best of all, quick.

Many of these directly involve your dog, so look forward to some good bonding time with him.

Helpful Kitty Massages Therapy Dog

"My main concern was keeping Daisy's spirits up, keeping her challenged, stimulated and occupied vs. lying in bed, so that she had something to live for. I was so incredibly proud of her for everything she had overcome all ready; it was easy to tell her how wonderful she was and to thank her for everything she's ever done, every day with the **Pledge of Thanks**! She helped me foster over 250 dogs during her life time. She selected the dogs we brought home from the kill shelters, and she helped reassure then, train them when they needed training (manners, house training, you name it). She corrected them, and made it so easy for me. She kept her brothers and sisters in line, she was a therapy dog, and she was always there for me when I just wanted to go for a walk and get away from everything. We did a lot of energy healing and a lot of massage therapy and touch therapy. Even our cat got involved and I found him curled up next to Daisy, both on their sides with his 4 paws massaging her back in a **Message Massage**! We kept Daisy a **Dynamic Dog**; stimulated and playful. We took her out to sit at the field and watch the sun set, and the other dogs play, and sniff the air, the grass, and the trees. She couldn't go far sometimes but just being outside with the other dogs and still keeping to her regular schedule really stimulated her! We also discovered something called the "Dog Brick" which I think is an amazing toy, especially for a dog going through cancer, provided they aren't nauseous. It is made by Nina Ottosson and has a number of sliding compartments where you can hide treats. The dog can sniff the treats and has to use their brain power to slide the doors open to find and get to the treat. Nina makes a number of toys like this with different levels of challenges for dogs. The great thing is the dog doesn't have to move much and it takes more brain power than physical power so it's a great stimulating tool!"

– Chris Shoulet, Bethesda, Maryland

My Dog Should Be a Dog ... Not a Sick Dog

"I had forgotten how important it was for my dog to enjoy being a dog... not being a sick dog. The few minutes of one-on-one play meant so much to each of us. When I became quiet and focused on him without distractions, our relationship deepened exponentially. Talking with him, feeling my love for him and his back to me at such a wonderful level, gave us a wonderfully expanded relationship. We knew that no matter what happened in the future, we were so much closer than we'd ever been before."

— Susan Harper, High Wycombe, England

Dealing with My Depression Helped Her Stay Happy

"The prognosis was devastating to me and left me with an overwhelming feeling of helplessness. By using the emotional management exercises I changed from a focus on the bad to addressing my depression. She didn't know "what" was wrong so by me being able to remain positive, in return it let her remain happy. It was a bond that I may have needed more than she, but I'm sure it helped both of us in regards to a feeling of love and the ability to keep living to the best of our abilities."

— Julian Trevino, Roseville, Michigan

THREE DEEP BREATHS

Duration: 2 minutes

Indication: any negative emotion

Studies have shown that breathing exercises like this one make you more focused, calmer and better able to handle new situations. Errors in thinking drop off, learning is enhanced and attention bandwidth is expanded to deal with critical information.

To illustrate just how quickly attention to the breath can make a difference, let's take two minutes right now.

Check a clock and notice what time it is.

Turn your attention to your body and see where you find discomfort. Maybe you have an ache in your heel, a slight headache or your wrist hurts. It doesn't matter how uncomfortable it is, or where it is. Don't try to do anything to solve the discomfort – just notice it. It may be easier to close your eyes, so that you can focus on the physical sensations.

Rate the discomfort on a scale of 1 to 10, with 1 being slight discomfort and 10 being extreme discomfort. Remember this number (write it down if you need to).

Now, turn your attention to the sensation of your breath's movement as you breathe in and out. You might feel it in your nose, mouth, throat, chest or belly. Close your eyes to help you focus

continued on next page

THREE DEEP BREATHS,
continued

there while you take three slow, deep, deliberate breaths. Let your lungs fill completely and then, breathe out completely. As you do this, pay attention to the physical sensations which the breath creates in your body.

Now, turn your attention back to the body part you noticed earlier. What do you sense there? Rate your discomfort on the same 1 to 10 scale. How does it compare to your first number?

Look back at the clock and notice how much time has passed.

The vast majority of guardians experience a decrease in their discomfort as a result of directing their attention to their breathing. For some, the discomfort disappears altogether.

In addition to relieving physical discomfort, this simple, two-minute exercise lowers stress levels, oxygenates your blood (and your brain), calms and relaxes you. By focusing on physical sensations, rather than emotional content or thinking, you are creating some distance between your emotions and your thoughts.

You are also cultivating your observational skills. Checking the clock before and after the exercise can affirm for you just how powerful your own breath is – and how quickly it can help you.

This exercise has a lot of impact. And if you do it again (feel free to repeat it right now), the effects add up. When you need quick relief, this is a good exercise to use. You can do it just before you go into the vet's office, at night before you go to sleep, or in the shower. Use it as often as needed.

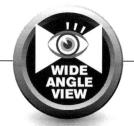

WIDE ANGLE VIEW

"The greatest mistake in the treatment of diseases is that there are physicians for the body and physicians for the soul, although the two cannot be separated."
—Plato

It's been over two thousand years since Plato wrote those words, and they're still true today. Matters of the soul are not generally addressed in conventional medicine … and we're slowly learning that we need to go beyond the "nuts and bolts" of anatomy. The body-mind connection is a focus of study in many different areas of medicine.

Paying attention to your dog's body, while ignoring his emotions, is like putting gas in your car, but never changing the oil: eventually, the engine will seize up and stop running. You can also consider the exercises in this chapter part of Step Five of Full Spectrum cancer care (see Chapter 15).

FIRE BELLOWS BREATHING

Duration: 15 seconds to one minute
Indication: for clearing the mind

This exercise is adapted from a breathing technique used by yoga practitioners. While slightly noisy, it can make you feel more alive and alert. It's also been shown to enhance thinking: in one study involving medical doctors, this exercise reduced errors in their daily work.

If you're feeling agitated, angry, restless, confused, or if you need a "pick me up," this exercise can help. Here are the steps:

Breathe in and out rapidly through your nose, with your mouth closed and your jaw relaxed. Placing the tip of your tongue just behind your front top teeth can help to relax the jaw. This will feel like controlled hyperventilation. Keep your breaths as short as possible, and don't worry about the snorting noise you're making.

The optimal rhythm is three breath cycles per second: in, out, in, out, in, out. Make each in-breath as long as each out-breath. You will find your belly and chest moving in and out, like a bellows.

On your first try, continue for fifteen seconds, if you can. Each time you do this increase your time a little, until you reach a full minute.

After you are finished, breathe normally.

It can be difficult to do this if your nose is stuffed up; although some find that it clears nasal passages quickly (have a tissue handy, if you need one). You may want to do this exercise in private, because you must make noise to get its full benefit.

MEDITATION

Duration: 5 minutes
Frequency: preferably daily

A daily meditation practice is a great way to connect to your dog, even if you can manage only five minutes. Depending upon your background, you might think of meditation as an esoteric or foreign practice. It's not. Some form of meditation is used in every culture and in every religion on the planet (in Christianity it's sometimes called "contemplative prayer"). Meditation is also used in stress management programs, although it may be called "breathing exercises" to make it sound more familiar.

My friend and business partner, James Jacobson, introduced me to the concept of meditating with your dog when he wrote an entire book about it. I must admit that, at first, I thought it was

continued on next page

MEDITATION, *continued*

pretty silly. After reading his book (*How to Meditate with Your Dog: An Introduction to Meditation for Dog Lovers*), however, I realized there was a good argument for meditating with your dog.

There are many forms of meditation. For our purposes I'm going to recommend a very simple practice: pay attention to the breath. Observing the breath as it naturally occurs helps the mind to develop focus, increase patience, and learn quickly.

Here's a quick dog meditation:

Set aside five minutes to sit quietly with your dog. Sit in a comfortable position, with plenty of support for your back. Make physical contact with your dog, even if it is just your hand on her head.

Focus on your own breath. Take a deep breath or two, and then let the breaths fall into your natural rhythm. Keep your attention lightly focused on your breath. If your attention wanders, gently bring it back. It may help to think, "I am inhaling" as you inhale and "I am exhaling" as you exhale.

Now focus on your dog's breath for a few breaths. To keep your focus, it may help to think, "My dog is inhaling," as he breathes in and, as he breathes out, think, "My dog is exhaling."

Stay focused on the breath (yours or your dog's) for five minutes (longer if you like). Other thoughts may crowd in and emotions might come up; this is normal. However, since you have chosen to focus on the breath, not on thoughts or emotions, simply return your attention to the breath. No matter how many times you lose focus, you are still meditating, as long as you remember to re-focus on the breath.

Most dogs enjoy sitting in calm with their guardians. If your dog is restless and moves away, you can choose to go get him and continue, or let him go and sit on your own, feeling your connection to him from afar.

Sitting in meditation with your dog can remind you of several important facts:

Your dog is still breathing. She is alive.

You are still breathing. You are alive.

You can connect to your dog.

You can manage your emotions, which helps your dog.

I recommend regular meditation practice to help cultivate a good mindset for dealing with dog cancer. As in most things, consistency is helpful to get the full benefit of this exercise. Short daily sessions give more benefit than do irregular, longer sessions. Meditating for five minutes is manageable for most guardians.

VENT IF YOU'RE BENT

Duration: 5-30 minutes

Indication: for anger and frustration

Some guardians dealing with dog cancer feel angry or "bent out of shape." This is normal, because anger often comes when we want a situation to change but feel incapable of doing anything to make it happen.

Regardless of how normal it may be, feeling angry is not helpful when you need to make decisions. According to research, a tendency toward anger promotes risky decision-making in many different areas of life. It also interferes with mental clarity in general. Plus, dogs can experience stress when their guardians are angry.

Anger is a powerful emotion that demands an outlet. Here's an idea:

Go to a place where you will not be disturbed: your room or a secluded spot in nature. It's best if your dog is not with you.

Vent in a way that feels good to you. Here are a few ideas:

Yell at a wall (not a mirror).

Scream into a pillow.

Run as fast as you can around a track.

Hit a punching bag at the gym.

Pound sand at the beach (stay out of the water, though).

Scribble angry words in a notebook.

Slash at a paper with crayons.

Turn up loud music and scream the lyrics.

Stay safe, of course. Don't hurt yourself or anyone else. This is about releasing the pent up anger, not using it as a weapon.

If anyone asks what you are doing, refer to this book and say you're following a vet's advice.

Keep venting until you literally run out of steam. You'll know when this happens: you'll feel exhausted, and the venting will peter out. You might find yourself sighing big sighs, crying a little (or a lot) or just staring off into space, void.

When you are finished, take three deep breaths to remind yourself that you are still alive.

Now that the emotional charge is gone, you may be able to see what you really want to do about the situation that triggered your anger.

How long it takes for you to run out of steam will depend upon many things, including how angry you are, whether other events from your past life come up, and how much permission you've given yourself for full expression.

MESSAGE MASSAGE

Duration: 10 minutes

Indication: sad feelings or anxiety

Some guardians dealing with dog cancer find themselves feeling terribly sad, guilty or numb. Giving your dog a massage can reconnect you to your dog and your shared love. This can ease your emotional pain, and it is also good for your dog; massage is now incorporated as a regular part of cancer care in human cancer centers like New York's Memorial Sloan-Kettering Cancer Center. (See chapter 15 for more information.)

Giving your dog a massage is a lovely, gentle, healing exercise. It's also a natural activity for dogs. Dogs living in packs care for each other by licking and massaging with their strong tongues. If your dog has ever licked you when you were sad or tired, you were receiving a "Message Massage" (I believe the message was "I love you").

You can send that message back to your dog. The length of time and timing of your massage should hinge on your dog's state of mind and being.

Here are some tips for giving your dog a loving Message Massage:

Start your massage when your dog is already relaxed, for example, sitting quietly or cuddling with you. If you start when the dog is playing, he may reject the massage (dogs don't massage when they wrestle and play).

Start slowly and very gently. Dogs seem to prefer light to medium pressure, much like what they would receive from another dog's tongue. If you think of your fingers and hands as tongues, it will help you to keep them soft and light. Use repetitive, circular movements, like you are slowly finger painting. Avoid pokey fingertips, knuckles or anything that has an edge.

Pay attention to your dog's comfort as you massage. If her muscles grow heavy and soft under your hands, you are likely doing a great job. If she shifts, edges away, or stiffens, you are probably going too deep or working an area too hard. Dogs with cancer can be extremely sensitive. Back off and see if she relaxes. If she does, continue with the massage. If she stays stiff, let it go for another time and give her a few gentle pets, instead.

There are certain areas that dogs really like massaged. You can try:
- the muscles on the top of the neck,
- the muscles on the left and right side of the spine,
- the muscles on the left and right side of the skull,
- the shoulders,
- the thigh and hamstring muscles on the thighs, and
- the muscles on the front and back of the calf and forearm.

Keep your distance from cancer tumors themselves as you massage. Sessions can last as long as your dog can tolerate and enjoy the massage.

continued on next page

MESSAGE MASSAGE, *continued*

This is one of the best ways to counter your feelings of numbness, sadness and guilt. It also helps your dog, by reassuring him that his pack cares for him. You probably cannot give your dog too many Message Massages.

PLEDGE OF THANKS

Duration: 10+ minutes
Indication: every feeling

Expressing gratitude can have profound positive effects. Studies have shown that expressing thanks on a daily basis makes us feel proud, hopeful, inspired, forgiving and excited. It directly increases our sense of satisfaction with life, makes us more optimistic and more likely to reach out for social support.

Our dogs pick up on our attitude and, the more positive we are, the better we can help our dogs. The Pledge of Thanks is very simple.

Set aside a time to be with your dog. Pick a quiet place where you can both be comfortable and feel safe.

Thank you dog for everything you can think of, big and small. Say "thank you for _____, and thank you for _____, and thank you for _____." Thank her for playing with you, eating her food, sleeping next to you, and for the time when she growled at the guy who came in the back yard. Keep going until you cannot think of one more thing for which to give thanks.

Do it out loud, because speaking out loud can prompt our mind to remember things we wouldn't if we are silent. While you speak, allow yourself to feel your gratitude. Tears are allowed – and smiles are, too. Don't hold back.

When you run out of specifics, you might still be "on a roll of gratitude." If this happens, you can say "thank you, thank you," until your urge to speak slows and the words stop.

This exercise often reconnects guardians to a sense of unconditional love. Once you are finished, take a moment to enjoy the feeling of love you have unleashed. Enjoy your recognition of the gifts your dog has given.

I would allow at least ten minutes for this exercise and that may not be enough time. Many readers have written to say that this one exercise is the most important one in this book.

DYNAMIC DOG EXERCISE

Duration: 10+ minutes
Frequency: daily
Indication: every feeling

As anyone who has raised a puppy can attest, dogs naturally love to play and learn. However, a dog with cancer may feel slow and depressed. Gently stimulating her with daily challenges can shake her "back to life" and raise her self-esteem. It can also serve as a reminder to you of just how powerful your dog's will to live can be.

Becoming excited or optimistic – about anything – directly improves your dog's state of mind. You can see this, for example, when you offer your dog a treat she really loves, and her whole body responds with a wiggle.

Challenges do not have to be big. In order to get the blood pumping and the nervous system firing, they should be manageable and achievable. Pick one thing each day to change, just a little, for your dog. When the task is achieved, even a little, create a big, celebratory commotion with a huge amount of cheering and praise. This recognition is a key to building your dog's innate strength.

Vary your walk route by a block or two, or go to a new place. Reward your dog with abundant praise for dealing with the new route.

Change the pace of the walk: slow it down, or speed it up a little. Praise your dog generously along the way.

Change your dog's feeding schedule. Feed her a little earlier, or a little later in the day. Once again, praise your dog at mealtime.

Remember puppy school and do some basic training exercises like "sit," "stay," and "come." When he does well, give him treats he's never had before. Don't forget to praise him extravagantly!

Teach your dog a new trick, giving lavish praise along the way.

A new toy can be very stimulating for a dog, even if she cannot take full advantage of it.

Go on short trips to new locations; give him lots of praise along the way.

If your dog is social, create new opportunities for her to interact with other dogs. Reward her for good behavior.

Introduce your dog to new people, and reward him for being nice.

Creating these rich life experiences boosts your dog's self-esteem. In addition to the health benefits, these small challenges to your dog can remind you both that you are a team and you are the guardian your dog needs.

CHEAT DAY

Frequency: every 5-7 days
Indication: every feeling

When you and your dog are dealing with cancer, it can feel like never-ending work. There are vet appointments, new foods, supplement regimens and, sometimes, painful treatments. When you need a break, it's time for a Cheat Day: time to spoil your dog.

I steal the term "cheat day" from a rigorous diet program my wife and I followed once. We ate according to strict rules ... but every once in a while we had a day where we could eat anything we wanted. These days helped us to stay motivated and to stick with the program the rest of the time.

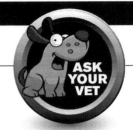

Depending upon which medications your dog takes, his other health issues and dietary needs, the treats I list here might not be appropriate for your individual dog. Always clear a new treat with your vet first.

A Cheat Day for your dog is a day when you give him an undeserved, unearned, delicious reward – just because he is your dog!

Dogs usually love Cheat Days. I recommend having one every five to seven days. On these days, give your dog a really yummy treat. Some examples are:

- Chicken breast cooked in low-sodium or slightly diluted bullion
- Lean hamburger, cooked in low-sodium or slightly diluted chicken broth (and strained)
- Turkey breast in diluted teriyaki sauce
- Human baby food from a jar (meat flavors are the favorites)
- Boneless fish cooked in a clear, low-sodium, slightly diluted broth or soup
- Lean lamb cooked in low-sodium or slightly diluted vegetable broth
- Peeled shrimp cooked in low-sodium or slightly diluted beef broth
- Lean pork cooked in slightly diluted chicken noodle soup
- Hardboiled egg whites chopped up in low-sodium or slightly diluted beef broth
- Tuna fish in water with a dash of Italian food seasoning

I hate to put any restrictions on Cheat Day treats, however, I recommend using low-sodium or salt substitutes, avoiding grains and sugars, avoiding cream-based soups, and avoiding carbohydrate-rich foods like potatoes, peas, or carrots.

The power of Cheat Day is that it is new and unexpected. This unpredictability helps your dog's mind stay optimistic, stimulated and excited. Keep Cheat Days coming and space them out, so that the element of surprise is always at work.

LIFE STORY

Duration: 30+ minutes

Indication: every feeling

This powerful exercise is an uplifting and freeing way to reconnect with your dog. I learned about it from my dog-meditating friend, James Jacobson. When his little Maltese, Maui, was very ill and near the end of her life, he received thousands of messages from fans of his book (*How to Meditate with Your Dog*). One of them offered this exercise, as a way to deliberately connect with Maui before she left this world. Setting aside the time to do this exercise gave James some relief from his fear and helped him to deal with Maui's illness. This is a simple exercise, but it can be very emotional. If you need to, go slowly or take breaks.

Have tissues handy.

Sit down with your dog and tell him his life story, out loud. Start at the beginning and go all the way through to the present.

Give as many details as you can. Starting with the first time you saw your dog, tell him as much as you can, including:

Who was there?

Who arrived and left?

Where were you?

What did you two do?

What were the good times?

What were the tough times?

Making physical contact with your dog while you tell him his life story can enhance your connection.

If your spouse, children, other family members or friends are close with your dog, you might want to include them in this exercise. Your dog will bask in the love that surrounds him.

Don't forget to tell your dog how you feel right now, sitting next to him and telling him his life story. Tell him what this is like for you.

This is a powerful exercise that can reveal just how deep your bond is with your dog. Once you reconnect with that bond in this conscious way, the motivation to be the best guardian possible may grow even stronger.

Amplifying the Effects of Positive Emotions

Up to here, I've been focusing on managing negative emotions and emphasizing how unhelpful those emotions are when dealing with your dog's cancer. The opposite is also true; your positive, good moods can be extremely helpful in dealing with dog cancer.

Your good mood makes your dog feel secure and content in her relationship to you. As a pack animal, she experiences a deep need for this kind of security. Your kind, loving, compassionate, open-hearted feelings can amplify your ability to deal with dog cancer, ease your discomfort, make you think faster and smarter, and change your perception of your experience.

Everyone's experience is different, and I do not want to put any undue pressure on you to "perform well" during this trying time. However, there are people who transform cancer from a nightmare into a beautiful, moving experience. I've seen this happen with human cancer patients, family and friends, and guardians dealing with their dog's cancer. If you open your heart and work through this time with your dog, you may be able to see the cancer as a "gift from God," as a client named Sarah said.

"At first, I felt terrible all the time," Sarah reported.

"But now, I feel so blessed to have this feeling of continuous, unbroken connection. I never gave myself the opportunity to open my heart this wide – even after three kids and my own personal

---

Nighty Night: Bedtime Stories for Madison

"Every evening before I go to sleep, while Madison is already resting comfortably on our bed for the night and the room is dark and quiet, I do the **Pledge of Thanks,** telling her all the reasons that I'm thankful she's in my life. Some nights I tell her the same reasons over and over, and other nights I think of even more reasons I hadn't already thought of. The list seems endless. All the while I also stroke her fur softly and the combination of these two activities helps to make me calm, ready for a good night's sleep."

– Christine Darg, Winnipeg, Manitoba

Talk It Out with the Best Listener

"The one I use daily is **Pledge of Thanks**. It allowed me to express and release my true feelings, after all your companion, your best friend has cancer which is extremely scary but you can talk it out and you have the best listener in the world. I would tell Uli, my boxer companion, how thankful I am for every new day and thankful that we have that time to do things we enjoy, thankful for God and the fact I was blessed to have such a wonderful companion to share each day with."

– Jon Marshall, Norman, Oklahoma

---

cancer scare. But somehow, for my Sunny, I could do it. Every day, I wake up grateful that she's alive, and grateful that she's in my life, no matter how long we have together. Living with that attitude of gratitude is a miracle, and I don't think I would have received it any other way. In the four months since she was first diagnosed, I have found more strength, stamina, courage, and hope than I ever thought I had in me. I will carry this with me forever. I wish she'd never gotten sick, of course, but I wouldn't trade my new attitude for anything. It's her gift to me, and I will always remember and honor her for it."

Sunny passed away a year after Sarah shared this, and sixteen months later than the statistics predicted – and when it happened, the whole family contributed to her hospice care as outlined in Chapter 25. Sarah reported that it was a terribly sad, but very loving and moving time for everyone.

I don't expect you to adopt Sarah's point of view immediately or even at all. I just wanted to show you another possibility. Knowing that some people come out of this experience stronger could give you hope on a dark day.

Dogs Pick Up on My Moods

"By re-establishing our daily walks we are all feeling healthier. The walks also keep us happier and we play more than we used to. I am ashamed to say I became really lazy in the past few months. I am also not as depressed about the cancer situation since we are all more active and I believe that Buddy and Jack both "pick up" on my mood change."

– *Debbie Granger, Chesterfield, Missouri*

Everything Is In Her Best Interest

"One of the first things I did was to try the emotional management exercises, and I found that they gave me a sense of peace, knowing that everything I would be doing would be in Sparkle's best interest."

– *Susan McKay, Winnipeg, Manitoba*

Thank Them Every Day

"I do the Pledge of Thanks just about every day (even with my older dog who does not have cancer). I feel that our dogs are "gifts" to us in life, and we need to thank them (every day) for being with us."

- *Sheril Allen, Austin, Texas*

At first, the exercises in this chapter might feel like that oxygen mask on the plane – necessary to help you, so you can help your dog. Perhaps they could also be used as amplifying devices to make your average moods good and your good moods even better. Every uptick in your emotional mood will help you, and help your dog.

Chapter 3:
Three Common Questions

There are three questions guardians tend to ask first when they get a cancer diagnosis. Because these three questions seem to weigh on the mind and could distract you from learning anything new, I am going to answer them as best I can.

How could my dog get cancer almost overnight?

Why didn't my vet catch this earlier?

Is my dog dying right now?

How Could Cancer Happen Overnight?

One of the hardest things for most guardians to grasp is how they didn't see this coming. Many times the dog seems healthy right before she's brought in for an evaluation. Sometimes dogs don't seem sick at all.

How did this grave illness escape your attention? The answer may surprise you: your dog may have hidden it from you.

Dogs have an old, genetic program that encourages them to conceal any sign of illness, a legacy from when they ran in packs. The pack mentality oriented them toward maintaining their position in the hierarchy and defending the pack from predators. Weak dogs slow down the pack and become predators' targets. As a result, they risk losing their rank in the hierarchy or being left behind, which is a terrible fate for a dog. A dog will do just about anything to avoid this – including behaving as if nothing is wrong for as long as she can.

Despite generations of domestication, dogs still think like wild animals when they feel ill. If your dog felt sick before his diagnosis, you can bet he did everything he could to make you think he was just fine.

When a dog can no longer hide his symptoms, he gives up trying and seems to get sick overnight. This is called **decompensation**, and it often occurs just before the guardian takes the dog to the vet. This leads me to the second reason that cancer seems to sneak up on us: our reliance upon sight.

Humans use sight as their primary information-gathering sense. We see our dog eating, walking, playing, sleeping, going to the bathroom, and wagging her tail when we come home. Over time, we use this visual information to create a picture in our mind of what is normal for our dog. As long as we see all of these things happening, we assume that nothing is off-kilter.

Dogs, on the other hand, use their sense of smell as their primary means of gathering information. When they sniff each other (a habit we often find funny or gross) they are actually gathering information. Is she in heat? Is he healthy? What did she eat for breakfast? All these questions and many more can be answered by decoding a dog's scent.

Our puny human noses cannot smell our dog's illness.

Because of our dog's ability to compensate for their symptoms, our eyes are blind, too. Given all of this, we cannot possibly blame ourselves for not discovering cancer before decompensation occurred.

"Wait a minute!" some guardians are thinking, "I suppose I can understand why I didn't catch this earlier, but what about my vet? Shouldn't he have seen this coming?"

Why Didn't My Vet Catch This Earlier?

This is a complicated question, and there is no one "right" answer. Let's start with the most obvious and least controversial answer I have.

Cancer Can Be Invisible

Some cancers simply are not visible to the naked eye, cannot be felt with the fingers, and don't

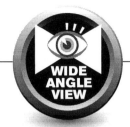

Early Detection Is Key

Cancer is an epidemic, but the veterinary community is not treating it as one. Dr. Ettinger and I both feel that this must change, and soon.

Vets can advocate for dogs by informing clients of the risks for cancer when they find a lump. Every lump must be checked for cancer as soon as it's found, using simple and minimally invasive fine needle aspirates and lab tests.

In addition, using simple imaging tests such as X-rays and ultrasounds during routine exams could make catching cancer earlier possible, just like mammograms do for human breast cancer.

Of course, there is a lot of debate amongst vets and oncologists about how much screening is too much. As we recently saw in human cancer, there can be costs associated with screening for cancer that outweigh the benefits.

You may remember when a task force analyzed the data on mammograms and human breast cancer and suggested that the guidelines be

continued on next page

Early Detection Is Key, *continued*

changed: instead of getting a yearly mammogram after the age of forty, women would get one only when their doctor felt they were at risk for breast cancer – otherwise, they could wait until fifty to get their first mammogram, and then get one every two years thereafter.

The proposed guideline change was to save the majority of women (85%) who do not get breast cancer in their forties from the discomfort of the test itself, the cost of the test, and the emotional toil of waiting for the results, false positives and unnecessary biopsies.

I don't want to advocate for unnecessary screening and I certainly don't want dog lovers to start feeling paranoid about their dogs' every little problem. We do not know how often to do screenings – a chest X-ray every year? Every two years? Only after age five? Six? Seven? How much cancer would this early screening actually catch?

There are a lot of questions that need to be answered.

And still, the problem remains: **cancer is epidemic, *and we're not taking action.*** Routine exams are not happening often enough. Fine needle aspirates – simple, non-invasive, and relatively inexpensive – and biopsies are not being used often enough. These tests are worth it. And Dr. Ettinger even recommends adding chest X-rays and abdominal ultrasounds to routine physical exams for middle aged and older dogs.

Realizing that cancer is here, and it's a big problem, we must open our minds to cancer treatments that come from other places, disciplines and therapies. Adding tools to our toolbox is imperative.

produce a noise that can be heard with a stethoscope. These cancers are often advanced by the time the dog decompensates and the guardian realizes something is wrong. This can be true for human cancers, too. In deep body cancers, we don't usually realize something is wrong until after symptoms start to show up.

Cancer can take a long time to develop; we'll talk more about this later. For now, it's important to realize that cancer does not appear overnight. It just seems to.

Cancer Can Start Before Birth

Some dogs are born with genetic mutations passed on from their parents' DNA, which can develop into cancer later.

This is a very complex subject, so I'm going to vastly over-simplify it. Cancer goes through many steps – for the sake of explanation, let's pretend it is ten steps – before it is fully developed and diagnosed. If a dog is born with a genetic mutation that pre-disposes her to develop cancer, she may already be on, say, step three of ten, at birth. If the cancer does develop, it may take years for recognizable signs to appear.

To the guardian, that cancer

may seem to pop up overnight when, in fact, it developed over the genetic history of the dog. If it were possible to trace the molecular history of that genetic mutation all the way back to where it began in her ancestors, you could even say that in some cases cancer develops over millennia.

Cancer Screening Can Be Difficult

It would be ideal if vets had screening tests that could catch cancer early, but, we don't. While some human cancers can be found by measuring certain markers in the blood, we can't do this for most dog cancers.

Routine physical exams can uncover suspicious lumps and bumps. Unfortunately, many dog lovers seem to think of the vet like they do a car mechanic: they take the dog in only when something is obviously wrong. Regular physicals are critical for finding cancer as early as possible, but, even they can't always catch cancers that start on a microscopic level, or are located deep in the body.

The Wait and See Approach

When some vets find a lump during an exam, they recommend taking a "wait and see" approach. They advise the guardian to look for changes or growth before testing the lump for cancer. However, waiting can be problematic. If a lump is cancerous and left untreated, it can spread, becoming much harder to treat later.

No one, not even my oncologist co-author Dr. Ettinger, can tell what a lump is without testing it for cancer cells. When I see or feel a lump on a dog, I can often make an accurate, *educated guess* about whether it is a malignancy. However, I can also make an *inaccurate*, educated guess.

If I believe a lump is benign, I tell my clients something like this:

"Nine out of ten times when I feel a lump like this, it turns out to be benign ... but if your dog is the one dog about which I'm wrong it won't matter to you that I was right about the other nine dogs. If you choose not to get this tested, keep in mind that your odds are good, but that you are still gambling."

Many vets are hesitant to recommend extensive or expensive testing procedures, because we are sensitive to guardians, who might be thinking that we're just "running up the bill." This is especially true if tests come back negative. *If you weren't going to find anything, why did you order that test in the first place?*

While it's true that there may be a few vets who run unnecessary tests, it's impossible to know for certain that cancer is present without at least a fine needle aspirate and/or a biopsy. Metastasis, or cancer spread, can only be confirmed with X-rays or some other imaging test, blood tests, urine tests, and other screening tools, depending upon the cancer's type. There is simply no way around it – in order to get a diagnosis, we must run tests.

So why don't vets push their clients harder to get lumps and bumps tested as soon as they are discovered? If this were another disease, such as heart disease or diabetes, most vets wouldn't even consider the cost of the tests. They would say, "We need to get this tested, so that if there is a problem, we can start treatment right away."

So what's different about cancer? Three things.

Some Vets Don't Realize Cancer Is Epidemic

Cancer is the number one killer of dogs (following euthanasia), according to organizations like the National Canine Cancer Foundation. This is not yet common knowledge among vets.

According to estimates, one in three dogs will get cancer, and this increases to one in two in dogs over the age of ten. Those are scary numbers, and not every vet believes they are accurate, because the data is coming from a foundation, rather than a systematic examination of every clinic's cases. This leads me to the second reason some vets don't push for early cancer screening.

Good Marketing Can Sway Opinion

Veterinary school teaches many wonderful things, but (usually) not how to assess a published paper for bias on the part of the authors. As a veterinary student, I was never taught to ask questions like:

What are the strengths of their study? Are there any weaknesses? Were enough animals included in the study to make the results statistically significant? What are they overlooking in their conclusions? Could they be manipulating the data to serve a particular agenda? How was their research funded? By drug companies? By the government? By themselves? Do they have any financial interest in the outcome of their work? Do they have personal bias that might influence their interpretation of the data? It's easy for vets to read their trade journals and assume that the authors are unbiased. It's also just as easy for some vets to be swayed by marketing.

If you've brought a new puppy into your life in the last few years, you may have received a "puppy kit" from your vet. Pharmaceutical companies, dog food companies, and pet product manufacturers regularly provide free "gifts" to veterinarians to hand out to new puppy guardians. Perhaps the folder that held your puppy's papers was also an ad for a heartworm medication. Perhaps the new doggy toy has the name of a popular dog food printed on the tag. I freely admit to using some of these gifts in my own practice.

While it's wonderful when vets save money and give their clients a gift at the same time, it's also an implied endorsement of the company's products. Does it create a potential bias toward using that company's products? Certainly. Is that bad? Not necessarily. The promoted products have a beneficial purpose that could be lifesaving. However, we should ensure that each vet is aware of her bias, does her own research, and asks those tough questions of the information presented by the companies involved.

Conventional Medicine Does Not Offer Complete Cancer Care

If your dog has heart disease, conventional vets have effective medications that can often control it for a long time. If your dog is diabetic, we can usually help manage the disease so that it doesn't affect her quality of life too much.

Was That a Dog in the Drive-Through Window?

"The Vent if You're Bent exercise helped me let out the anger about my young dog being diagnosed with a disease that was going to rob us of many years together. Cheat Day was for Apollo: on chemo days we started adding a trip to McDonalds or A&W on the way home. I would buy him a single cheeseburger and let him have the meat and cheese. Most of the time he was very happy to get it."

– Sandy Miller, Palo, Iowa

Unfortunately, when it comes to cancer, we have just a handful of conventional tools: chemotherapy, radiation, and surgery. In many cases, guardians consider those tools too expensive and not good enough at extending life, enhancing the quality of life, or providing comfort to the dog. Some vets agree, even if only on a subconscious level. The cure for systemic dog cancer has not been found, at least not yet, by conventional oncology.

In general, vets are animal lovers who entered the profession so they could be around animals all day long. Limited tools and dispiriting, confusing statistics make dealing with cancer a frustrating experience for most vets. It is profoundly unsatisfying not to be able to cure a dog with cancer.

This helplessness can cause vets a great deal of stress. The vet might try to avoid that feeling, without realizing it. He might go numb and make an insensitive comment. He might be unaware of the latest options for cancer treatments, and give up too soon. He might tell you "There's no point in doing anything now, it's too late. Take your dog home and prepare for the end."

Vets can be sabotaged by stress, just like any other person. This is another reason why you must step up and advocate for your dog by becoming a fierce dog guardian.

You will probably never *really* know why the cancer wasn't caught earlier. Perhaps we didn't look hard enough or often enough, we didn't use our existing diagnostic tools early enough, or we simply need better tools. Or, perhaps we could have done more, and we still would not have found the cancer.

Let's turn ourselves to the last question.

Is My Dog Dying Right Now?

No, he's not. He's alive right now, and the healthy cells in his body are operating as they always have. They are living right now. Many of them are even fighting the cancer.

There is another way to look at it, of course. Here's another, equally valid answer: this may be a tough pill to swallow, but yes, in a way, your dog is dying right now. Death is inevitable, and always has been. It's an unavoidable part of life on our planet. From this point of view, nothing has really changed, but you may now be more aware of your dog's eventual death than you were before you received the cancer diagnosis. Or, you may understand that death is inevitable, but are feeling that death is coming too soon. I think most dog lovers feel this way about the possibility of their dog's death.

Whichever perspective feels most comfortable for you, the chances that your dog is going to expire as you are reading this are low. You have time.

You may know a woman who had breast cancer, one of the most common human cancers. Perhaps she had no idea that she was sick until a doctor found a spot on her mammogram. Her body appeared healthy, and indeed most of her cells were normal. She didn't actually feel sick; she had time to get treatment and live a good life. Maybe she even beat the cancer into remission.

This could be the case for your dog, as well. It is possible that your dog could beat cancer. I cannot guarantee it. I cannot assess your dog's condition through the pages of this book, and I cannot directly treat your dog, however …

———— • ————

"Remember, cancer is not an immediate death sentence. Cancer is a living process that happens in a living body."

———— • ————

I have seen some recoveries that can only be described as miraculous, and I take nothing for granted when it comes to a dog's ability to heal.

There is no way for you to know, right now, that your dog will definitely die of cancer, any time soon. Each dog, each case, is different. That's why I am so glad that you are taking the time to educate yourself, so you can make decisions that will lead to the best outcome.

As you'll learn, your dog's body is already hard at work, fighting the cancer cells. Remember, cancer is not an immediate death sentence. Cancer is a living process that happens in a *living* body.

And your dog's body might be better equipped than most to handle the challenges of cancer, just because she is a dog.

Chapter 4: Super Dogs

*C*anis familiaris is one of the most incredible species on the planet. My guess is that every human who has lived with a dog has noticed that dogs are capable of unconditional love. You'll learn later that love is a healing attitude and the foundation of good health. Your sense of shared love with your dog can be the driving force behind his healing.

Sealy, the mattress manufacturer, conducted a survey that reported 67% of Americans sleep with their pets. This intimate habit has been around since we domesticated dogs at least 15,000 years ago (which some say happened even earlier — 30,000 years ago). During those centuries of living together, dogs have developed into wonderful companions.

> *Love is a healing attitude and the foundation of good health. Your sense of shared love with your dog can be the driving force behind his healing."*

Dogs display sensitivity to our gestures and speech that other species seem to lack. For example, dogs tend to automatically follow the most subtle gestures and body language. They have an uncanny sense of when we'll return home. They seem to offer us comfort when we're in pain. And some guardians admit that their dogs seem to listen more closely to their troubles than any human companion does.

Despite our close contact with our dogs, we are often completely in the dark about what our dogs' life is like or what their true capabilities are.

Did you know that …

… the lining of a dog's nose is twenty to forty times more sensitive to smell than the lining of a human's nose?

… dogs can hear ultrasonic frequencies that are five times higher than those that humans can?

… dogs can smell their owner's scent from a mile away?

… dogs can detect cancer by smell alone? In a recent study, trained dogs correctly detected lung cancer samples 99% of the time. They correctly detected 88% of breast cancer samples.

… dogs can sense where someone has been, even days after he has left the area? This is why police often use hounds to find missing people.

… dogs seem to be able to tell if someone wants to harm you? Remember that time when your dog stood between you and someone else and growled at them for "no reason"?

… dogs and other animals seem to know when an earthquake or other natural disaster is coming?

… some dogs can detect pending epileptic seizures in people before they begin and can warn them to prepare?

Dogs are, in one word, remarkable. Keep their "super powers" in mind as you read this book. One of the most important things I have learned from dogs is that they can do almost anything – especially when they have the love of a calm, balanced human to sustain them.

Part II:
What You Should Know About Dog Cancer

In this Part, we'll look at dog cancer from a bird's eye view, starting with defining some common cancer terms, and then briefly going over how cancer begins and how it spreads in the body. We'll see how veterinarians diagnose cancer, what tests they use, and why they're important. We will learn about a very important and basic body process called apoptosis. We'll also look at the possible causes of dog cancers, including carcinogens, genetic factors, and vaccinations. This background material will help you to understand Full Spectrum cancer care and, later, make decisions about how to treat your dog's cancer.

Chapter 5: Dog Cancer Phrases, Words and Meanings

This chapter defines some common terms you may hear from your vet, oncologist, or other practitioner. I've expanded most of the traditional definitions to include information

Reading through these definitions now will give you a birds-eye-view of cancer. Later, you can use this chapter as a glossary, referring back as needed.

Acupuncture: The use of needles to stimulate certain points on the body. The model used in this system involves regulating the energy flow ("chi" or "ki") in sites or pathways in the body ("meridians"). Acupuncture is a branch of Traditional Chinese Medicine (TCM), a complex medical system with thousands of years of history. Some conventional and many **alternative** veterinarians use acupuncture for cancer treatments, pain relief, reducing nausea, and its many other benefits. TCM is very different from western medicine, so I recommend finding a veterinarian who has been licensed to perform acupuncture if you want to explore this system's benefits.

Alternative Medicine: Any treatment that is not within the bounds of conventional veterinary medicine is labeled "alternative." Some vets embrace this label for themselves and may even reject many conventional treatments. In this way, an alternative veterinarian can be just as dogmatic in her thinking as a conventional veterinarian. In addition, as treatments once labeled alternative – supplements, for example – become more popular, they themselves become conventional treatments.

Angiogenesis: Angiogenesis means "creating new blood vessels." Cancer tumors form new blood vessels out of existing vessels, so they can access nutrients and oxygen in the bloodstream. These new blood vessels shunt nutrition to the tumor at the expense of healthy body parts. They also serve as transportation routes for cancer cells to metastasize to other parts of the body.

Apoptogens: Agents that induce **apoptosis** in cells (the supplements discussed in Chapter 12 are apoptogens.) Inducing apoptosis in cancer cells is a way to get the cancer to actively kill itself.

Apoptosis: Apoptosis is the completely natural body process that causes cells to destroy themselves at the end of their natural lifespan. Also known as "programmed cell death" or "cell suicide," apoptosis can also be triggered when a cell sustains irreparable damage, becomes infected, or starts dividing uncontrollably. In an average healthy human adult, somewhere around fifty to seventy billion cells die each day due to apoptosis and then quietly exit the body to make room for new, healthy cells. In most types of cancer, apoptosis genes "turn off," which leads to lower apoptosis levels. When this happens, cancer cells do not die naturally. Diminished apoptosis is a hallmark of most types of cancer, and is one of the major ways for a tumor to expand. Forcing cancer cells to commit suicide, via apoptosis, is one of the central goals in **Full Spectrum** cancer care. Although many people pronounce this word "ay-POP-toe-sis," the most correct pronunciation features a silent second p: "ay-po-TOE-sis." Substances that turn on apoptosis are called **apoptogens**.

Benign: A tumor with a very low potential to spread to other areas is generally not dangerous and is called benign. Even benign tumors can cause problems, however, if they press on an internal organ, interfere with normal movement, are prone to injury, or if they burst open to cause bleeding or infection.

Bioavailability: The relative amount of a drug or agent that reaches the circulation (and therefore has a better chance to reach the cancer cells). Theoretically, an agent that is given through injection has higher bioavailability because it is 100% intact when it first enters the blood (although it may later be broken down or otherwise cleared by the body). Supplements, nutraceuticals, and pharmaceuticals administered by mouth, on the other hand, may break down in the digestive system so much that they enter the blood stream at only a fraction of their original intensity. The more intact an agent is when it reaches its target, the better it works *in vivo*.

Biopsy: A surgery that removes a tumor, or a sample of a tumor, for the purpose of cancer diagnosis. The specimen is submitted to a **pathologist**, where special processing and examination of the tissue yields a classification of the cancer (or lack thereof). Because of the time it takes to properly prepare and examine biopsies, the results are usually not available for at least five days, and often not for as long as ten days.

Cancer: Cancer is an uncontrolled growth of cells in the body. Cancer can form tumors, invade surrounding healthy tissues (called **local invasion**), and slip into the circulation to start new growths in distant sites (**metastasis**). Cancers are usually named for the body part or type of cell in which they arise. Cancer that has spread is sometimes called **systemic cancer**.

Carcinogens: Carcinogens are cancer-causing agents, which can be found anywhere – in our food, in our water, in our air, and in our soil. Carcinogens are discussed in some detail in Chapter 8.

Cell: Cells are the tiny "building blocks" of the body. They are so small that over 10,000 can fit on the head of a pin. Until a few years ago, science believed that once a cell committed to being a certain kind of cell – a heart cell, a liver cell, and so on – it could never change into any other kind. Recent evidence shows us that perhaps this is not entirely true.

Chemotherapy: Historically, the word chemotherapy referred to the use of any chemical in any medical treatment. Today, it is used to describe the use of pharmaceuticals in a cancer treatment. Chemotherapy kills cancer cells in a variety of different ways, including: increasing damaging free radicals within cancer cells, damaging DNA, blocking cell division, interfering with cell metabolism, and increasing apoptosis. Often there is a blend of different processes leading to **cytotoxicity**. Chemotherapy drugs are usually administered intravenously or by mouth, depending upon the drug. Typically, the goal is to give the dog the **maximum tolerated dose**, although lower doses are used in **metronomic chemotherapy**. Dogs do not usually require sedation or anesthesia during chemotherapy treatments.

Chronotherapy: Literally, "time therapy." Most compounds (chemotherapy drugs as well as other agents) seem to have a time of day when they are at their most potent, with the fewest side effects. For example, one drug may be best at 10am, while another is best at 3pm. Chronotherapy is in its infancy in the U.S., but we're learning more every day.

Clean Margins: A biopsy is said to have "clean margins" when the pathologist does not see evidence of tumor cells in the margins of normal tissue examined during the **comprehensive margin evaluation**.

Complete Blood Count: A very common test used to assist in diagnosis. It measures many aspects of the blood, including the numbers and types of white blood cells, red blood cells, and platelets. Also known as a CBC.

Complete Remission: All measurable signs of cancer are gone. However, due to the inherent nature of systemic cancer, measurable signs are likely to return at some point in the future. See **remission**.

Comprehensive Margin Evaluation: An examination performed by a pathologist to see if there are cancer cells along the margins of biopsied tissue. If there are cells on the edge of the tissue sample, there are likely some left in the dog, and another surgery or other treatment may be in order. If cells are present, the results are called **dirty margins** or "incomplete margins"; if the pathologist doesn't find any microscopic tumor cells, the results are called **clean margins** or "complete margins." Despite the use of the word "comprehensive," a pathologist only looks at a couple of areas along the margins, not the entire margin. This is why **wide margins** are so important to prevent malignant tumor regrowth.

CT Scan: CT stands for computed tomography, which is a medical imaging technique using two-dimensional **X-rays** taken in a series and digitally computed, or manipulated, so that a three-dimensional image of the inside of the body is formed.

Each image shows a "slice", also called a tomograph, of the body and provides more detail than X-rays or ultrasound. CT scans are usually only available in large veterinary or specialty hospitals. It's important that the dog remains still during a CT scan, so heavy sedation or general anesthesia is usually required.

Cure: When cancer is completely absent from the body, and is not expected to return at any time in the future, the patient has achieved a "cure." I have seen dogs live long years past their prognosis, and I have also seen cancer disappear from bodies and never return. Unlike other areas of veterinary medicine, where we can say "this can be cured" or "this can be managed forever," we cannot say this yet for **systemic cancer** cases. Until that day, I rely on conventional and outside-the-box treatments, in the hope that something – or more likely, many things together – will work for your dog. In the meantime, Dr. Ettinger and I both agree that it may be helpful to think of your dog's cancer as a treatable, chronic condition, rather than a curable disease.

Cytotoxic: Literally, "toxic to cells." This word is used to describe cancer treatments that are toxic to cancer cells. Unfortunately, these same treatments may also be toxic to other living cells, such as bone marrow cells, hair follicles and the cells of the gastrointestinal tract. Conventional veterinary cancer care seeks a successful balance of cytotoxicity between cancer cells and healthy cells in the body. Drugs, radiation, and even some supplements can be cytotoxic in the body. This word implies that the cells would not have died without the use of the agent or treatment.

Decompensation: When a dog can no longer hide or mask the signs and symptoms of disease and suddenly becomes very obviously sick. Dogs have a talent and instinct for compensation, or hiding their symptoms, which is why they can seem to get sick "overnight" when they finally decompensate.

Dirty Margins: A biopsy is said to have dirty margins when the pathologist sees tumor cells in the margins of normal tissue examined during the **comprehensive margin evaluation**. Dirty margins indicate that cancer cells are likely still in the body around the surgical incision or scar.

Double-blind, Placebo-Controlled Study: The preferred way that conventional medicine evaluates treatments. In this type of study, at least two groups of identical (or as near as possible) patients are given treatments. One group receives the actual treatment being studied (the treatment group) and the other does not (the placebo group). Neither the doctor nor the patient knows which group is getting which treatment (double-blind). The treatment is evaluated by comparing its effectiveness with the placebo. While this can be useful, it is not the only way to thoroughly and thoughtfully evaluate a treatment. Using only treatments "proven" by this kind of study excludes many that may be just as – or more – effective. There are treatments proven by historical use, from other systems, or even those that may be untried, but worth a shot in a last-ditch effort to treat the dog. Other countries, including Japan and several European countries, rely more on historical use and the experience of practitioners. Some researchers consider the use of placebos to be cruel, and instead choose to compare a group of patients receiving the new treatment to a group of patients receiving the current best treatment. While some clinical researchers in American western medicine are using this approach, most scientists still feel the double-blind, placebo-controlled experiment is the gold standard.

DNA: Deoxyribonucleic acid (DNA) is a chain of molecules that contains the genetic instructions for any living organism. DNA is like a blueprint, a recipe, or a code. It stores information about how the body will develop and function throughout its life. DNA has segments, called **genes**, which carry this genetic information and help cells develop, live, and die, all according to the instructions in the DNA.

Durable Remission: This diagnosis is achieved when there are no measurable signs of cancer, and there have been no signs for a reasonable length of time. Most oncologists consider a remission durable after fourteen to twenty-one days. If a patient cannot stay in remission between treatments, it is typically not an effective treatment.

Fine Needle Aspirate: This is an initial screening procedure which vets use to test a tumor or other site in the body for malignant cells. A skinny needle is inserted into the site, which draws up a small sample of the cells and fluids inside the tumor. The sample can – in many cases – confirm the presence and type of cancer. Fine needle aspirates cannot be used to grade a cancer, and their results can sometimes be inconclusive. This type of aspirate can also be used to sample lymph nodes, the liver, the spleen, the kidney, or other sites. This procedure typically does not require sedation or anesthesia and is often relatively inexpensive.

Full Spectrum: This is my phrase to describe an unbiased, results-oriented, strategic approach to cancer care. The goal is to optimize life quality and increase longevity. As a Full Spectrum vet, I consider and treat all aspects of cancer, including diet, lifestyle, and the psychological well-being of both the patient and the guardian. Conventional tools (chemotherapy, surgery and radiation) are part of Full Spectrum cancer care, as are many alternative treatments and others, never previously considered for canine cancer care.

Gained Life Expectancy: How long do we expect a dog to live if he does not get treatment for his cancer? How long do we expect him to live if he does? The difference between those two numbers is the gained life expectancy of that treatment. For example, if we expect that a dog has two months to live, but with treatment could live six months, the gained life expectancy is four months. Knowing the gained life expectancy can be helpful when making treatment plan choices.

Genes: Genes are segments of DNA, which carry codes for specific proteins, functions, and cell processes in the living organism. A gene usually contributes to the control of a small segment of what happens in a cell or in a body. Altogether, genes manage every facet of life on the tissue, organ and body level. Genes behave like microscopic cell managers, while making sure that everything happens according to their instructions.

Grade: How aggressive a cancer is can be predicted by its grade. To grade cancer, a pathologist examines a biopsied tumor under a high power microscope and notes special characteristics of the cancer cells, which can indicate how aggressively they may behave in future. Sometimes, veterinarians and oncologists use words such as "angry" or "hot," to describe very aggressive tumors. Different grading systems are used for different tumor types, but generally the more aggressive a tumor is the higher is the number assigned. "High grade" tumors are more aggressive and "low grade" tumors are less so.

Historical Use: This term suggests evaluating treatments by looking at their use over time, rather than using clinical studies. Some drugs, like aspirin (pain relief) and phenobarbital (anti-seizure), were used before the Food and Drug Administration (FDA) started regulating pharmaceuticals. These drugs, which have strong historical evidence of working in the body, are grandfathered into the system and do not need to go through the lengthy (ten to fifteen years) and extremely expensive (millions of dollars) approval process. Since 1938, new drugs undergo safety and efficacy trials to prove to the FDA that

they work for the purpose for which they are intended. Drugs are usually approved for one, fairly narrow use, although their action may be useful in other diseases. Once approved, doctors and veterinarians can prescribe them for their approved purpose, or for any other purpose they judge to be safe and appropriate. A classic example of this is using phenobarbital – grandfather-approved for seizures – as a sedative. This practice, called off-label prescription, is very common, especially in veterinary medicine. Using off-label prescriptions, vets can prescribe a drug approved for humans for use in any other species. Vets may also use a drug approved for a condition in one species in a totally different species, and even for a different condition. There are two chemotherapy drugs approved for use specifically in dogs; both are approved for some types of mast cell tumors: Palladia and Kinavet CA-1. Many, but not all, other chemotherapy treatments used in conventional care have been reviewed for safety and efficacy in dogs, but do not have specific FDA approval. If a treatment (drug or not) has been in use for a long time and is successful, it is considered valid, even if there are no FDA studies "proving" its validity. Most pragmatic vets agree with this point of view, although a few demand more proof.

Homeopathy: An alternative medical practice started in Germany in the late eighteenth century, homeopathy uses extremely diluted substances to stimulate symptoms similar to what the patient is already experiencing, according to the principle of "like cures like." For example, if the patient is coughing, a remedy might be given that would cause coughing in a healthy person. Despite this counter-intuitive reasoning, homeopathy has been shown to be useful for certain forms of brain cancer, in combination with drugs. It may also be useful for other cancers. I recommend consulting with a veterinarian trained in homeopathy, if you are interested in using it.

Immune System: The body's defense against external microbes and viruses, and also the body's "clean-up crew" for deranged and mutated cells. Incredibly complex, it can be strengthened or weakened by nutrition, emotional states, sleep (or lack of it) and stress. A strong immune system deploys cancer-fighting cells to destroy cancer, but if cancer overwhelms the system (which it can), immunity is suppressed. This creates a higher risk for secondary infections. There is even evidence that cancer can recruit certain immune cells to help the cancer spread or metastasize. For more details on how the immune system operates, see the vaccination discussion on page 87. Strategic boosting of the immune system is an important part of Full Spectrum cancer care.

In Vitro: Means "in glass" and often refers to a treatment that is tested in a test tube, a petri dish, or in other equipment in a lab. Many promising cancer therapies work very well *in vitro*, but not *in vivo*.

In Vivo: Literally translated as "in life," this often refers to a treatment that is tested in a living body. If a tested cancer treatment works *in vivo,* it is more promising.

Inflammation: This refers to a protective response of body tissues to injury or irritation. There are many factors involved in creating inflammation; the main characteristics are pain, warmth, swelling and redness. But if inflammation becomes chronic or excessive, it can become problematic; arthritis, asthma, allergies, and other diseases are associated with inflammation. Inflammation is also implicated in cancer promotion, which is why managing it is an important part of Full Spectrum cancer care.

Initiation: According to the genetic mutation theory of cancer, initiation is the first stage of cancer development. In this stage, a cell's **DNA** is damaged beyond repair, often including the DNA involved with **apoptosis** (natural cell death).

Local Invasion: When cancer tumors spread to the healthy tissues immediately surrounding the tumor, we call it local invasion. Local invasion is therefore different from **metastasis**, which is cancer that has spread to distant locations in the body.

Lymphatic System: The lymphatic system is a type of circulatory system that runs throughout the body. A vast network of tubes that are connected to body organs and tissues, the lymphatics carry a clear fluid called lymph. The lymph carries white blood cells, making it a crucial component of the **immune system**. A map of the lymphatics resembles a busy subway system, with the tubes, the tracks, and the lymph glands or nodes (filters that catch viruses, bacteria, and other invaders so that white blood cells can destroy and dispose of them), the stations. Because the lymphatics reach nearly every organ, cancers that occur in the lymph cells – lymphomas – are by definition **systemic cancers**. Other types of cancer may also use the lymph system as a means to **metastasize**. For this reason, lymph nodes are often aspirated or biopsied during cancer diagnosis, to check for spread.

Malignant: A tumor, which is dangerous and growing uncontrollably, is called malignant. This word is a synonym for cancerous. Another word used to refer to a malignant tumor or a cancer is malignancy.

Margin: This refers to the area of normal-seeming tissue surrounding a tumor that has been removed during a biopsy or other surgery. This area may contain microscopic cancer cells, so, a pathologist examines it during a **comprehensive margin evaluation**. If the margins are narrow (one or two millimeters), malignant tumors are more likely to recur. For this reason, **wide margins** of two to three centimeters are preferred.

Maximum Tolerated Dose: In conventional treatment, this phrase is used to describe the highest dose of **chemotherapy** that can be given without the patient's having unacceptable, severe **side effects** or dying from the treatment. The higher the chemotherapy dose is the more cancer cells are killed; therefore, the aim of chemotherapy is to give as high a dose as possible with the fewest (manageable) side effects. There is a great deal of information on chemotherapy side effects and how to manage them in Chapter 11.

Measurable Disease: This refers to a tumor that can be measured for size with calipers or imaging techniques; also called macroscopic disease. You can see these tumors with the eye, unlike microscopic tumors, which are too small to see without magnification.

Median Survival Time: The time, from either diagnosis or treatment, at which no more than half of the patients with a given cancer are expected to be alive. For example, if a group of dogs all have lymphoma and all start the conventional chemotherapy protocol that Dr. Ettinger recommends, she would expect half of those dogs to be alive after fourteen months, and half of them to have passed. It is useful for the guardian to know this number, but it is also important to remember that it is only a guide. It does not apply directly to any particular dog. Some vets use the term "median overall survival" or the term "median survival."

Metastasis: When cancer spreads to distant sites in the body by slipping tumor cells into the circulatory system (the blood or the lymph), we call it metastasis.

Metronomic Chemotherapy: A relatively new approach to chemotherapy, which doesn't attempt to kill cancer cells directly (like **maximum tolerated dose** does), but instead attempts to cut them off from their supply of oxygen and nutrition. Low doses of drugs are given on a regular basis to target the lin-ing of the blood vessels feeding the tumor. This can stop the tumor from building new blood vessels (**angiogenesis**). Some tumors may stop growing, while others may shrink. The low doses mean that the normal tissues of the body are rarely affected, and side effects greatly reduced. See page 137 for more details.

Micrometastasis: This is the spread of very small numbers of cancer cells to distant sites through the circulatory system. Micrometastasis is usually undetectable (or undetectable with our current diagnostic tools), due to the small numbers of cells that have spread when the diagnostic tool is applied

MRI: MRI stands for magnetic resonance imaging, which is an imaging technique that uses powerful magnets to generate electromagnetic fields. These fields pick up information in the body and broadcast it to a radio antenna. The resulting image is a series of "slices" much like what is seen in a CT scan, with much more detail. MRI is an advanced imaging device and is typically only available in very large veterinary hospitals or specialty hospitals. Dogs usually require general anesthesia while the MRI is conducted.

Natural: This indicates not synthetic: originating from a source found in nature. While many guardians have a bias towards using natural substances in cancer treatments, it is important to remember that not all natural substances are safe. There are naturally occurring deadly poisons in mushrooms, a form of cyanide in peach pits, and toxins in frogs in the Amazon that can cause paralysis. All natural substances are not necessarily effective, either. While there are many natural substances recommended for **Full Spectrum** care, Appendix B lists natural remedies that are less effective than their proponents often claim.

Nutraceutical: Originally, nutraceutical was defined as any substance from dietary ingredients that could yield health benefits. Today, the word's meaning has been expanded to include purified agents from many sources, including botanical (plant) sources. For example, a nutraceutical agent in Apocaps, luteolin, comes from peanut hulls. Most people who eat peanuts (dietary) do not eat their hulls (botanical). Another familiar nutraceutical is glucosamine chondroitin, a popular joint supplement. A nutraceutical tends to have higher concentrations of the agent than are commonly found in nature, and therefore more potent effect. Generally, the intensity of a nutraceutical's effect on the body is somewhere between that of a supplement and a pharmaceutical. While pharmaceuticals – usually purely synthetic agents – are assumed to be fast acting, nutraceuticals can take a little longer to build up in the system and produce their full effect (usually a week or more).

Non-resectable: This word refers to a tumor that cannot be removed with surgery. Non-resectable tumors, also called inoperable tumors, must be treated with other methods.

Normal Life Expectancy: The general expectation for a given dog's natural lifespan, this number is based on the breed and/or weight of the dog. In general, small dogs live longer than big dogs. Taking exceptions into account, knowing your dog's *general* life expectancy can be helpful when making treatment plans.

Oncologist: A veterinary oncologist is a veterinarian who has completed additional specialized training in conventional oncology. A general medicine and surgery internship is required, plus a residency in their chosen focus: chemotherapy (oncologist), surgery (surgical oncologist), or radiation (radiation oncologist). Once the internship and residency are complete – which can take three to five years – the oncologist must pass special exams to become certified by their college. For example, Dr. Ettinger is Board Certified by the American College of Veteri-

nary Internal Medicine, with a subspecialty in oncology. Oncologists focus exclusively on cancer and become very skilled at using their tool of choice. According to the Bureau of Labor Statistics, in 2008 (the last year for which data is available) there were 59,700 veterinarians in the United States. As of this writing only about two hundred of those are board certified veterinary oncologists, most of them located in large urban centers.

Oncology: Oncology literally means "the study of cancer." This word is commonly used to describe the conventional veterinary approach to cancer care. Three primary treatment tools are used: surgery, chemotherapy and radiation. Other possible tools include some nutritional support and more recently, genetic therapy and immunotherapy. While oncology has some success with certain kinds of cancer at certain stages, outcomes are generally not as desirable as those associated with other medical conditions (for example, treating infections).

Pain: During cancer and/or cancer treatments, pain can have several sources, including tumors pressing on organs or tissues such as bones and nerves, tissues stretched beyond their normal lengths, blocking of circulation, inflammation resulting from cancers, and surgical incision healing. A dog in pain may isolate himself, seem apathetic, or limit his movement. Some dogs may vocalize. Some treatments may cause temporary pain (such as surgery) – but, in the end, if the treatment prevents more pain than it causes, there can be higher overall life quality. Unmanaged or chronic pain, however, can cause a decrease in life quality. Pain management is part of a Full Spectrum cancer care plan, and is addressed in Chapter 17.

Palliative: A palliative treatment is one that alleviates symptoms associated with the illness. It improves the quality of life, but does not extend survival time or cure the illness. A familiar example is the use of painkillers, which do not treat the cancer, but do help to reduce discomfort. Another example is palliative radiation therapy, which aims at slowing tumor growth and, more importantly, decreasing pain and improving quality of life. While most oncologists do not think of conventional treatments as palliative treatments, I do, because they usually do not provide a "cure" for systemic cancer at this time. This is why I have come to think of cancer as a chronic disease to be managed, rather than a disease that can be cured. We'll talk a little more about this later.

Partial Remission: This is said to occur when some of the measurable signs of cancer are gone. Most oncologists call a remission partial when they see between 50% and 100% **response** to treatment.

Pathologist: A specialist in pathology (the study of disease), pathologists examine and evaluate cells, tissues or organs in order to come to a diagnosis. They usually work in pathology labs or very large hospitals. When your vet or oncologist submits a **biopsy**, for example, a pathologist is the one who actually examines the tissue under a microscope.

Primary Health Advocate: In **Full Spectrum** cancer care, I urge every guardian to take this leadership role (discussed on page 254). I do this because we do not yet have a cure for systemic cancer, and vets and oncologists are usually unable to provide a treatment recommendation that will yield a cure. With this sad fact in mind, it's logical that the guardian needs to be active in decision-making. After all, only the guardian can take into account what may be gained with treatment and balance it against life quality concerns, age of the dog, personal values, available time, and financial resources. As primary health advocates, guardians have the eventual final responsibility for all health care decisions. Reading this book will prepare you to become your dog's primary health advocate and conduct your own **Treatment Plan Analysis.**

Prognosis: The overall expected outcome of the cancer case under consideration, prognosis can include the median survival time, a description of how life functions will be affected, and whether the disease will cause a lingering decline, a sudden crisis, or neither of these. A prognosis is usually classified somewhere along the continuum of "excellent" to "poor." It is useful to note that "prognosis" means "prediction." While it is very helpful to know your dog's prognosis, it is neither a promise nor a sentence; it is an educated guess. The more information your vet or oncologist has, the more accurate the prognosis tends to be.

Progression: The final stage in cancer development (after **promotion**), when cancer cells have multiplied to become full-fledged cancers and can now divide uncontrollably, invade normal tissues, and may metastasize.

Promotion: This is the second stage in cancer development (after **initiation** and before **progression**). If the **immune system** is unable to dispose of damaged cells, and if **apoptosis** genes fail to induce cell suicide, damaged cells persist. They also begin to grow and replicate, forming tumors or cancers.

Pyschoimmunoneurology: This field of study examines the complex connections between mental function (stress, depression, anger, happiness) and body function and disease. It brings together the fields of endocrinology, psychology, immunology and physiology to elucidate how the body interacts with itself and its environment. In short, this is the scientific study of a facet of the mind-body connection. Full Spectrum cancer care incorporates pyschoimmunoneurology into treatment plans because it has been documented that supporting the mind-body connection helps to battle cancer in humans.

Quality of Life: How enjoyable is life for the dog? Sometimes treatments may extend longevity, but also increase the number of side effects a dog experiences. If side effects can't be managed or become too severe, life quality may go down. On the other hand, life quality can also be deliberately increased. Paying attention to the optimal balance of life quality *and* longevity is discussed in the Making Confident Choices section of this book.

Radiation Therapy: Radiation therapy is a conventional medical treatment that sends high-energy particles, usually photons or electrons, into tumors. These particles interact with the atoms in the DNA of the cancer cells and destroy them. This, in turn, destroys the cancer cells. Radiation also kills cells by increasing the amount of harmful free radicals within the cell. Healthy cells that fall in its path, especially rapidly multiplying cells such as those in the skin, can also be harmed. Dogs must be immobilized to receive radiation, so each session requires general anesthesia.

Remission: This term indicates that the cancer has responded, or gone away, to some degree. Vets usually modify this with words like **complete** or **partial**, to indicate the degree of remission. In common use, remission is usually synonymous with complete remission.

Rescue Protocol: If a dog has gone into remission, but then has a relapse, another course of treatment may induce a second remission. That second treatment is called a rescue protocol.

Residual Disease: This phrase is used to describe cancer cells that remain after attempts to remove them have been made.

Response: The cancer "responds" to treatment, or

gets better. You may hear "her response so far is good" or "he isn't responding to this treatment." Sometimes response is also used as a synonym for complete or partial remission.

Side Effect: In any given treatment, a certain effect is desired; for example, a desired effect of surgery might be tumor removal. Any effect other than the desirable effect is called a side effect. Side effects can range from harmless (loss of hair) to harmful (a life-threatening staph infection). Sometimes side effects increase with higher intensity treatments – for example, the higher a chemotherapy dose, the more likely a dog is to vomit. Sometimes, however, side effects are "idiosyncratic." Idiosyncratic side effects are (non-allergic) side effects where the severity of the reaction is not in proportion to the dose of the treatment (how much is given). Idiosyncratic reactions, not seen in large numbers of dogs, seem to be caused by individual variation. In other words, one dog reacted badly to that medication, although the vast majority of dogs would not, even at the same dose. It is important to keep in mind that side effects can happen for several reasons, and cannot always be anticipated. It is, therefore, important to ask about the possible side effects of any treatment you are considering.

Staging: Staging is the evaluation of a cancer to determine how far it has spread or metastasized. Diagnostic tests used to stage cancer may include lymph node aspirates, lymph node biopsies, chest X-rays, abdominal ultrasounds, CT or MRI scans, and occasionally bone marrow or internal organ aspirates and/or biopsies. Generally, the lower the stage number (stage one, for example), the more likely the cancer is to respond to treatment and therefore have a better prognosis.

Supplement Hierarchy: Many supplements are discussed in this book, and some guardians ask which are most important. For this reason, I created a hierarchy that lists supplements in their order of importance. Starting with the supplements at the top of the hierarchy and adding others as time, budget, and the dog's preference or tolerance will allow, is a good strategy (see Appendix A).

Surgery: Surgery is a conventional treatment that removes tumors by cutting them out of the body. While the ideal goal is complete removal, this is not always possible. In these cases, **palliative** surgery may be recommended: removing some, but not all, of the tumor (also known as debulking). Surgery is generally done under anesthesia, and may require post-operative recovery care, such as wound cleaning, changing of bandages, physical therapy, and limiting movements to allow incisions to heal.

Systemic Cancer: This is cancer of any type that has spread to and/or affects the entire body. Some cancers, such as lymphoma, are systemic by default because they occur in cells that circulate throughout the entire body. In other cases, a cancer is called systemic if it has **metastasized** to distant locations from the primary tumor or if it has invaded the surrounding tissues via **local invasion**.

Touch Therapies: Touch therapies include massage, Reiki, T-Touch, and other energy healing modalities that involve hands-on, physical contact with the patient. Memorial Sloan-Kettering Cancer Center in New York City has integrated several touch therapies into their standard menu of cancer treatments because their research shows that touch therapies may help with outcomes like pain reduction, chemotherapy tolerance, and a variety of other issues related to cancer.

Treatment Plan Analysis: At this point, there is no cure for systemic cancer, so there is no "one right plan" for cancer treatments (the right plan would be the one that cured the cancer). Treatment plan analysis is the process of looking at all of the available treatments for your dog's cancer and making a plan based on your values, your dog's age, your desired quality of life, your budget, and other factors. Often guardians leave the planning to the vet, but, the vet may not know enough about the guardian to make a good plan. Taking on the responsibility of treatment plan analysis empowers you to make conscious choices and know you have done everything possible to help your dog. Part Four of this book is dedicated to treatment plan analysis.

Tumor: A growth, mass, or bump made of benign or malignant cells is a tumor. Tumors can be technically classified as benign (generally not dangerous) or as malignant (dangerous, cancerous). In common use, however, the word is usually used only when the tumor is malignant. If your vet refers to a growth as a tumor, she likely means it is a malignant tumor.

Ultrasound: Ultrasound is a diagnostic medical imaging technique that can help get a picture of the deeper areas of the body. While this tool's most familiar use is to check on human baby development during pregnancy, it can also produce an image of the interior of any other soft-tissue organ. In contrast, an x-ray image often just shows a silhouette or shadow of internal organs without revealing their internal architecture. The heart, eye, muscles, tendons, and many internal organs in the abdomen can usually be seen with ultrasound imaging. The technique is non-invasive, has no known risks for the patient, and is available at many veterinary hospitals. Dogs typically do not need sedation during ultrasound.

Wide margin: Margins of at least two to three centimeters (sometimes more, and sometimes less, depending upon the case) that surrounded the cancer and were removed from the body during a biopsy or other surgery. Malignant tumors are more likely to recur if they are removed with narrow margins, so wide margins, if possible, are preferred.

Wild Diet: Dogs are not designed to eat dry kibble, just like we are not designed to eat crackers as our main food source. Dogs in the wild eat freshly killed animals. While the wide availability of pre-packaged commercial dog food in the last half century has led us to think of it as the dog's natural diet, it is decidedly not so. According to human cancer research (including that done by Sir Richard Doll, a British epidemiologist who was knighted, in addition to receiving several other honors for his work), about one third of human cancers can be prevented by improving the diet alone (see Appendix E for references). The wild diet is the basis for the dog cancer diet featured in Chapter 14.

X-rays: X-rays are a form of electromagnetic energy, which can be used to take images of the interior of the body by projecting them onto a film sensitive to their wavelength. Because X-rays are flat, two-dimensional films and the body is three-dimensional, the area being imaged is usually X-rayed from two 90° angles. These two images are then compared, which allows for a more complete image of the interior of the body. When the chest is being imaged, however, two X-rays may not give a complete picture. In these cases, three-view X-rays are usually taken: one while the dog lies on her right side, another on her left side, and a third while lying on her back. Most veterinary hospitals have X-ray machines. Depending upon the area being filmed and the individual dog, dogs may need some sedation or anesthesia to get an X-ray.

Chapter 6: How Cancer Begins and Spreads

T here are a few certainties if your dog has cancer: one, there is a serious problem in her body, and two, her cancer probably started some time ago (certainly before she decompensated and started showing obvious signs of illness). As an oncologist once told me, "Beyond that, it's complicated."

As unbelievable as it might seem – and as frustrating as it is when you want answers now – scientists do not (yet) have one single explanation for cancer development that includes every piece of data. Much like the search for the "theory of everything" in physics, the one theory that accounts for all of the evidence is the goal of some cancer research. More is being learned everyday – but we're not there yet.

Understanding how cancer starts and spreads is important: if we know how it starts, we can understand how to treat it. Because of the complexity of this subject, we'll skip most of the details and focus on the basics – just enough for you to understand why I include certain treatments in Full Spectrum cancer care and exclude others.

Mindset Matters

Most cancer researchers have what is called a "reductionist" mindset. Reductionism is the theory that every complexity can be understood by looking at how individual components of the problem interact. Reductionists assume that in order to understand cancer, it must be broken down into smaller and smaller parts. The interaction of those smaller parts (which may have smaller parts, which may have smaller parts, which may have smaller parts, and so on) can explain everything, this theory says. Understanding and solving the "one problem" at the lowest level can also solve the larger problem. In other words, to reductionists, the whole is just a sum of its parts.

This mindset has led to the prevailing view of cancer development: it begins at one of the smallest, most basic levels, with mutations in the genes in the DNA. Fix (or destroy) these mutations, this view says, and you can cure the cancer.

There are a few who don't subscribe to this point of view. These researchers point out that the reductionist approach has resulted in few substantial gains over the last sixty years of cancer research, especially when compared to other areas of medicine. These experts want to widen the lens we use to focus on cancer, and view it as a system with many seemingly independent parts. Maybe, they postulate, we don't have to understand how cancer operates on a cellular level. Perhaps, if we looked for patterns on broader levels, we could control cancer – even if we don't fully understand it. These experts are interested in looking at how changing the internal environment in the body (through lifestyle and other treatments that don't directly "attack" the cancer cells) can either support cancer's development or diminish it.

In other words, perhaps the whole is more than a sum of its parts.

For a clear presentation on this newer kind of thinking, I recommend starting with Dr. David Agus' speech to the TED Medical conference. It is called A New Strategy in the War on Cancer, and you can find it at www.Ted.com.

For our immediate purposes, both mindsets have yielded important information that may help you understand your dog's cancer and evaluate treatments. We've already noted that cancer and its development is a complex topic; a thorough discussion of it is beyond the scope of this book. The good news is: you don't need to know everything in order to make some treatment decisions.

Genetic Mutations

Broadly stated, the genetic mutation theory of cancer development posits that cancer begins when mutations form in a cell's genes and the cell grows and multiplies to form a tumor (or cluster of cancer cells).

Genes are found in segments of the DNA, the mysterious stuff that regulates the body and contains all of the blueprints – or job descriptions – for each cell. Genes control each body cell from birth to death. If the genes are normal, the cell behaves normally; if the genes are abnormal, the cell may behave abnormally, too.

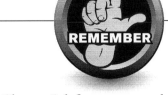

Chapter 5 defines common dog cancer phrases and words, so remember to refer back to it, if you need help.

Different genes control different cell functions and processes. For example, one set of genes controls cell growth: when these genes are activated, cells grow and multiply, or make new cells. When your dog was a puppy, these genes were very active, and today, when your dog sustains an injury like a cut, some of these same genes activate new cells that close it up.

Another set of genes controls cell death, or apoptosis. These genes activate when growth is complete; for example, when your puppy has reached full size, or when the cut is fully healed. If the growth genes are like the gas pedal, the apoptosis genes are like the brake pedal. They can stop the cell from multiplying and they can shut down the cell's life processes so that it dies a natural death (apoptosis is discussed in more detail in the next chapter).

In the case of cancer, trouble starts when one or more errors, or mutations, occur in the genes. This could happen for many reasons, some of which we'll discuss in the next chapters. According to researchers, genetic mutations happen all the time — as many as 10,000 times every day, in the typical mammal. In the vast majority of cells, the genes can withstand the mutations. Often they can repair the damage. If they can't repair it, the apoptosis genes can force the cell to commit suicide.

When the cell is damaged enough (or often enough), the genes that control cell growth and cell apoptosis can also become damaged. Then, apoptosis might not happen, leaving the mutated cell alive in the body. This lowering of apoptosis is considered one of the hallmarks of cancer cells.

This stage of cancer development is called **Cancer Initiation**: cancer has not yet begun, but there is at least one cell whose growth genes are becoming deranged, setting the stage for future growth at will. In this cell (or in these cells, if more than one cell is affected), the gas pedal is jammed to the floor and the brake pedal is broken.

Once a single cell or cluster of cells has become cancerous, it starts broadcasting biochemical signals to alert the immune system that something is wrong. In response, the immune system deploys

What We Learned with Shadow Helps Keymos Today

"Shadow was one of the true loves of my life. When he was diagnosed, and we then fought the cancer that had attacked him, we came to know that winning the ultimate fight was not as important as the days we shared. Living in the moment really came into its own. While I would always choose to still have Shadow with me in physical form, he opened doors and brought realizations to my life that would not have happened without his illness. I know for certain that it was his path and ours together, to learn. When he friend, Keymos was diagnosed only a year after losing Shadow, at first I couldn't believe that we had another diagnosis. But, we were already armed. Keymos was already on a wonderful diet, and he began Apocaps immediately. Thought he is older at 13 than Shadow was at only 9 years, Keymos is fit and sturdy. But without the lessons learned from Shadow, we may not have had the tools in place to help Keymos be this well. There is no evidence of cancer in him anymore, and he revels in every day, teaching the younger dogs what he knows."

- Susan Harper, High Wycombe,

specialized cancer-killing cells. If they are successful (and sometimes they aren't), those cells destroy the cancer cell and the body eliminates it naturally.

Sometimes the immune system cannot detect or destroy the cancerous cell because it has been compromised. This can happen for many reasons, some of which we'll talk about in this and the next few chapters. If the immune system fails to kill the cancerous cell, it will continue to live.

If conditions in the body favor cancer growth – for example, if inflammation is present, or if sugar is readily available – the cancerous cell becomes stronger. If the cancerous cell or cells evade destruction, they move to a new stage called **Cancer Promotion**. The single or few pre-cancerous cells have now become full-blown cancer cells, ready to "promote" themselves by changing the body's environment to suit their own needs.

Cancer cells change the body in several ways. They can recruit local blood vessels to steal nutrition from normal neighbors, which is called angiogenesis. These new blood vessels can also be used to launch new cancer cells into the circulation so they can metastasize in distant locations.

The cancer cells also make special enzymes, which they use to tunnel between neighboring normal cells, so they can make room for their own growth.

Cancer cells also shift the body's metabolism. Normal body cells use oxygen to extract energy from sugars in a process called oxidation; cancer cells use very little oxygen. Instead, they break down sugars using a completely different method, glycolysis, followed by a secretion of acid. This is called the Warburg effect, and, like reduced apoptosis, it is another hallmark of cancer cells. The secreted acid lowers the pH of the surrounding tissues, which creates a lot of inflammation, further favoring cancer's growth.

Cancer cells also send themselves chemical signals that stimulate their own growth and even recruit other types of body cells to do the same. Once the cell starts dividing and replicating itself, it has reached the next stage, **Cancer Progression**. Now the growth genes are working overtime: tumors, large lumps of millions of cancer cells, form and spread.

Assuming that everything goes smoothly during replication, new cancer cells are clones of the first. Each carries the same genetic blueprint as the mother cell, including the switched off apoptosis genes. This means that tumor cells tend to multiply exponentially.

Cancer cells are often genetically unstable and may continue to change over time, possibly even becoming stronger and more resistant to treatments.

This very broad overview of an incredibly complex process gives you an idea of how cancer is believed to start on the cellular level, and explains why some Full Spectrum treatments target cancer cells there.

Now let's take a look at cancer development from a completely different angle.

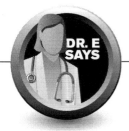

DR. E SAYS

We typically find tumors once they measure about one centimeter in diameter. This may not seem large, until you realize that a tumor this size contains 10^9, or **one billion**, cancer cells.

Tissue Environment

The theory of genetic mutation assumes that a cell's natural state is rest: the cell does not want to grow and is content to stay the same size, doing what it does naturally according to its genetic instructions.

There's another theory, however, which assumes the complete opposite. According to the century-old tissue environment or "epigenetic" theory, which is only now gaining acceptance, a cell's natural state is one of growth and replication.

(By the way, the word environment in this case refers to the internal environment of the body, which is also called the extracellular matrix. It does not refer to the external environment.)

This is an important distinction, because if a cell tends to grow and replicate if left on its own, then what stops it from doing so?

Tissue environment theory posits that growth decisions are not controlled by the genes *inside* the cell, but by the *neighborhood* of the cell – including fluids and connective tissue, also called the matrix. The matrix, which surrounds each cell and connects it to all the others, is one decision-maker; and every other cell in the neighborhood is also a decision-maker.

According to this theory, the cells and the matrix are like a community, constantly engaged in conversation. Biochemical and neurological "talk" whizzes around the community, keeping each cell informed as to its function, whether to induce apoptosis, or whether to replicate. This community regulates and limits the growth of each individual cell.

Cancer starts when the communication between cells is interrupted and an individual cell loses its sense of purpose. As it loses touch with its cellular neighbors and the matrix, the cell falls back into its default state. Apoptosis genes are shut down, growth genes are turned on, and the cell starts to multiply, because that is what it does if left in its natural state. If this continues, a tumor can form and grow.

The assumption that the basic nature of cells is growth and replication is already accepted in some areas of medicine. For example, it has been proven that bacteria cells replicate when they are fed nutrients. If they are starved, they either die off completely or send out spores, hoping that those little seeds will find a place to grow. Plant cells share this inherent tendency for growth, and, according to researchers, so do animal cells.

The cell that has been cut off from its environment and has reverted to its natural state of rapid replication is not *genetically* faulty – it's just out of touch with the environment and behaving badly. It could, especially if it is caught early enough, be cajoled back into good behavior.

This theory does not discount the fact that genetic mutations may *also* be present in cancer cells; it argues that these mutations simply do not cause the cancer. The cellular environment – and the many factors that influence it – is more important.

Gardeners will tell you that poor quality soil, or soil that is not deep enough, yields unhealthy plants. To get healthy plants, a deep layer of topsoil that has the proper pH, nutrients and water is needed. The tissue environment theory proposes that if the "soil" of the matrix is improved, this may be able to affect cancer – even though it does not directly address it on a cellular level.

The idea of supporting the body has become a popular catchphrase in alternative medicine; this theory gives it a scientific backbone. The tissue environment theory shows that nurturing the surrounding tissues and re-establishing healthy cell-to-cell communication – targeting the matrix – is as important as attacking the cancer cell directly. Later on you'll see that several Full Spectrum cancer care treatments target the matrix, or internal cellular environment, in the body.

Cancer Spread

Once a tumor is established, it can use many mechanisms to spread locally and/or distantly. The body's first line of defense against tumor spread is the immune system, one of the most

It Empowered Me

"Dietary benefits aside, making Gordon's food was cathartic. It empowered me. When we found out he had cancer, I felt absolutely helpless. Making his food gave me the opportunity to have some control in what felt like a hopeless situation. I didn't have to just stand back and watch; I could fight it for him. I was doing something that had real potential to heal him. For the base mixture I primarily used turkey. I'd usually cook and debone a whole turkey (I eventually went to boneless skinless turkey breasts). Sometimes I would add a pound or two of ground beef. I always used all the recommended cruciferous vegetables, the red/yellow peppers, Shitake mushrooms, and low-fat cottage cheese. Beef or chicken liver depending on what was available; same with turkey necks until I found out I could order them in bulk from the grocery store and could always have some in the freezer. I chose brown rice over the oatmeal at my vet's recommendation. At each meal we'd add some combination of garlic, ginger root, parsley and other recommended herbs, sardines in olive oil, blueberries (he picks them out if he can) and coconut oil. In the evening meal only, we'd add fish oil. Lastly, I changed all his in between meal treats to only freeze dried or dehydrated chicken, beef, or fish. He got nothing with flour or starch or carbs."

- Kim Gau, Stow, Ohio

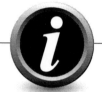

Macrophages Turn Traitor

Cancer is sneaky and smart, and tumors can use many mechanisms to evade the immune system. While talking in detail about these and other methods of progression is beyond the scope of this book, for the purposes of illustration, I will share how one particular immune system cell, the macrophage, can be recruited by cancer to help its spread.

Macrophages are large, blob-shaped cells, and their primary job is to eat (the name is Greek for "big eater"). They eat things that don't belong in the body, including bits of broken-down tumor cells. Like hulking bouncers in a nightclub, they're often on the scene of trouble and they can send out a system-wide signal to alert other immune cells that there is a problem.

Macrophages are often attracted to tumor cells because they sometimes grow so fast that they die from a lack of oxygen. Low oxygen areas are a sign of trouble, so macrophages often show up on their own. They may also come to a tumor because the tumor actually broadcasts recruitment signals, which can convince a macrophage to help the tumor. Cancer biologists call these traitorous macrophages "tumor-associated."

Once a macrophage has turned bad, it helps the tumor in several ways: by breaking down the surrounding cell matrix so it can invade neighboring tissue; by helping to create new blood vessels, so that it can get the oxygen it needs to grow; by releasing proteins that prevent other immune system cells from destroying the tumor; and by providing a growth factor that helps the tumor find existing blood vessels, so it can spread to distant sites.

If this weren't bad enough, traitorous macrophages have one more trick up their sleeves. They start producing inflammatory chemicals – among them, tumor necrosis factor. These bad macrophages form a halo around the tumor and continue secreting inflammatory compounds, creating the perfect environment for more cancer growth and spread.

Research has shown that chronic, low grade, microscopic levels of inflammation have a clear link to cancer (and to other diseases of civilization such as diabetes, Alzheimer's, heart disease, and depression). One reason inflammation could be linked to cancer is that it provides cells with a higher risk of mutating. When cancer cells change, they can also develop resistance to medications and supplements, rendering cancer treatments ineffective. Inflammation also switches off apoptosis genes.

Exactly how to fight these macrophages directly is not yet fully understood. Just shutting down the whole immune system – which is already compromised by cancer – can result in secondary infections and worsening cancer. Instead, we can strategically reduce inflammation using anti-inflammatory Full Spectrum treatments, which may help to check tumor growth and spread. Studies have shown that, in some cases, eliminating inflammation through daily management can decrease the signs of cancer and help lower cancer rates and cancer progression.

complex systems in the body.

The immune system's duties include fighting off foreign invaders such as viruses and bacteria, destroying deranged body cells and helping to heal wounds. There are also special immune cells, called natural killer cells and cytotoxic T-cells, which destroy cancer cells. Many guardians wonder why the immune system doesn't manage to kill cancer earlier, and others believe that if the immune system is restored to health, it could eventually kill the cancer naturally.

While it's true that a healthy immune system has mechanisms which deal with cancer, if your dog already has cancer, the system has failed or been overwhelmed. Cancer suppresses immune function in general, and some lifestyle choices can further suppress it. Oddly enough, certain immune system cells can even actively help cancer to spread (see the sidebar about macrophages on page 64). Tumors actually have several ways to evade the immune system's cancer-killing strategies, making this a very complex topic. A full discussion is beyond the scope of this book, but what's most important is this: the immune system's interactions with cancer are complex and intricate. There are many different types of cells doing many different jobs, and they intersect with cancer at several levels. Several Full Spectrum treatments aim to boost the immune system in specific and strategic ways, as covered in later sections.

In addition to strategic recruitment or disabling of the immune system, there are several other mechanisms cancer uses to spread in the body. It can cause inflammation, shift the body's metabolism, start breaking down sugars without oxygen, and use enzymes to destroy neighboring connective tis-

Chemo for the Rest of His Life?

"Finding out your dog has cancer is devastating, especially if your dog is only 7 like my Charlie. There are so many decisions to make and so much research to do, but with the news of cancer, also comes strong motivation to find out everything you can to save your dog's life. I talked to our chemo specialist here in Kelowna and found out that Charlie would be on Chemo for the rest of his life - once a week for the first six months, and then if the dog is still around the chemo would be reduced to once every two weeks. The side effects can be horrific and we just felt we couldn't bear to see our beautiful dog become extremely sick from such an ordeal. So we chose the healthier route. I changed the diet drastically. I began giving most of the supplements Dr. Dressler recommends. I do massage and exercise and talking healing every day. I enjoy my daily moments with my dog and know that I am doing everything I can to keep his as healthy as possible for as long as possible."

- Audry Arnall, Kelowna, British Columbia

sue, to name just a few. How cancer spreads, also known as "cancer progression," is a complex subject, and a thorough discussion of each of the mechanisms tumors use to grow and metastasize deserves its own book. You'll encounter more information about progression throughout the rest of the book, both in the next section on cancer-causing agents and in the Full Spectrum treatment section.

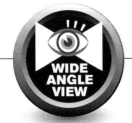

Scientific Mindset or Dogma? Why All This Matters to You and Your Dog

In case your veterinarian looks at you strangely when you mention the treatments you find in this book, I want to explain why I've come to distrust some of the assumptions the mainstream veterinary community makes about cancer and how to treat it.

As the philosophically minded cancer researchers, Dr. Anna De Soto and Dr. Daniel Sonnenschein of Tufts University point out, some cancer researchers have lost the scientific mindset and started believing in their own theories. Busy vets, too, who don't have time to do their own research, could be falling victim to the dogma.

Scientists of all kinds are schooled in the scientific mindset during their training. This mindset forces us to analyze our own assumptions and discover how we may be right, and also how we may be wrong. Here's a rough outline of the method we use to analyze a scientific theory:

1. Look for patterns and regularities in nature, such as repeated events and common structures.

2. Build a hypothesis to explain those patterns. This hypothesis is not "the truth." Instead, it is a first guess at what the truth may be.

3. Test the hypothesis. If it is accurate, future events will be predictable. Set up an experiment or watch natural events, and see if the hypothesis predicts what actually happens.

4. Compare the results to the original hypothesis. If the new data does not fit, revise the hypothesis and test again. If the hypothesis is accurate, events will be predictable, repeatable, and accounted for by the hypothesis.

5. A hypothesis that has undergone enough testing of this sort turns into a "theory." A theory is a plausible explanation that has been tested and found accurate. It is still not "the truth;" it must continue to be tested.

Scientific Mindset or Dogma? *continued*

6. Consider other possibilities. Are there any other explanations for what is happening? If so, can the theory be expanded to include those explanations, or do they directly contradict the theory?

7. If data does not fit, and cannot fit, the theory is considered invalid. A brand new hypothesis must be developed, based on the new data.

8. Repeat testing, based on the new hypothesis.

The scientist who commits to this mindset knows "truth" is elusive, and is open to new information that contradicts her hypothesis or theory. Even if she firmly believes her theory, she must keep in mind that she could be wrong. She might not like having to start over if contradicting data appears, but she is committed to finding the truth.

Unfortunately, some scientists — including some in the field of medicine and oncology — start to believe in their theories (or in theories believed by their mentors). They stop in the middle of step four, close down their minds, and become dogmatic. When evidence that contradicts their theory shows up, they ignore it and continue operating as if they were correct.

According to De Soto and Sonnenschein, this tendency to ignore contradictory evidence has been happening in the field of cancer research; the genetic mutation theory has become a dogma. Anything that directly contradicts it is often dismissed, in spite of published evidence worth contemplating.

This could be disastrous for patients. Who knows how many new treatments there are, which do not fit into current thinking, and therefore will be ignored?

If oncologists insist that genes are the main problem in cancer, while ignoring evidence that cancer might start due to environmental or lifestyle issues, or might not spread without the active cooperation of the immune system, they may be missing new avenues to a cure.

To paraphrase the popular television counselor Dr. Phil, "Would you rather be right, or would you rather cure cancer?"

Perhaps a cure for cancer will come out of the reductionist methods used by many cancer researchers. Perhaps it will come from a much broader approach that looks at body systems as a whole. I personally don't care where it comes from. Do you?

This may seem like an academic discussion to you. I include it because, while many vets are pragmatists like I am, and don't care where a treatment comes from as long as it works for your dog, other vets are more dogmatic.

If you have a dogmatic vet, it's helpful to know. His bias may be informing his treatment

continued on next page

Scientific Mindset or Dogma? *continued*

recommendations. If he's conventional, he may be emphasizing those methods, while minimizing, leaving out, or refusing to consider "outside the box" treatments – even though the treatments he recommends don't give desired results. If he's an alternative vet, he may be dismissing surgeries, chemotherapy, or radiation treatments, even though they have a history of really helping your specific dog's cancer type.

I hope that this description of the scientific mindset – and knowing that not all scientists are blindly dogmatic – will help you to discern whether your support team is open to new ideas. There is more information on how to talk to your vet in Chapter 22.

PS: I don't want you to accept what I write as dogma, either. If anything in this book is ever shown to be wrong, I will work hard to overcome my personal disappointment, as I start over. As new evidence comes up, I change my recommendations, as this second edition of the book demonstrates to readers of the first edition.

Chapter 7: Apoptosis

Apoptosis, nature's way of clearing the body of old or damaged cells, is often diminished when cancer is present. Restoring normal apoptosis levels is an important goal in Full Spectrum cancer care.

In the normal course of events, cells are born, grow, live, and finally die to make way for new cells. Apoptosis genes activate when the body no longer needs the cell or when the cell has reached the end of its usefulness – when it is time to create what scientists call "programmed cell death" and occasionally "cell suicide."

Apoptosis is not only a completely normal cellular process, it's also vital for a normal life. One of my favorite examples of how apoptosis helps us on a grand scale is the human finger. When you look at images of babies developing in the womb, you can see that they have flipper-like hands early on. Later, they have fingers – and that is because their apoptosis genes activated to carve out the excess tissue and separate the flipper into five digits.

Apoptosis can happen when a cell reaches the end of its natural lifespan or when a cell sustains irreparable damage. If the cell cannot repair the harm caused by, for example, radiation, oxygen depletion, infection or DNA damage, the apoptosis genes direct the cell to die. In other words, the cell kills itself if it can't repair itself.

Apoptosis happens on a regular basis; it's estimated that somewhere between fifty and seventy billion cells undergo apoptosis every day in the average adult human body.

Apoptosis is a very controlled cellular process. A detailed description of the complicated series of steps apoptosis genes take to shrink and finally disintegrate the cell is beyond the scope of this book; the important thing for our purposes is for you to understand that once a cell's life is over, the body disposes of the waste debris quietly, naturally and safely.

There are other ways for cells to die. For example, another kind of cell death is called necrosis, which is uncontrolled death, as when the body is injured accidentally. This traumatic cell death can lead to inflammation, especially when many cells die at the same time. Apoptosis, on the other hand, does not usually create inflammation in the body.

A consistent hallmark of cancer cells is that they evade apoptosis: instead of dying a natural death, they divide, divide again, and divide some more, and keep on proliferating. If we could get apoptosis levels back up, we might be able to manage cancer.

Dr. Robert Gerl and Dr. David L. Vaux said in their paper *Apoptosis in the Development and Treatment of Cancer,* "One of the few areas in the cell death field that everyone does agree upon is that having cancer cells undergo apoptosis would be a good thing."

> *"One of the few areas in the cell death field that everyone does agree upon is that having cancer cells undergo apoptosis would be a good thing."*

You may have never heard of apoptosis before you read this book, because it usually gets about two paragraphs in high school biology texts. I like to think about it because I choose to take a wide-angle view for problems like cancer. Apoptosis is a clear pattern we can examine for clues, as most normal body cells undergo apoptosis, most cancer cells evade apoptosis, and most experts agree that getting cancer cells to undergo apoptosis would be a good thing. For these reasons, boosting apoptosis levels in the body is an important theme in Full Spectrum cancer care, no matter what the diagnosis or tumor location.

The idea of using apoptosis to fight cancer has been around since the late nineteen-nineties and it is beginning to gain real traction. Pharmaceutical companies are starting to research synthetic apoptogens (compounds which cause apoptosis), and according to a pharmaceutical market research report from the United Kingdom, the apoptosis market is already worth billions of dollars. In a few years, most people will know about apoptosis, as they now know about DNA.

While programmed cell death was first described nearly two hundred years ago, it wasn't called apoptosis until 1972, when a landmark paper was published in the *British Journal of Cancer.* The paper's authors wanted to make a clear distinction between natural programmed cell death and cell death that results from trauma, so they consulted a Greek language professor to help them find a new name for cell suicide. He suggested the word apoptosis. The first part, *apo* means from, off, or without, and the second part, *ptosis* means falling. In the original Greek, the word is used to mean the "dropping off" or "falling off" of leaves or petals from

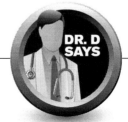

DR. D SAYS

The traditional and most correct pronunciation is the Greek, which features a silent second p: "ay-po-TOE-sis," although many people pronounce the word in English as "ay-POP-toe-sis." I prefer and use the original pronunciation.

plants or trees (the dropping of leaves from trees in the autumn is *apoptosis*). The researchers used it in their seminal paper, and the name has stuck. The image of petals falling from flowers or leaves drifting from trees is certainly lyrical, and a good metaphor for this normal, natural body process.

Chapter 8: Cancer Causes

As you have probably gleaned by now, it is nearly impossible to untangle a dog's history and get down to the one single cause of cancer. Even the idea of a single cause for cancer – just like the idea of a single cure for cancer – is probably a myth. Cancer is more complex than that; it's a living system.

We can plant an acorn in the ground; whether it grows into a towering oak depends upon soil conditions, the rain, the wind and other factors. The same is true for cancer: to grow, it must have the right conditions.

This chapter will cover a few of the most implicated causes of dog cancer: carcinogens, chronic inflammation, bad breeding, spaying and neutering, excess sunlight, and viruses. Stress, depression, and improper sleep patterns, plus, a much-hyped cause of cancer – free radicals – and their much-hyped cure – antioxidants, will be discussed, too (the story beyond the hype is more complicated than what's in the media and on vitamin bottles).

Carcinogens

A carcinogen is any substance capable of causing cancer by damaging healthy cell DNA. Carcinogens can be found everywhere: in our food, our water, our air and our soil. Familiar examples include: tobacco smoke, asbestos, industrial chemicals and certain pesticides.

In general, the more industrial development anywhere, the more carcinogens are present, which naturally leads to higher cancer rates. For example, it has been shown that canine cancer rates increase in an urban, industrialized environment. It's interesting to note that some researchers who study the impact of the environment on human health are paying close attention to the health of dogs and other pets because they can be sentinels (warning signs) for human disease. In other words, they look at our pets, whose shorter life spans can give more information faster than our own longer life spans, for warnings about what we might be facing ourselves.

Not every exposure to carcinogens causes cancer, of course, but, every exposure could increase the *risk* of developing cancer. There is also evidence that the DNA in cancer cells is unstable, or prone to changing in unpredictable ways. Because of this, carcinogen exposure may worsen existing cancers by increasing mutations, possibly causing them to change into more aggressive forms. This is why reducing your dog's exposure to carcinogens is critical – and the place to start is his food bowl.

Plastic

There is an organic compound found in polycarbonate plastics called Bisphenol A, or BPA for short, that can leach into food and water. BPA, once in the body, acts like the hormone estrogen, interacting with cells through a lock–and–key process (in which estrogen is the key, and receptors on cell walls are the lock). Because of its similarities to estrogen, BPA can enter estrogen receptors, causing those cells to start multiplying. There is a theory that low levels of BPA and other estrogen–like compounds may promote cancer through this mechanism.

Many plastics manufacturers no longer use BPA in their polycarbonate products (for example, baby bottles and water bottles). However, BPA can still be found in food and beverage containers, carbonless shopping receipt paper, the lining of canned goods, white dental fillings, and more. It could also be in your dog's plastic food and water bowl.

There are Environmental Protection Agency (EPA) limits on the amount of BPA used in these products, of course, but according to the most recent safety studies, even exposure within what is considered safe parameters might be disruptive.

Public concern about BPA and other estrogen–mimicking chemicals found in plastics has shifted us away from using plastic for food storage and children's toys and other items. It's logical that we do the same thing for our dogs: use ceramic or glass food and water bowls, and avoid plastics in general.

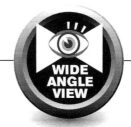

How Safe Is Safe? (Don't Ignore Synergy)

Regulatory agencies, like the Environmental Protection Agency in the U.S., conduct safety studies for known carcinogens, which help the agencies decide what a "safe" level of exposure is for each agent.

The problem is that most safety trials look at each carcinogen in a vacuum, while most of us – and probably your dog, too – live in the real world. Out here, in the real world, we almost never encounter one substance at a time. We may be drinking, eating, or inhaling one agent, while other chemicals are consumed or already present in the body. This combination of carcinogens can create synergy (when two or more agents working together have amplified effects, beyond what each would cause alone).

One example of synergy features two familiar non-carcinogens, prednisone and aspirin. If your dog had arthritis, you might think it's a good idea

continued on next page

How Safe Is Safe? *continued*

to give him a dose of the anti-inflammatory, prednisone, along with aspirin for pain relief. Both of these drugs are generally safe to use, but the synergistic effect of the two together puts your dog at a much higher risk of vomiting, diarrhea, digestive tract inflammation, stomach or intestinal bleeding, and intestinal ulceration (holes).

It is impossible to construct a safety study for any agent that accounts for every single combination of substances. As you'll see when you read about nitrites and nitrates, even harmless substances can be converted to carcinogens when they're combined in the right circumstances. It's also impossible to test all of these combinations over time. Real life exposure to carcinogens may last years, but most safety studies take place over a much shorter time. Because of this, the long-term effects of carcinogen exposure are largely unknown.

The bottom line is that safety studies cannot accurately predict all the cancer-causing effects of carcinogens. It is possible to nail down what is *definitely* carcinogenic, but not possible to say what *could* be carcinogenic. This is why it is important to limit carcinogen exposure when you can, and counteract its negative effects whenever possible.

Carcinogens in Commercial Dog Foods

Commercial dog food is convenient and relatively inexpensive, but most of it – including some "scientifically-formulated" and "premium" brands – is not particularly good for your dog. I want to be clear that I am not condemning every commercial dog food, but I do think you should watch out for commercial foods that have been processed at high temperatures, or those with nitrites and nitrates or ethoxyquin.

You have probably heard of **nitrites and nitrates,** the food preservatives found in many processed meats and some brands of dog food. Although these preservatives do a great job of extending food's lifespan on the shelf, they can be harmful once they're in the body. According to studies conducted in rats, dogs and people, nitrates and nitrites can combine with naturally occurring amines (which mainly come from protein in the diet) in the stomach to form N-nitroso compounds, known carcinogens. This is a good example of synergy.

Because of the potential for synergistic carcinogen formation, I do not recommend feeding your dog food that contains nitrites or nitrates. This includes some commercial dog foods, but also many human foods, such as hot dogs. Dog snacks with meat flavoring may have these chemicals as well; check the ingredients on the product label.

Ethoxyquin is a preservative that may be in some commercial dog foods. It has been shown to increase the effects of some carcinogens in rodent studies, and to cause kidney damage and pre-cancerous changes in the kidneys in humans when given in high doses. It does not seem to be carcinogenic by itself at the levels found in dog foods, but I am concerned about the possibly synergistic effects for dogs with cancer (see the synergy discussion on page 73).

You might not find this preservative listed on the label of your dog's food, but you might see "fishmeal;" federal law mandates ethoxyquin is packed along with fishmeal for shipping. For this reason, I recommend avoiding any food made with fishmeal.

To make most dry dog foods, a mixture of meat or fish, fat, grains (and in some cases, animal remains) is heated to an **extremely high temperature** (sometimes as high as 392°F) after being pushed through a machine called an extruder (which creates the uniformly shaped kibble). Many dog treats are also made this way.

The high temperatures produce chemicals called **heterocyclic amines**, which are known to be extremely potent carcinogens. If the food is starchy, like the corn found in many commercial dog foods, **acrylamide** may also be created, particularly when the starch is cooked with oils. Acrylamide, a potent carcinogen that can be found in many processed food items (french fries and potato chips, for example), has recently become the subject of intense study. While results for non-lab animal species have not yet yielded a consensus, acrylamide has been proven carcinogenic in lab animals.

Both heterocyclic amines and acrylamide likely remain in the kibble, even after it cools off, as they do with human foods. Neither compound

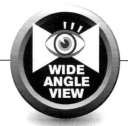

Does Civilization Cause Cancer?

Human cancer rates have increased by 27% since 1950, and that number does not even include cancers caused by cigarette smoking. Some cancer researchers have noted that disease rates rose as modern life conveniences increased (for example, processed foods and electronics).

This is interesting, because there are places in the world — we often call them undeveloped countries — which enjoy a much lower rate of cancer than we do. Studies show that when people migrate from these countries to more developed countries, their cancer rates rise to match the rates in their new home. Could cancer, which is sometimes called a "disease of civilization," have a direct relationship to life style choices and diet?

You bet it could. One study shows that 85% of human cancers are a direct result of diet and lifestyle choices, and that roughly 30% of cancers can
continued on next page

Does Civilization Cause Cancer? *continued*

be avoided by improving diet alone. Because of our physiological similarities (remember, many human cancer studies use dogs as test subjects), if this is true for us, it may also true for our dogs.

Taking steps to reduce the impact of civilization on your dog's body is an important part of Full Spectrum cancer care. Changing your dog's diet and other specific recommendations for accomplishing this are included in the next section of this book.

has to be listed on the manufacturer's product label; they are not present before the mixture is processed, so they are not considered ingredients by regulatory agencies.

Whether they are listed on the label or not, the high-heat processing of many dry dog foods and treats probably creates carcinogens. In Chapter 14, I will recommend a home-cooked diet, prepared at relatively low temperatures, to avoid creating acrylamide and heterocyclic amines.

(Cooking at or below 212° Fahrenheit avoids both acrylamide and heterocyclic amine formation, and cooking below 302° Fahrenheit avoids heterocyclic amine formation.)

All kibble is cooked at high temperatures, and I suspect that other, non-kibble commercial dog foods are, too. Second only to a home-cooked diet, I recommend doing the best you can with high quality brands such as Halo, Solid Gold, Orijen, Blue Buffalo and Taste of the Wild. Dehydrated brands are also a good idea (Honest Kitchen, for example), because they do not heat the food at all, and you use warm water to reconstitute it at home. You might also consider partially cooked or frozen brands.

Pharmaceuticals in the Water

In 2008, investigative reporters from the Associated Press (AP) published a series of articles about our drinking water. They found that at least 46 million people in two dozen major metropolitan areas are drinking water that contains minute amounts of pharmaceuticals, including still-active hormones from birth control pills, chemotherapy agents, and antidepressants.

How did these drugs get into our water supply? One way is through the sewage system. If an individual takes a pill — let's say a heart medication — and the body does not completely absorb it, the excess is released through the bowels and the urinary tract. Sometimes, breakdown products (metabolites) that still have activity are released, also. These flow into the sewage system, where the water is treated to make it drinkable, then piped back into household faucets for normal use.

Water treatment facilities can remove bacteria and protozoa, but, according to the water suppliers interviewed for the AP series, the technology to remove pharmaceuticals is not in place and/ or is not definitively working. Therefore, the drugs and active metabolites may remain, even in the treated water.

According to the AP, this inadvertent dumping of prescription drugs is not the only problem. Some hospitals across America dispose of unused medications by flushing them down the toilet! In these cases, the drugs enter the sewage system at full strength. Our dogs ingest these small doses of pharmaceuticals in their water, over the years. A medical doctor would never recommend taking random pharmaceuticals all mixed together, and neither would a veterinarian. The synergistic results are unpredictable and could, at least theoretically, set the stage for cancer development in some dogs.

The federal regulation of prescription drugs in drinking water is complex. For example, pharmaceutical waste from private homes is not currently regulated. Some drugs are classified as medical waste, not hazardous waste, which makes them subject to different regulations. According to the AP investigation, the EPA acknowledges the problem, and some water suppliers are working on it. I have a suspicion that we will be hearing more about this as time goes on, because it's too big a potential danger to ignore for long.

Lacking direct control over our water supply, I recommend giving your dog water that has been purified through filtration or reverse osmosis. To be sure you are removing as many unwanted pharmaceuticals compounds as possible you will likely need to use an ozonation system; water filtration technology is always changing and improving, so as this danger becomes more known, systems will likely improve and become less expensive.

Fluoride in Drinking Water

There is a large (largely ignored) body of evidence that fluoride in drinking water likely increases the risk of bone cancer in growing boys and in rats. Since osteosarcoma is more common in dogs than it is in humans, fluoridated water could be a problem for dogs.

Many public water suppliers add fluoride as a health treatment, which may be one reason why

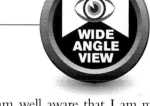

WIDE ANGLE VIEW

I am well aware that I am more concerned and cautious about water quality than most vets and oncologists are, including my co-author. However, if a more widely accepted and definitive link between osteosarcoma and fluoride is someday found in dogs, you will be happy that you received this information when you did. If not, there is little (or no) harm done by filtering drinking water! Some of my top filter picks are available at www.DogCancerShop.com.

some of this research has been deliberately suppressed. An expose in *The Washington Post* reported that a Harvard School of Dental Medicine epidemiologist told federal officials that he didn't find any significant links between fluoridated water and osteosarcoma … but later they learned that he had supervised a doctoral thesis just a few years earlier which concluded the exact opposite: boys exposed to fluoridated water at a young age *were* more likely to get osteosarcoma.

I have not found direct evidence for fluoridated water's causing bone cancer or other cancers in dogs. However, dogs and humans are very similar, physiologically. Since there is some evidence that fluoridated water may be a risk factor for bone cancer in other species, my recommendation is to at least consider avoiding it if your dog is a breed prone to osteosarcoma. You can filter your water (most filter systems remove fluoride) or use distilled water. This is one area in which Dr. Ettinger and I disagree – she feels I am overly cautious.

I advise avoiding bone meal (a common ingredient in commercial dog foods), and oyster shell calcium supplements, also, both of which often contain high levels of fluoride.

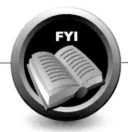

Water Safety Information for Your Region

Check the with the Environmental Protection Agency's (EPA) to find out exactly what's in your drinking water and what you can do to improve it. They have an excellent website to start your research: www.epa.gov/safewater/faq/faq.html

The EPA also hosts a Safe Drinking Water hotline at 1-800-426-4791.

For more information, you can contact your state's Department of Health, or call the Community Right to Know Hotline at 1-800-424-9346.

Asbestos in Drinking Water

Asbestos is a common name for six naturally occurring minerals with heat and sound insulation properties. After using asbestos for centuries, to insulate homes and for a host of other applications, its use is now restricted in the United States, and totally banned in the European Union. A potent carcinogen, asbestos can cause lung cancer and mesothelioma.

A few decades ago, we worried about breathing in airborne asbestos only. Recently, it's been found in a new place: our drinking water. According to the Environmental Protection Agency (EPA), seven million "long" fibers per liter of drinking water are considered safe – but 10% of the population uses water with more than ten million fibers per liter, and 18% uses water with more than one million fibers per liter.

The possible synergistic effects of asbestos are sobering, and one spokesperson from the Department of Health and Human Services argues that the repeated ingestion of even low levels of asbestos, will likely result in a substantial number of cancers.

If you knowingly work with asbestos, I recommend leaving your dog at home, and showering and changing your clothes before playing with your dog. Even if you do not work with asbestos, it is worth reading about it on the EPA's website to ensure that you are aware of any problems in your home, work, or water.

Carcinogens in the Air

There is a large sugar processing plant on my home island of Maui, Hawaii. The first step in processing sugar is burning the cane, so, when it's time to harvest a particular field, workers go out in the very early morning and set the sugarcane on fire. Cane smoke blows over the island, leaving a brown streak in the sky that takes hours to disperse. As a result, some residents wake up with headaches, sinusitis, and difficulty breathing.

Like it or not, many of our modern manufacturing processes release carcinogens into the air – and not all of them are as visible as cane smoke. There are many documented airborne cancer-causing chemicals, including those from kerosene, coal residue from household heaters, chemical solvents, engine exhaust, paint fumes and industrial wastes.

Second-hand tobacco smoke is a very well-

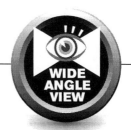

Marketing Spin

Manufacturers always try to present their products in the best light possible, even when those products present a health risk. For example, in 1965 the federal government required cigarette manufacturers to label their product with these words: "Caution: Cigarette Smoking May Be Hazardous to Your Health." This phrase indicates a risk to your health, but not a direct link to a specific illness.

However, decades later when scientists proved a direct link between cigarette smoking and cancer, emphysema, and heart disease, the government required the following label: "Smoking Causes Lung Cancer, Heart Disease, Emphysema, and May Complicate Pregnancy."

The reason for the change was that the government wanted to clarify that cigarettes don't pose a risk for illness; they cause it.

known airborne carcinogen. As it undoubtedly causes cancer in humans, there is mounting evidence linking it to malignancies in dogs (and other pets). It is strongly associated with nasal cancer, particularly in older dogs with long noses like Collies and Dachshunds, and it's likely that future studies will reveal even more associations. If you smoke, and your dog has cancer, it's wise to stop smoking, both for your own health, and for his.

Pesticides and herbicides used in home and lawn care can be a source of airborne carcinogens. The use of 2,4-D, an herbicide found in over 1,500 weed-killers, was found to increase lymphoma rates (the study was later refuted, but even mixed evidence concerns me). Lawn pesticides have also been found to be associated with transitional cell carcinoma, the most common type of bladder cancer.

Researchers do not fully understand how high voltage power lines create airborne carcinogens, but an increased incidence of cancer (particularly childhood leukemia) is associated with them, and slightly more so downwind. The cause could be magnetic fields or their generation of a carcinogenic particle (called a corona ion) in the air around the lines, or other factors. This is another area of research where initial evidence was later disputed and yet is once again a topic of interest. Despite the mixed response of the medical community, you as a guardian will want to be aware of the higher incidence of cancer associated with high voltage power lines.

If you take the air we breathe for granted, this information may feel a little overwhelming. As most of these airborne carcinogens are invisible, how can you be certain you're avoiding them? It's not possible, or desirable, to put your dog in a bubble, but it is worth thinking about ways to keep her air as clean as possible.

For example, keep your dog away from areas (inside or outside) that have been treated with pesticides or herbicides, for at least six hours after application. If you smoke, consider making her area a smoke-free zone. If your house needs a new coat of paint, wait to do the interior walls, or remove your dog from the home while you do. The same goes for the use of solvents. If your dog spends a lot of time in or near the garage, consider moving her away from the area to reduce her exposure to car exhaust. Try to avoid walking your dog on busy streets. The same advice applies if you use kerosene in heaters, stoves, or lamps, and also coal heaters. Be sure to ventilate well, when using these appliances.

Carcinogens in the Soil

Industrial manufacturing processes usually produce by-products, and this waste does not always go up in smoke. Sometimes it goes into the ground, where it can stay for years, spreading carcinogens into the soil, and even the water table that feeds wells and reservoirs.

We didn't always understand just how hazardous industrial waste is to our health. Entire communities have been built on top of landfills, packed with industrial waste. One of the most famous of these is a neighborhood in Niagara Falls, New York, named Love Canal. Twenty-one thousand tons of chemical waste, buried in drums, started leaking and caused a public health emergency and a national scandal in the late 1970's. The Environmental Protection Agency (EPA) classifies sites like Love Canal as National Priority Sites – also known as "Superfund sites." As of this writing, there are 1,279 such sites in the U.S.! Obviously, human health problems are higher in locations contaminated with toxic waste. I haven't seen a study specifically looking at cancer rates in dogs living near Superfund sites, but I would guess that their health likely suffers as well.

To find out if you are close to a Superfund site, go to the EPA's website: www.epa.gov/superfund/sites.

Chronic, Microscopic Inflammation

Inflammation is a natural response to bodily injury. If you are stung by a bee, have acid indigestion, or suffer a cut, inflammation brings extra blood and lymph to the injury. These fluids make the tissue warm, red, and swollen with cells that help fight infection and repair the injury.

In acute situations like these, inflammation is an immediate and helpful response; much like the fire department's showing up when your house is on fire: you may be relieved and thankful they can put it out, but if they are still spraying water after it is extinguished, they would be causing damage to your home, not preventing it.

The same is true of inflammation. If inflammation lasts for too long, or if it becomes a chronic, low-level (often undetectable) condition, inflammation can wreak some pretty serious damage.

As we've already discussed in Chapter 6, inflammation can help cancer to metastasize by destabilizing DNA, helping the tumor build new blood vessels, and even by stimulating tumor growth. My own clinical experience agrees with this; when I examine a cancer patient's history, I often find factors that could have led to microscopic levels of long-term inflammation. For example, diets with high levels of omega-6 fatty acids and not enough vegetables are common. Obesity is another common culprit; obesity is related to low-grade body inflammation in humans, and has been shown to pose a cancer risk for dogs.

You'll read more about overfeeding, omega-6 fatty acids, and the importance of vegetables in Chapter 14. The dog cancer diet can help reduce the possible presence of chronic, microscopic inflammation in your dog.

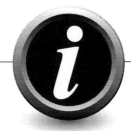

Some Examples of Dog Breeds with Higher Cancer Rates★

Breed	Common Cancer Type
Arctic breeds	Perianal adenomas, perianal adenocarcinoma
Beagle	Transitional cell carcinoma, perianal adenomas
Basset Hound	Lymphoma, nasal tumors
Bernese Mountain Dog	Histiocytic sarcoma (aka malignant histiocytosis)
Boston Terrier	Mast cell tumor, gliomas (brain cancer)
Boxer	Lymphoma, mast cell tumor, brain cancer, skin hemangiosarcoma, gliomas (brain cancer)
Chow Chow	Oral melanoma (especially tongue)
Cocker Spaniel	Anal sac carcinoma, mammary cancer (along with other Spaniel breeds), oral tumors including melanoma, perianal adenomas
Collie	Transitional cell carcinoma, meningiomas (brain), nasal tumors
Doberman Pinscher	Osteosarcoma, oral tumors, brain tumors

Breed	Common Cancer Type
English Springer Spaniel	Mammary cancer, anal sac adenocarcinoma
	Sublingual squamous cell carcinoma, oral tumors
German Shepherd	Hemangiosarcoma, mammary cancer, nasal and oral tumors, osteosarcoma, and anal sac adenocarcinoma
Golden Retriever	Osteosarcoma, hemangiosarcoma, lymphoma, brain, mast cell tumor, anal sac adenocarcinoma, oral tumors including fibrosarcoma
Great Dane	Osteosarcoma
Keeshound	Nasal tumors
Labrador Retriever	Hemangiosarcoma, lymphoma, mast cell tumor, oral fibrosarcoma
Poodle	Mammary cancer (toy and miniature breeds), oral melanoma
Pug	Mast cell tumor, gliomas (brain cancer)
Rottweiler	Osteosarcoma, heart hemangiosarcoma

continued on next page

Breed	Common Cancer Type
Scottish Terrier	Oral tumors including melanoma, transitional cell carcinoma, brain
Sharpei	Mast cell tumor
Shetland Sheepdog	Transitional cell carcinoma, acanthomatous ameloblastoma (oral tumor)

Breed	Common Cancer Type
St Bernard	Osteosarcoma
West Highland White Terrier	Transitional cell carcinoma

*Note: This lists some common examples of breed-related cancers, but it is not comprehensive

Inherited Bad Genes

Certain dogs have been bred over many hundreds, and in some cases, thousands of years. Human intervention has strengthened certain traits, including intelligence in herding dogs, acute smell in hounds, and cooperation in sporting dogs. Sometimes less visible traits have been passed down as well, including DNA encoded for cancer development. This is why some breeds are more prone to cancer overall and why certain breeds are more prone to certain cancers.

For example, if two individual dogs with the same cancer-causing mutated gene are mated, their pups may have a much higher probability of developing cancer than the parents.

There are also entire breeds with a very high probability of developing cancer. Both Boxers and Golden Retrievers have exceptionally high cancer rates, and 75% of Goldens *die* of cancer.

Responsible breeders can help improve bloodlines by avoiding breeding dogs whose parents or grandparents developed cancer. If a tendency to develop cancer is in the historical breed line, it will always be a potential hazard in descendants. This is probably why mixed breed dogs have much lower cancer rates than purebred dogs.

Spaying and Neutering

Mammary cancer is the second most common form of dog cancer, and it can be nearly completely eliminated by spaying a female dog before the first heat, probably because removing the ovaries and uterus reduces the production of sex hormones and keeps breast tissue from developing. On average, the first heat arrives at six months of age and recurs approximately every six months until late in life.

Spaying provides less protection with every passing heat. Studies have shown that dogs spayed before the first heat have a 0.05% risk of developing mammary cancer, when compared to intact female dogs, which means the risk is almost completely eliminated by the surgery. If the spay happens between the first and second heats, female dogs still have quite a bit of protection, with only an 8% risk, compared to their intact sisters. If the spay happens between the third and fourth heat, female dogs have a 26% risk, compared to intact dogs (and some oncologists cite a paper that puts this risk at a much lower 6%). Clearly, spaying a female dog reduces her risk of mammary cancer. It also removes all risk for ovarian and uterine cancer.

For a male dog, neutering (removing the testicles) decreases the risk of benign perianal adenomas and also eliminates his risk for testicular cancer.

If you just look at these factors, spaying and neutering might seem like an obvious choice. It's not. There is actually evidence that spaying and neutering increases the risk for other aggressive cancers.

The following data may create a negative reaction among some (maybe even most) practicing veterinarians. This information has not been widely publicized in veterinary circles, even though it is from published, peer-reviewed papers with respected authors. It represents a very inconvenient truth for us vets. How will we reconcile population control and the euthanasia of unwanted pets with the associations between spaying, neutering, and cancer development? These are murky ethical waters for animal lovers. (The scientific references for this are located in Appendix E.)

Purebred dogs who have been spayed or neutered are *twice as likely* to develop osteosarcoma (bone cancer), and the risk is even higher for Rottweilers. One study showed that both male and female Rotties, who were surgically sterilized before the age of one year, had an approximately one in four risk for developing osteosarcoma during their lifetime, while intact Rotties were much less likely to develop the disease.

Spaying has also been shown to increase the risk of lymphoma, and other studies show that castration increases the risk for developing transitional cell carcinoma (bladder cancer) by three to four times. Spaying and neutering also increases the risk of prostate cancers and hemangiosarcoma of the heart.

Osteosarcoma, transitional cell carcinoma, hemangiosarcoma of the heart and lymphoma are generally more aggressive than mammary cancer; one in four of which is cured with surgery alone. These factors should be considered when we decide whether to spay and neuter dogs.

The prevailing opinion in the veterinary community is that sterilization is good, and keeping dogs intact is bad. There are some good reasons for this, one of which is the huge population of unwanted dogs in this country. Sterilization also helps to reduce uterine infections, and, in some cases, unwanted behaviors like humping and marking. It can also reduce aggression in some dogs. It's also worth mentioning that spays and neuters are a profit center in many vet practices, mine included.

Because the increased cancer risks from spaying and neutering are serious, guardians should consider the big picture when evaluating the timing of these procedures. Most dogs reach sexual maturity at about twenty-four months, approximately at the fourth heat in females. At this point in their development, dogs have received the protective benefit of adult sexual hormones and are at a decreased risk for the cancers mentioned above. If you choose to spay or neuter your dog, my general recommendation is to spay females sometime between the third and fourth heats – which will have the added benefit of reducing the risk of mammary cancer – and neuter males sometime between the ages of eighteen and twenty-four months.

There are other health issues related to spaying and neutering that are beyond the scope of this book, and all of these factors should be considered. There may be a reason why you should spay earlier in life – as always, this decision should be made on a case-by-case basis, in consultation with your vet.

Sunlight Exposure

The sun is essential to life. In addition to providing light, warmth, and energy, there is new evidence that sun exposure in the right amounts – just fifteen to thirty minutes per week – can actually protect us from cancer by stimulating the body to generate the active form of vitamin D.

Excessive sunlight exposure, however, can increase cancer risks in some dogs, particularly dogs with light skin pigmentation. The two dog cancers associated with sun exposure are skin hemangiosarcoma and squamous cell carcinoma. Oddly, canine melanoma is not associated with sunlight, as it is in humans.

I see a great deal of skin hemangiosarcoma in Hawaii, where we get lots of equatorial sun all year round, and mostly in breeds that are already prone to develop it. A colleague from South Africa, Dr. Crewe, sees much more squamous cell carcinomas than skin hemangiosarcoma. She believes that this is because the ozone layer is so much thinner in the southern hemisphere than it is at the equator, allowing stronger rays to pass through and affect the skin.

It is probably rare that sunlight directly *causes* cancer, but it can tip the scales in favor of cancer, when other risk factors are also present. If your dog has a cancer linked to sun exposure, using sunscreen (making sure to keep it out of her eyes and nose) and keeping your dog indoors, especially during midday hours, is a good idea. Dr. Crewe even recommends a Lycra full-body suit, made just for dogs (also available at www.DogCancerShop.com).

Viruses

Viruses can cause growths on the body: warts, for example. Usually benign, these growths can be contagious, or transmitted through physical contact.

One type of benign growth that you may see on your dog is called a papilloma. These are small, fleshy, wart-like growths that often show up on young dogs. They are mainly a cosmetic issue, although if they are large and occur in the mouth, they can create problems.

There are also venereal tumors, some of which can spread during mating. These tumors can interfere with fertility if they're in the wrong location. Sometimes dogs chew or scrape them, which can lead to bleeding or infection.

Very rarely, a venereal tumor can be cancerous. Because these tumors are suspected to be caused by a virus, this cancer, known as canine transmissible venereal tumor (TVT), may be transmitted to other dogs through physical contact, such as copulation.

Low Melatonin Levels

Mothers, throughout the millennia, have implored their children to get a good night's sleep, and those children have often ignored this excellent advice, risking their health as a result. Perhaps because we're unconscious during sleep, we often don't realize just how many essential body processes happen during those hours; many of them can't happen unless we're asleep with the lights out.

One of those crucial processes is the manufacturing of melatonin, a hormone that, among many other helpful body activities, fights cancer. One way it does this is by blocking a dietary fat, called linoleic acid, from entering cancer cells (linoleic acid stimulates some cancer cells to grow).

There are numerous studies showing that melatonin can lessen the risk of cancer development and progression. In one, higher rates of breast cancer were found in women working the night shift, and in another, higher rates of breast, uterine and prostate cancer were found in men and women with low melatonin levels.

Correcting a melatonin deficiency in cancer patients has been shown to lessen cancer cachexia (weight loss), reduce metastasis, lessen the side effects of chemotherapy and radiation treatments, help with sleeplessness, and even extend life expectancy.

Melatonin is generated by the pineal gland, a pea-sized gland located between the eyes, deep in the skull. The pineal gland does not generate melatonin in the presence of light, especially blue light, which is why complete darkness at bedtime is essential. And just turning out the lights and blocking out light from outside is not enough. Televisions and computer screens throw off a lot of blue light, so reducing their use in the evening can help to generate more melatonin.

Our dogs generally sleep when we sleep. Making sure that your dog has a dark place to rest, and goes there early in the evening (perhaps by going to bed yourself), can boost his melatonin levels and give him an edge on cancer. Some dogs may also tolerate melatonin supplements (the doses are on page 185).

Vaccines

I've given vaccines to thousands of dogs over the course of my career, so when I first heard that vaccines could be linked to cancer development in dogs, I was absolutely sure that was not true. Even the word "vaccinosis" sounded made up to me, as if

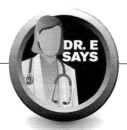

There is a well-known soft tissue sarcoma tumor associated with vaccines and other injections that develops in cats at the injection site, but this syndrome does not occur in dogs.

it were created by someone with an axe to grind, someone who wanted to vilify vets who vaccinate dogs.

It turns out that vaccines may, at least theoretically, be linked to cancer development in dogs, as is shown in studies conducted in rodents and humans. To understand how, let's quickly look at how the immune system works.

To defend the body against pathogens (viruses, bacteria and other microorganisms) and against damaged or mutated body cells (cancer), the immune system deploys several layers of defense.

Barriers physically protect the body by blocking pathogens. An example is the skin, which almost completely seals the body off from the outside. Another barrier is mucus, which entangles pathogens in slime so they can't enter the body. Another is the lungs, which can initiate coughing or sneezing to eject pathogens. There are also barriers inside the body, which help defend cells from microbes that succeed in reaching them. For example, cells have outer membranes, which are like a skin and have chemical barriers, which can neutralize or block pathogens.

The **innate immune system** activates if viruses, bacteria, or other microbes make it through barriers and enter the body. This system takes immediate and massive action to deal with problems. One example of many innate immune responses is inflammation. If a tissue is damaged, it sends chemical signals to alert the immune system, which immediately responds with extra blood flow to the area, and an increase in the concentration of immune cells, which can destroy foreign cells and repair tissue, among other tasks. Natural killer cells are also part of the innate immune system. These cells can recognize and target cancer cells and cells that have been infected by a virus.

The **adaptive immune system** is more sophisticated than the innate system. This part of the immune system has a "memory." When certain cells from this part of the immune system encounter a pathogen, they develop a response (antibody) that is specific to that pathogen. Once they have destroyed it, the system can "remember" it in the future, and respond to it much more quickly than the first time around. This process is called humoral immunity.

In general, the purpose of a vaccine is to stimulate immunity. When an injectable vaccine is used, a tiny amount of a pathogen (a modified virus, for example) is injected: not enough to cause a full-blown infection, just enough for the cells involved in humoral immunity to learn about it and develop a method of destroying it. If the body is exposed to the real virus later in life, the adaptive immune system "remembers" it and eliminates it before it can do any damage.

Vaccines are very useful, because they use the immune system's natural actions to protect the body. When everything works perfectly, it is very unlikely that the vaccinated disease will ever develop. Vaccines are a miracle of science, and they have prevented many very serious diseases. However, after decades of using vaccines to immunize humans, especially infants, against specific diseases, the picture is not entirely rosy.

According to researchers, early vaccinations in human infants stimulate humoral immunity at the expense of another function of the adaptive immune system, called cell-mediated immunity. Cell-mediated immunity includes cells such as natural killer cells and cytotoxic T-cells, both of which target cancer cells for destruction. As fewer natural killer cells and cytotoxic T-cells are produced, more pre-cancerous cells go undetected, which could mean cancer has more opportunities to develop. By immunizing our infants at a young age, we may be making a trade-off: increased humoral immunity against specific diseases that come from outside the body in exchange for decreased cancer-killing cell-mediated immunity.

This is called a polarity shift, and studies in mice have found that once an immature immune system has made this shift, the effect tends to last well into adulthood. So, a choice made in childhood may raise the risk of cancer development later in life. We don't yet know whether infant vaccines actually increase the overall cancer rates – but the question is certainly worth closer examination.

I am well aware of the contentious debates in the public arena over vaccine use, and this information is not meant to throw oil on the fire. I am not anti-vaccine, and I admit that there is no study yet that proves vaccinated dogs are more prone to cancer than unvaccinated dogs. What we do know is that the polarity shift is real in vaccinated human infants and mice, and we know that its effects last into adulthood in vaccinated mice.

So what does this imply for vaccinating our dogs? It's tricky. We obviously should exercise caution when vaccinating infant dogs, but unfortunately, it is hard to determine exactly when infancy ends and childhood begins. Still, I have changed my policy in my own practice to take these studies into account. I no longer recommend vaccinating puppies at six weeks of age; instead, I suggest holding off on the first vaccination until the dog is ten weeks old. This gives the dog's cancer-patrolling cells a little more time to mature, and hopefully preserves their functions into adulthood. In the meantime, puppies can be quarantined at home until after the last vaccination is given, so their exposure to infectious diseases is minimized. When I first graduated from veterinary school, we gave booster shots every year; now, I prefer to give them every three years (now the standard of care). I don't give booster shots after the age of seven unless a titer test shows one is needed. Also, I don't recommend vaccinating against anything that does not directly threaten the dog. For example, rabies is nonexistent in Hawaii, so I do not administer rabies vaccines to dogs who will never leave the islands.

Many readers cringe when they read this section, because they may have been vaccinating their dogs throughout their lifetimes. Keep in mind that I am cautious due to my research, and some vets, even after hearing my reasons for starting the puppy series at ten weeks, may think I am overly cautious. Even so, the studies I've seen make me believe that our current policy of "infant" vaccination for puppies will eventually change.

Stress and Depression

The link between chronic stress, depression, and illness in humans is clear; so much so that there is an entire field of science devoted to exploring the interactions between psychology, illness, and immunity. I'm interested in psychoneuroimmunology (known in popular culture as the mind–body connection) because the emotional bond between dogs and their human companions is undeniable. Since dogs are often models for scientists who study human cancer treatments, it's logical to think that there may be some value to applying mind–body tools to canine cancer.

One of the most important insights I've gleaned from this field is the recognition of how important overall attitude is when it comes to health. According to a French study involving human patients with head and neck cancer, optimists live 10% longer than pessimists. Optimism is not just a more pleasant state of mind; it actually gives you a significant edge over your cynical neighbors. It is logical to think the same may be true for our dogs.

Another important insight I'd like to share is how human children who have cancer experience illness symptoms. According to researchers, children with cancer don't describe their symptoms as if they are separate issues. They don't say "I have a headache," or "my stomach hurts." Instead children report global feelings: "I feel bad" or "I hurt" or "I feel sick." No matter what individual symptoms they may have, their overall disposition could be summed up in two words: bummed out. I suspect dogs feel the same way: sick "all over."

If dogs are similar to kids in the way that they respond to illness, then I have another insight from pediatric medicine to share with you. There seems to be a parent-child emotional feedback loop that plays a big role in cancer care. Children can pick up on their parents' attitudes about their illnesses and adopt them without question. If, for example, a mother acts very upset when her child vomits, the child may automatically become upset the next time he vomits. As you'll see in a moment, emotional upset and depression actively interfere with the body's ability to heal. When parents take a calmer, more "let's get it done" attitude, children seem to be calmer and get over their pains and symptoms more quickly.

In my experience, the dogs who live the longest and have the best quality of life are the dogs whose guardians take this "matter of fact," pragmatic approach to treatments. Your expectation that your dog can handle the challenge of cancer sets up a positive feedback loop between the two of you.

Contributing positive emotions to the feedback loop is not just about maintaining an optimistic outlook or keeping your mood up. Positive emotions actually affect the body on a physical level. When it is calm, the human brain sends signals to the digestive tract to process food, relax the muscles, and keep the heartbeat normal. The body gets to "rest and digest."

When stress comes, the human brain releases an avalanche of hormones and chemical signals to help the body deal with the problem. For example, epinephrine, norepinephrine, and cortisol are released in levels high enough to raise blood sugar, open the lungs, make the heart beat faster and stronger, and send more blood to the major muscle groups. These activities organize the body for "fight or flight."

Any stressful event can trigger a fight or flight response. A saber tooth tiger can trigger this response, but so can financial hardship, relationship issues, or dealing with dog cancer. Over the long term, these reactions have serious detrimental effects on the body.

In a study involving children with cancer, those with feelings of low self-worth had higher levels of the stress hormone, epinephrine, and children who lacked social support from friends had higher levels of norepinephrine. These children also showed a weakened immune response to cancer, possibly because stress and depression is associated with decreased activity in the immune system's cancer-fighting cytotoxic T-cells and natural killer cells. The stress hormone epinephrine has also been shown to switch off apoptosis in cancer cells. In other words, if the mind is under stress, cancer cells have a better chance of multiplying out of control. If your dog is under emotional stress, there is a chance that the cancer-fighting cells in his immune system are being suppressed and that apoptosis is being switched off!

There is more than enough evidence available in human medicine to convince me that managing stress and depression are a crucial component of cancer care in every species. The more confident and relaxed your dog feels, the fewer stress hormones are released, the more cancer-killing immune cells are able to do their work, and the fewer apoptosis genes are switched off. Best of all, many activities that boost your dog's self-esteem are free and fun for you both. Giving your dog lots of opportunities to feel good is my reasoning behind several of the emotional management exercises in Chapter 2 and Step Five in Full Spectrum cancer care, Brain Chemistry Modification, which is covered in Chapter 15.

Free Radicals

You may have heard of free radicals (molecules which react with and injure other molecules until eventually they change DNA enough to cause cancer), because they've been mentioned in the press many times over the last several decades. The hype about free radicals partly inspired the huge jump in sales of antioxidant vitamins (A, C, E, etc.), which neutralize free radicals in test tubes.

As is often true, what works in test tubes (*in vitro*) does not always work in the complicated real world of the body (*in vivo*). To understand how and why to use antioxidants to treat your dog's cancer – and how and why *not* to – it is important to understand just a few of the technical molecular details.

You probably remember from high school science courses that cells are made up of molecules, each of which is made up of even tinier atoms. Atoms have a center, called a nucleus, and minuscule electrons, which surround the nucleus. Every type of atom (oxygen, carbon, hydrogen, etc.) has a fixed number of electrons it needs in order to be stable. Usually, this number is an even number, and most molecules are made up of two or more atoms "sharing" an even number of electrons so they can be stable together.

If a molecule is missing an electron, or has an extra one, it becomes unstable and reacts easily with other atoms, often in unpredictable and almost imperceptibly fast ways. This unstable, reactive molecule is called a free radical. A free radical seeks to regain stability, so it either gives an electron to or steals an electron from, a neighboring molecule. Typically it will steal an electron. If it succeeds, the now-stable free radical has created a new free radical in its neighbor. This new free radical now pursues stability and creates another free radical, and on and on. This molecular activity, if left unchecked, can lead to damaged cell DNA and genetic mutations. For this reason, free radicals are thought to cause cancer, along with a host of other illnesses.

Although this may seem like a logical conclusion, some research leads us to question whether it's really that simple. It's true that carcinogens that enter the body can be free radicals or can cause increases in free radicals inside cells. In theory, those free radicals could cause mutations in cells, which could lead to cancer. Unfortunately, some of the real world evidence just doesn't fit.

Free radicals are a normal part of everyday living in the body. When normal cells need energy, they burn body fuel stores using a process called oxidation, and free radicals are a by-product of oxidation. At any given time, normal cells are creating free radicals in this way, and the more energy that's needed for a given task (a mile run, for example), the more free radicals are generated. Normal cells are able to clear out these free radicals, using several different methods.

Cancer cells generate free radicals, too, but in far greater numbers, because of their tremendous growth rate. They are engaged in nearly constant metabolism: multiplying, growing, building new tissue, building new blood vessels, and metabolizing energy. All of this activity creates far more free radicals, and they are not as good at clearing them out.

Free radicals are unpredictable by nature, and when enough accumulate, they can do something quite impressive: switch on apoptosis genes and cause a cell to commit suicide. Ironically, cancer cells pose a danger to themselves by generating so many free radicals!

Some immune system cells create free radicals to target cancer cells in this way, and this is the mechanism behind some conventional chemotherapy agents and even some nutraceuticals, such as high doses of luteolin and apigenin (see Chapter 12). These **pro-oxidant therapies** introduce even more free radicals into an already unstable environment. The result can be that apoptosis genes kick in and kill the cancer naturally.

I hope it's clear by now that free radicals *could* theoretically cause cancer, as we once thought, but they can *definitely* help kill cancer, when enough accumulate within a cancer cell. They're not always bad.

This distinction is important, because there has been a tremendous amount of media hype around free radicals, in part because vitamin manufacturers wanted to sell more antioxidants (which neutralize them). Saying that a vitamin helps to prevent or cure cancer by neutralizing free radicals is a powerful selling point. The problem is that antioxidant supplements don't always prevent cancer, and in some cases, may even help cause it. Let's take a closer look at antioxidants.

Antioxidants are stable molecules; so stable that they can afford to donate an electron to a free radical. Once the free radical takes the electron, it becomes stable and stops creating new ones. The sooner antioxidants arrive on the scene the sooner free radicals are neutralized.

Vitamin C and vitamin E are well-known antioxidants, as are several other vitamins. The body can also produce antioxidant enzymes that neutralize free radicals in the same way dietary antioxidants do, but instead of using vitamins, these enzymes use minerals such as copper, manganese, and selenium. These are the body's natural antioxidant systems. If you have run a mile, it would be a great thing to have enough of these vitamins, minerals, and enzymes in your body to counteract all those extra free radicals and keep you in balance.

Vitamins and minerals are found in food, especially in brightly colored fruits and vegetables. Studies have shown that people who eat a lot of fruits and vegetables have a lower risk for cancer. We used to think this was because of the high level of antioxidants in these foods, but researchers have recently found that other substances in fruits and vegetables – such as naturally occurring anti-inflammatory compounds and chemicals that modulate genes – may have a much *bigger* role in cancer prevention than the antioxidants.

Antioxidants may even hurt the body, under certain circumstances. Ingesting mega-doses of certain antioxidants – which once seemed like a good "natural" strategy to fight cancer – now seems like a bad idea. "Boosting the immune system" in a body that is severely compromised by cancer may not work out as well as it can in the sanitary environment of the test tube.

One long-term study (seven and a half years) looked at the use of dietary levels of antioxidants (vitamins A, E, selenium and zinc) in humans, and found that there was no benefit in cancer prevention or increase in longevity. A secondary analysis looked at the data and found that there actually was a reduction in cancer development, but only in men.

In another study, smokers who took high doses of antioxidants (vitamin A and alpha tocopherol) actually experienced higher lung cancer rates. This mystifying result really punched a hole in the theory that antioxidants always help prevent or manage cancer. Clearly, dosing with mega-doses of certain antioxidants could do more harm than good. It seems that grouping all antioxidants into one category is not helpful and leads to faulty assumptions. It is preferable to look at each antioxidant independently and evaluate its effects separately.

Am I saying that antioxidants should not be used? No. Mega-doses may be counter-productive, that's true. But low, supplemental doses of antioxidants such as vitamins A, C and E can have a good effect on the body. For example, in one study, (human) cancer patients were given antioxidants in addition to their regular chemotherapy treatments for six months. Although the doses were lower than the recommended dietary allowance for these vitamins, they still had a statistically significant effect on the patients. After six months, those taking low doses of vitamin C had less toxicity and spent less time in the hospital. After three months on vitamin E, patients experienced lower rates of infection. After six months on B-carotene, patients had a lower risk for chemotherapy toxicity.

These results are remarkable. If *supplemental* low doses of antioxidants can help a cancer patient experience less toxicity from chemotherapy, and fewer days in the hospital, that is an excellent (and relatively inexpensive) outcome.

Many people, including some vets, make the mistake of thinking that if a low dose is good, a bigger one is better – or better yet, a mega-dose. There are many proponents of mega-doses of antioxidants during cancer treatments. I strongly advise against indiscriminate mega-dosing. As we've

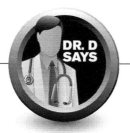

This chapter will be upsetting to some guardians. I remember feeling startled and a little guilty when I first started my research. I have dramatically changed the way I care for my own dog, and my patients, as a result of this information.

If you're feeling down, I hope that you will be gentle with yourself. This is not common knowledge, and it's all right that you were not aware of it earlier.

It helps me to remember that my dog is always living in the present moment, where the past is past, and the future isn't here, yet. Just like a dog shakes water off his coat, you, as guardian, can master your emotions, take your new insights, and use them to help your dog now.

seen, it may actually be desirable to give cancer cells pro-oxidants, which create free radicals, which could push the cell toward apoptosis, or natural death. In these cases, introducing antioxidants to neutralize free radicals may be counterproductive to healing the cancer.

(The one exception may be intravenous doses of vitamin C, given during and after treatments, which have helped a handful of human cancers go into remission, likely because the large doses of vitamin C actually caused a pro-oxidant effect in the body. I have not *personally* found large doses of vitamin C helpful enough to recommend them across the board, but I am not against their use if your vet has had success with them and they are carefully worked into a comprehensive plan. If this is something you are interested in, please consult with your vet about your dog's case.)

The bottom line is that mega-doses of antioxidants or potent antioxidant formulations could interfere with pro-oxidant therapies that use free radicals to target cancer cells. Supplemental levels, however, have been shown to be helpful with side effects from conventional treatments. Since eating vegetables has been shown to definitively help prevent cancer, using the cancer diet outlined in Chapter 14 for dietary antioxidants seems to be the wisest course of action, supplemented by a commercial multivitamin that contains regular, low, dietary levels of antioxidants.

Chapter 9: How We Diagnose and Stage Cancer

*E*ven the most experienced and skilled on-cologist cannot tell you for sure whether a lump is cancerous, just by looking at it or feeling it. To get a **diagnosis** (determine if cancer is present) we must run at least one test.

Depending upon the diagnosis, we may also need to look for evidence that it has spread, because sometimes it has by the time of diagnosis. What we find will determine the **stage** of the cancer.

Depending upon the cancer type, several different tests may be used to diagnose and stage your dog's cancer. Please see Dr. Ettinger's section of this book for details on the typical diagnosis and staging tests for the most common dog cancers.

Diagnosing Cancer

In order to determine whether a mass is cancerous, we have to run at least one test. A fine needle aspirate may confirm a tumor, and a biopsy is usually necessary to get an accurate diagnosis and enough information to plan treatments.

Fine Needle Aspirate

The first test for malignancy is usually the fine needle aspirate. The vet inserts a very thin needle into the tumor, to draw up a sample of the cells and fluid inside. If the aspirate is taken from an internal

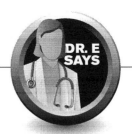

"Isn't there a blood test for cancer?"

This is one of the most common questions I hear from dog owners, and it sounds like a great idea. We would all love a practical, simple way to detect cancer much earlier than we typically do. It would be good to have a screening tool we could use in high-risk breeds, to make a diagnosis, determine a prognosis, and monitor remission during or after treatment.

The ideal test would be very accurate. It would measure markers in the blood, which are only produced by tumors, or by the dog's body, in response to the presence of tumors. Ideally, a positive result would occur only

continued on next page

"Isn't there a blood test for cancer?"*continued*

with patients who have cancer, and never with patients who don't. On the flip side, a negative result would always occur with patients who do not have cancer, and never with patients who do.

Getting a very accurate test like this is not easy. Inaccurate test results can occur when other, noncancerous health conditions create false positive or false negative test results. If the test doesn't reflect the state of cancer in the body accurately, it loses some of its value. "False-positive" test results can lead to additional testing or even to unnecessary treatments. False-negative results are also problematic; the patient might go without treatment.

We have not found a tumor marker that has met this ideal standard, which is why we do not yet have a blood test for cancer in dogs. No specific marker has been found which can be used as a practical screening tool for generally healthy dogs and/or for high-risk dogs.

This is a hot topic for researchers, so, hopefully, an accurate and relatively inexpensive test can be developed soon. If or when such a test becomes available, its use will still need to be evaluated on a case-by-case basis, because any test costs money, and the value of the information gathered must be weighed against a whole host of other factors.

There is one blood test available, which detects canine lymphoma markers in the blood, but I recommend its use only in certain cases. You will read about it in the lymphoma chapter, which starts on page 297.

organ, the surface area might need to be shaved and disinfected first. The procedure is often done without sedation or anesthesia, because it is usually only slightly uncomfortable for the dog. The entire procedure takes about two minutes, and the needle is only in the dog for a fraction of that time.

The vet cannot tell, just by looking at the sample with the naked eye, what kind of cells are inside, so the fluid sample is put on a slide and examined under a microscope by the vet or a cytologist (someone who studies cells). The sample can often confirm that, yes, cancer cells are present (and sometimes what kind) or, no, cancer is not present, at least not in that sample. The sample might also reveal signs of infection or inflammation.

Lymphoma, mast cell tumors, histiocytomas, and cysts are usually easy to diagnose with a simple fine needle aspirate. Other growths may be harder to diagnose this way because some tumor cells clump together so tightly that the vet can't create enough vacuum inside the needle to pull them apart and up. Other tumors, especially some connective tissue tumors, don't shed cells easily, so the sample contains only fluid, and no cancer cells. If there are no tumor cells in the sample that does not mean that the tumor is not cancerous. In these cases, the cytology report will label the test inconclusive, and another method will have to be used to diagnose the cancer.

A fine needle aspirate cannot be used to stage cancer (tell how far it has spread) or grade cancer (predict how aggressive it is) with precision. It only shows whether cancer is present in the collected specimen. This is why we so often need to do a biopsy.

Biopsy

A biopsy is a surgery, typically a small one, which removes tumor tissue for examination by a pathologist. It is more definitive than a fine needle aspirate, and can show the type of cancer and its grade (how aggressive it is). All biopsies are done under anesthesia or heavy sedation with pain control, so that the dog cannot feel the surgery.

Most biopsies are incisional, which means they don't remove the entire tumor and some tumor cells are knowingly left in the body. There are several tools that can be used, depending upon the nature and the location of the tumor. These include a scalpel, which takes a wedge shaped sample, or a core punch, which takes a disk shaped sample. Occasionally, an excisional biopsy is done, which is when the entire visible tumor is removed (with a scalpel).

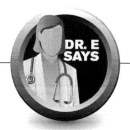

Biopsy reports are extremely useful because they give the diagnosis and a detailed description of the cancer cells. They will also often report the tumor type, grade and sometimes a margin evaluation (which tells you if the entire tumor was likely removed). The lab may also include comments about the cancer's likely prognosis – but these comments, unfortunately, could be viewed as facts. Keep in mind that the biopsy report is only one part of the story, and your dog's prognosis is not based solely on this one item.

For a more complete and reliable prognosis for your dog, it's best to have a discussion with an oncologist who has examined him, reviewed his medical history, and staged his cancer for spread. Putting that information together with the biopsy report creates a more complete picture.

If a tumor is deep in the body (for example, in the liver), a wide needle might be used to do the biopsy. If an even deeper biopsy is needed – for example, a bone sample – a very long core biopsy needle is used. Imaging tools, like ultrasound, are often used to help guide the needle during fine needle aspirates or biopsies of sites deep in the body.

Internal organs can also be biopsied using an endoscope: a small tube is threaded into the organ,

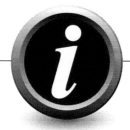

Can a Biopsy Get It All Out?

Many clients think vets can "get it all out in the biopsy." It's important to remember that biopsies are not usually curative surgeries for aggressive cancers, and almost never "treat" the cancer.

The point of a biopsy is to discern the type of tumor and to figure out how aggressive it is. The type and grade of the tumor determines the treatment plan.

Sometimes an entire lump, the visible part, anyway, is removed during a biopsy. This is usually because the tumor is discrete and easy to remove. It may look to us like the tumor is "gone" after the biopsy – but if the cancer is aggressive, there may be invisible and microscopic cancer cells still left in the region.

Occasionally a vet may biopsy a lump as if it is a curative surgery (often under pressure from guardians who try to squeeze two surgeries into one). She will remove the visible lump, plus a wide margin of tissue, hoping that even invisible cells are removed. The problem with this approach is that if the biopsy report finds the tumor benign, your dog has undergone a bigger surgery for nothing, and if it is a malignancy, your dog may still need another surgery or other treatment.

Careful planning usually saves money in the end, so if you hope to save money by reducing the number of surgeries, and insist upon attempting a curative surgery with a biopsy, I strongly suggest a fine needle aspirate first. Often, an aspirate will help your vet identify what type of cancer is present so that the surgery can be more effectively planned.

It is best to think of a biopsy as a test that is accomplished with a surgery. Just like a blood test does nothing to treat cancer, a biopsy usually doesn't, either. It's frustrating, but better to wait until after we get the biopsy report to plan a curative surgery.

and then a tiny machine with a fiber-optic camera is sent through the tube. The machine also has little arms that can grab and cut tissue samples, which are then pulled back through the tube.

Once the biopsy specimen is removed, it is sent to a pathology lab in a preservative, where it is prepared and embedded in a clear plastic. The specimen is sliced very thin, stained, and then examined under a high-powered microscope. The pathologist looks for several things, including the cancer type and grade. Knowing this can help us decide whether and where to look for cancer spread. It can also help us to plan how wide and deep an incision to make during a curative surgery.

Because of all of the steps involved, it usually takes five to ten days to receive your biopsy report after the actual surgery is performed. As you may have already experienced, it feels like ten years.

Despite the expense, the anesthesia, the recovery time, and the stress associated with a biopsy, it is a good idea to get one. Without it, you and your team are in the dark about the true nature of your dog's specific cancer case, or whether your dog even has cancer. Without a biopsy, it is hard to tailor a treatment plan.

Get a Biopsy after a Curative Surgery

In addition to their usefulness as an initial diagnostic tool, biopsies are done after curative surgeries, also. In these cases, the removed tumor will be sent to the pathology lab and examined along the margins, or edges, to see if there are cancer cells present. This is called a comprehensive margin evaluation. This type of examination can help a vet to know if another surgery or another treatment is in order, because, although some tumors seem very distinct from the surrounding tissue, they may have microscopic cancer cells spreading out in a halo. If the pathologist doesn't find any microscopic tumor cells, he pronounces the margins "clean" or "complete."

Clean margins in a sample may mean that the cancer is cured or unlikely to recur. If the patholo-

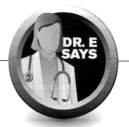

How Clean Are Those Margins??

Owners whose dogs have had a recurrence (regrowth) of a tumor in the same location often ask me how this could have happened, when the margins were pronounced clean after the first surgery. When I review the pathology reports in these cases, I often notice that while the tumor had "clean" margins, those margins were also very narrow, often only one millimeter. In these cases, the tumor cells were probably in tissue beyond that margin. Those cells, which were left in the dog, caused the recurrence.

For benign tumors, a one or two millimeter margin is probably adequate to prevent recurrence, but for most malignant tumors, *much* wider margins are required to prevent recurrence – from one to three centimeters!

Wide margins are doubly crucial in curative surgeries, because during a comprehensive margin evaluation the pathologist looks at a couple of areas
continued on next page

gist finds cancer cells on the border of the removed tissue, he pronounces them "dirty" or "incomplete," because it is very likely that cancer cells are left in the dog, too. In these cases, your vet or oncologist may suggest another surgery or some other treatment to target the remaining cancer cells.

Staging Cancer

Once a diagnosis is made, your vet or oncologist will probably want to stage the cancer, or check for spread. Not all cancers spread, but most do.

Cancer cells can spread in two ways, and the first type of spread is local invasion, sometimes called local involvement or local spread. To visualize this, picture a crab (cancer is actually the Latin word for crab). The body of the crab is like the tumor.

How Clean Are Those Margins??

continued

along the margin only, not the entire edge. If I see a very wide margin of one to three centimeters on a biopsy report, I have more confidence in the pathologist's conclusion that it is "clean."

The aggression of the tumor and its location are also important to note. For example, if your dog had a three centimeter, high grade, soft tissue sarcoma removed from the wrist, where there is not much room for wide margins, I would be very concerned about recurrence if the resulting scar only measured four centimeters. In this case, a one centimeter margin might be too narrow.

This is why planning curative surgeries is so important. Knowing what the tumor type is and planning for wide excisions increases the odds that the first surgery will be successful. If it's not, second surgeries, also called scar revisions, are trickier, and the dog's prognosis worsens.

The long crab legs are tumor cells reaching into normal tissues that surround it. These legs burrow through cell walls, create new blood vessels to steal oxygen from the bloodstream, and secrete acid to lower the pH in the surrounding tissues. Tumors hijack normal tissues and replace them with more tumor cells. This is how a tumor which begins in the nasal cavity can spread next door into the bones of the skull.

The second way that cancer spreads is by metastasis, also called distant involvement or distant spread. In this kind of spread, the tumor releases cancer cells into the circulation (bloodstream or lymphatics), so they can sail away and find distant places to live. This is how a cancer that begins in the spleen can also be found as close as the local lymph nodes, or as far away as the liver, lungs, or bone marrow.

Finding out what a cancer's stage is, or how much it has spread, will tell you and your vet how advanced your dog's case is. It will tell you what to expect over the course of the disease, and the

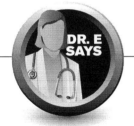

Do You Need an Oncologist to Supervise Testing?

Bringing a specialist like me onto your dog's team can seem like an added expense, but, in reality, it can help you to spend your money wisely. That's because, unlike many general practice vets, I only think about cancer. I can read tests with a more experienced eye than most general practice vets. My experience can be really helpful in deciding which tests to run for your dog with his particular cancer.

All too often, an owner comes to me with a thick folder, full of tests her vet has ordered, some of which turn out to be unnecessary. Each test represents an added expense, and some people have spent over $1,000, without even treating the cancer itself.

Unnecessary tests waste both time and money. Some owners would rather spend that extra money on conventional treatments, but now have to accept less aggressive treatments – or skip them altogether – because of limited funds.

Other owners, who make an educated decision to skip conventional treatments in favor of an alternative protocol, probably do not need all of those extra staging tests.

There is no doubt that comprehensive testing is helpful, no matter what methods are used to treat cancer. Testing establishes a diagnosis, helps us form a prognosis and gives us a baseline from which to measure progress. If budget is an issue for you, I recommend consulting with an oncologist before too many tests are run, especially if you are considering conventional treatments.

The best time to bring a specialist on to your team is just before you do a biopsy, or after you get the biopsy report. If there is no oncologist in your area, ask your vet to consult with one via phone or email. Search for an oncologist, using the specialist search tool at www.ACVIM.org.

prognosis. All of this information can really help you decide which of the available treatments to use.

Depending upon what the biopsy report shows us, we may need to look for spread with an ultrasound-guided aspirate or biopsy, X-rays, ultrasound, CT scans, urinalysis, various blood tests, or a bone marrow biopsy. To find out if the cancer has entered the lymphatic system, the lymph nodes may also be checked with a fine needle aspirate, or even a biopsy.

The tests will vary depending upon the type of cancer, its stage, and your own treatment and budget preferences. As Dr. Ettinger points out, a lot of money can be wasted on tests that you may not need, so be clear with your vet or oncologist about your budget. Reading the rest of this book, including the tests Dr. Ettinger uses for the most common canine cancers, will give some guidance about how far is far enough for you and your dog.

Micrometastasis

No matter how many tests we run, we don't yet have tools that can detect micrometastasis. In micrometastasis, a very small number of cancerous cells spread throughout the body, using the circulation system; they do not form tumors right away, but have the potential to bloom into full cancers later on. These cells may not be found in testing, even with our most sophisticated imaging tools. Their invisible spread is one of the reasons I recommend so many "outside the box" therapies in Full Spectrum cancer care. By using as many non-invasive therapies as possible, we may increase the odds of reducing micrometastasis.

Part III:

Full Spectrum Cancer Care

In this part of the book I will take you through Full Spectrum cancer care, step by step. We'll start with a short discussion about the Full Spectrum mindset, and then move on to Step One, Conventional Treatments, Step Two, Nutraceuticals, Step Three, Immune System Boosters, Step Four, Diet, and Step Five, Brain Chemistry Modification. By the end, you will have a solid overview of the things you can do to help your dog, starting immediately.

Chapter 10: An Overview of Full Spectrum Care

*F*ull Spectrum cancer care is based on the assumption that, no matter how much time you may have left with your dog, you can make the best of it … or, as medical professionals say, optimize it. There are many steps you can take, right now, to help your dog, no matter what stage or type of cancer she has – and a lot of these steps are free.

If you are like most guardians, your relationship with your dog is precious. Cancer doesn't change that. Your love for your dog can be a tremendous asset for you, motivating you to make high quality decisions. Full Spectrum cancer care is based on your loving relationship with your dog.

Every cancer case is unique, every dog is unique, and every guardian is unique. No two dogs need the exact same care; you may not choose to use all of the tools available. Even so, it's important that you consider each one. That's why I've broken my approach into five steps, each of which is outlined in detail in the next five chapters.

After reading those chapters and considering your own dog's case, you will have a very good framework, from which to design your own Full Spectrum plan. The next part of the book, Making Confident Choices, will

Your love for your dog can be a tremendous asset for you, motivating you to make high quality decisions.

help you to fine-tune your thoughts and make a real plan based on your values, your budget, your time and, of course, your dog's cancer case. Executing this plan with your team's expert help can give you an edge on your dog's cancer.

Let's go over the basics of the Full Spectrum mindset.

Full Spectrum Mindset and Cancer

I have great respect for cancer's ability to wage war on the body. As you've seen, cancer is a sneaky foe and a formidable enemy. Like any smart warrior, cancer attacks on more than one front. Here are the five ways cancer attacks your dog's body:

1. Cancer tumors grow larger and spread wider, crowding and even injuring neighboring body tissues. They metastasize, creating new tumors in new places, sometimes far from the original tumor.

2. Cancer suppresses your dog's immune system, which lessens her natural ability to fight cancer, leaves her vulnerable to outside infections, and slows wound healing.

3. Cancer robs your dog of nutrition, causing weight loss (cachexia) and muscle weakness; even when your dog is eating adequate calories.

4. Cancer steals resources meant for normal body functions causing otherwise healthy body systems to falter or even fail.

5. As cancer wreaks this havoc, life quality and happiness can take a nosedive. This leaves the body even more defenseless and increases the chances that the brain chemistry will change to "fight or flight." This, in turn, creates more stress, and the cycle continues.

Don't Accept the Standard Line

"Don't just accept the conventional thinking that most vets and vet oncologists will give you. It will be the same as human oncologists — cut it out, burn it out with radiation, poison it with expensive chemo drugs. As Dr. Andrew Weil said in Spontaneous Healing – ten or twenty years from now conventional cancer treatments will be considered barbaric. Unless it is a tumor that hasn't metastasized, it's likely to be an expensive and unsuccessful route. Instead, help bolster your dog's immune system so his immune system can cure his cancer or extend his life. Improve his diet with whole and unadulterated foods. Only give him purified water to drink. Start him on K-9 Immunity and Apocaps right away until you can figure out a supplement protocol. If you can't afford the Apocaps and K-9 Immunity, you can get herbs and supplements such as turmeric, green tea, fish oil capsules, milk thistle, quercetin and astragalus from many reputable online vendors (subscribe to Consumer Labs to make sure you're buying from a good vendor). Do your best to find a vet who gives credence to alternative therapies. Even if you want to utilize conventional chemotherapy, alternative therapies can be used in a complementary fashion. Read Andrew Weil. Subscribe to Dr. Russell Blaylock's newsletter and read all the back issues on cancer. Read the *Dog Cancer Survivor Guide*...and when you're finished read it again. Don't accept the line that alternative therapies are not "evidence-based" because gold-standard double-blind clinical trials have not been done. This does not mean that there is no evidence that alternative work; it just means that FDA-style clinical trials are simply too expensive to run on natural substances that cannot be patented. Love you dog every day. Give him a reason for living. And then maybe you'll actually see him in Heaven."

- Al Marzetti, Raleigh, North Carolina

Typical conventional vet care defends the first front by removing tumors and/or reducing their size. This makes sense, of course, and is also the first step in Full Spectrum cancer care. We don't stop there; we defend on all five fronts.

Full Spectrum Mindset and Cancer Treatments

Imagine that your house is under attack by a gang of five men. There's one who's climbing in the garage window, another is sneaking in the back, another one is taking a crowbar to your cellar door, another is shimmying up a drainpipe, and a fifth is throwing a rock through a plate glass window. You wake up, aware that someone is entering your home, but not sure who it is or what he wants with you.

To defend yourself, you have an alarm system, a cell phone that speed dials the police, a knife in your kitchen, and a gun under the bed. If you had to pick just one of these defenses, which one of them would you use?

That's kind of a silly question, isn't it? If you were really in this situation, you would at least *consider* using all of your defenses. And no one in her right mind would tell you not to be ready to use any and all means — the Full Spectrum — to stop the intruders from harming you or your family.

The same could be said of cancer treatments. When we face cancer we are often insufficiently armed, so if a treatment has been shown to help dogs get an edge on cancer, the Full Spectrum mindset demands it be considered for use. In Full Spectrum cancer care, therapies with a solid rationale for being safe and effective are always considered, regardless of their origin.

Not every Full Spectrum treatment we discuss is supported by multi-center, double-blind, placebo-controlled studies. So, why am I recommending them? Because I have carefully researched them, evaluated them, and concluded that they are safe and may help. There is no doubt that today we have an increased need for managing dog cancer and an increased urgency in treating it effectively. Just as human cancer patients are more likely than ever to be open to outside-the-box therapies, guardians are both more willing to treat their dog's cancer and more inclined to explore all of the options. I'm not willing, and neither are many guardians, to wait, when it comes to cancer.

If the treatment is safe and may help, it should be adopted, without waiting many years for the gold standard studies to be completed. As I've pointed out elsewhere, even some of the conventional therapies used by oncologists today don't have this "gold standard" support.

Dogs do not have much time; we should move with sense of urgency and be assertive. When fighting to stay alive, we cannot always do things perfectly or follow all of the conventional rules. We vets and oncologists should allow increased leeway for treatments which may help — and if it feels right to the guardian, we should go for it.

Few people used omega-3 supplements for their dogs when I was in school. Now, vets regularly prescribe them for dry skin, kidney disease, arthritis, allergies, and cancer. The same is true for glucosamine and chondroitin supplements, which are now used for arthritis, and for SAM-e, which is now used for liver and joint disease.

Even the Food and Drug Administration recognizes the need for speed, when it comes to new cancer therapies. It has instituted a "fast track" drug approval process, which allows therapeutics that may help advanced cancer cases to enter clinical trials much earlier than usual. Oncologists also recognize this need for speed when they use chemotherapy drugs off label. As long as it is safe and may help, let's apply this same method of thinking to every available tool.

Treatments from conventional medicine, alternative medicine, holistic medicine, and any other medical system – no matter how esoteric – can be used in a Full Spectrum cancer care plan, as long as the treatment has:

scientific studies supporting its effectiveness, and/or …

… a strong history of common clinical use supporting its effectiveness, and …

… minimal and/or tolerable side effects given the potential benefits.

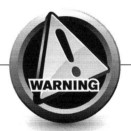

It may be tempting to read this and think "This is great! If I do everything here, my dog will beat cancer!"

While I have certainly seen dogs go into remission, or experience extended longevity and life quality, I cannot in any way guarantee that these recommendations will definitely help your dog with his particular cancer.

I'm sure you can understand why I must point out that it is impossible for me, or Dr. Ettinger, to diagnose or treat your dog through the pages of this book. ***Our recommendations are for your information only, and do not constitute veterinary advice for your dog.***

As always, you are the one in charge of your dog's cancer. If any Full Spectrum cancer care treatment resonates with you, I hope that you will check it out with your vet. Her expertise and ability to evaluate it, in the context of your dog's cancer diagnosis, other health conditions, age, and other factors, is invaluable. All decisions about your dog's care should be made with veterinary supervision and guidance.

With this advice and your vet's input, you can make an informed decision about what your next steps are … and be confident that you will have no regrets later.

The treatments outlined in this part of the book meet these criteria and, therefore, should be considered for your dog's cancer care. In the next chapters, you will find out how each treatment works and why I think it might help your dog. Many of them are universal treatments, which can help *any* cancer case.

Full Spectrum Mindset and Your Vet

Many of the treatments Dr. Ettinger and I recommend – whether they are chemotherapy agents, other pharmaceuticals, dietary changes, botanical nutraceuticals, or brain chemistry modifications – have potent effects on the body. For this reason, I strongly urge you to check out treatments with your vet and/or oncologist.

Be aware that some vets may not be open to hearing about Full Spectrum treatments. They may not believe that anything unconventional could work for cancer, and some may worry that even discussing these treatments is offering you "false hope."

If you encounter this resistance, my best advice is to remain calm and kind. None of us really knows what will work for your dog – including Dr. Ettinger and myself – so getting upset or deciding that your plan is "the right one" is counter-productive and not in the spirit of Full Spectrum care.

If your vet can't support the treatments you want to use, because he doesn't believe they will work, you can refer him to Appendix E for references. Every recommendation made in the pages of this book is backed up by thorough and extensive research. Sometimes, seeing real-world research helps to loosen up a resistant mind.

If your vet gives you a concrete reason not to use a treatment – for example, because it will interfere with another drug your dog is on, or because it will harm him due to some other factor – then, by all means, take your vet's advice. Dr. Ettinger and I cannot offer you advice which

Every recommendation made in the pages of this book is backed up by thorough and extensive research. Sometimes, seeing real-world research helps to loosen up a resistant mind.

replaces that of your vet or oncologist, and we did not write this book with that intention. Your vet or oncologist is going to have the fullest picture of your dog's health from a medical perspective.

(There is value in a second opinion, too. If you and your vet are in disagreement, bringing in another opinion can help you to decide what to do. I include lot of advice about how to work with your vet in chapter 22, including a long list of questions to ask your practitioners.)

Full Spectrum Mindset and You

You have probably heard of Lance Armstrong, the champion bicyclist, who not only fought cancer and won, but also, went on to win the Tour de France. Lance is an icon of persistence, courage, and belief in self. That's why I find it so interesting that Lance looks up to children for their ability to face the odds. He once said about cancer, "If children have the ability to ignore all odds and percentages, then maybe we can all learn from them. When you think about it, what other choice is there but to hope? We have two options, medically and emotionally: Give up or Fight like Hell."

Whether Lance faced cancer or the Tour de France, he encountered several obstacles at once, just as you are, with your own dog's cancer. It may help you to remember that dogs – much like children – have no interest in or knowledge of their odds.

Dr. Ettinger put it perfectly when she said that helping dogs is easier than helping the guardians, because dogs – bless their hearts – don't know they have cancer. They don't know they're supposed to be scared. They don't have to obsess over whether a treatment will cause side effects, or whether they will outlive statistical survival times.

> *"If children have the ability to ignore all odds and percentages, then maybe we can all learn from them. When you think about it, what other choice is there but to hope? We have two options, medically and emotionally: Give up or Fight like Hell."*
>
> – Lance Armstrong

You may have heard words as devastating as "two weeks" or as relatively hopeful as "one year" – but your dog has no worry or fear about his prognosis. He simply exists.

Part of him is gloriously, gorgeously *alive*.

To the degree that you can adopt Lance's child-like, hopeful, flexible, open-minded attitude, your Full Spectrum mindset will benefit immeasurably. It's what got Lance through cancer and kept his feet spinning and his heart pumping in those long, grueling bike races.

Five Steps to Full Spectrum Cancer Care

To fully address your dog's cancer, I advise systematically working through five separate steps. It may seem a little involved, but it's worth your time and effort. Here are the five steps, each of which is covered in detail in the following chapters:

Step One: Conventional Treatments (and how to manage their side effects)

Step Two: Nutraceuticals

Step Three: Immune System Boosters and Anti-Metastatics

Step Four: Dog Cancer Diet

Step Five: Brain Chemistry Modification

Depending upon many factors, you may ultimately choose to use tools from each step, or only from certain steps. For now, I recommend you become familiar with each step, so that you can make informed decisions later.

Making Confident Choices ... Later

As you read through the next five chapters, your Full Spectrum plan will start to take shape. No matter how urgent it seems for you to take action immediately, I recommend holding off until after you have read the final part, called Making Confident Choices. In that section, you'll find more information about life expectancy and life quality, and I will help you walk through the decision making process in a step-by-step fashion. There are many medical and personal factors to weigh, and approaching this in a systematic fashion usually results in a plan you fully understand and can follow with confidence.

Chapter 11: Step One, Conventional Treatments

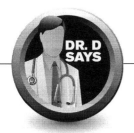

This chapter provides a general overview of surgery, radiation and chemotherapy treatments, including how to manage their side effects. For specific information on conventional treatments for common dog cancers, look in Dr. Ettinger's "From the Oncologist" section. Here, she describes the most common dog cancers in detail, including how each affects the body, what diagnostic tests are usually run, and prognostic factors. She also gives her advice about the best-of-breed conventional treatments for each cancer. Make it a point to read her introductory remarks and her chapter on your dog's cancer. Also, if she mentions specific chemotherapy drugs, be sure to look them up in the chapter on chemotherapy, Chapter 41.

According to studies, conventional medical cancer treatments usually cost between $5,000 and $8,000 – which is often reason enough for guardians to walk right out the door. Much depends, of course, upon what treatments are used. Single treatments, like surgery, may cost $2,000 (or less), while multiple or multi-modal treatments that include surgery, chemotherapy and radiation might soar to $10,000.

(Some readers may be tempted to skip this chapter altogether, but, even if you don't have that kind of budget or you don't think you'll choose conventional treatments, I recommend reading this chapter as part of your research. There is some financial assistance available (see chapter 24), and even the most die-hard alternative medicine adherent will find useful information here.)

Even guardians who can afford multiple hospital visits and expensive conventional treatments may find the words chemotherapy, radiation and surgery emotionally loaded. If this is you, take Three Deep Breaths (page 24) before you continue, so that you don't dismiss these options before you really consider them. It may also be helpful to know that, after discussing these three treatments, some conventional and natural methods for managing their side effects will be offered.

Surgery

Vets and oncologists often consider surgery first, because, if a tumor can be completely removed from the dog's body, the cancer may be cured. This can feel like a miracle, and it is. If a solitary tumor can be removed with surgery and has not yet spread locally or metastasized to other areas, surgery is a very hopeful option. But, as you'll see below, no surgery is minor when you consider all the factors.

When to Consider Surgery

The best candidate for surgery is a single, minimally aggressive tumor with no metastasis and limited local invasion. Unfortunately, many dog cancers are not diagnosed until after a tumor has already metastasized extensively into the area neighboring the tumor. In these cases, surgery may be used to remove the primary tumor, followed by chemotherapy and/or radiation protocols to "clean up" any invisible cancer cells. Depending upon the type and behavior of the tumor, radiation may also be used before surgery to shrink the size of the tumor and make it easier to remove.

Also, surgery may be used if an aggressive or metastatic tumor is causing pain or difficulty with movement – for example, when a tumor is pressing on a joint, or blocking the airway. In this case, surgery may be used to reduce the tumor's size (this is called debulking), even though cancer cells will still be left in the body. This is an example of palliative surgery, or surgery which is done with the intention of making the dog feel better, rather than curing him.

Sometimes, a tumor has not spread, but is impossible to reach, or is hopelessly entwined with vital structures. In these cases, the tumor is called inoperable or non-resectable, and other treatments must be considered.

Planning a surgery requires some investigation; just like you probably can't randomly knock down a wall to make your house bigger your vet can't just charge into an unplanned surgery. Investigation and planning may take anywhere from an hour to a few days, depending upon how much information your vet already has. Your vet may need to do a biopsy to determine what type of cancer is present, test lymph nodes for metastasis, or run other staging tests like blood work, urinalysis, ultrasounds, X-rays, CT scans, etc. Once your vet or oncologist knows what he's dealing with, he can come up with a plan for the surgery itself.

In some cases, surgery may not turn out to be the best option – but this can usually only be revealed once the right tests are run.

What Happens During Surgery

In general, every surgery has three stages: preparation, the operation itself, and recovery.

Preparation: You will likely need to withhold food, and possibly water, on the morning of the surgery. To prepare your dog for surgery, the vet and his staff bring him into a room that's been kept scrupulously clean. All of the linens and tools have been sterilized, and everyone has scrubbed hands and forearms. With the recent emergence of drug-resistant germs, including Methicillin-resistant Staphylococcus aureus (MRSA), most vets now require that everyone in the operating room wear a face-mask. Drug-resistant germs can hang out in the nasal passages (without causing symptoms) and be passed to others through the air. Since medical personnel are exposed to many infectious agents, they have a higher risk of carrying these unseen germs. Masking the surgical team protects your dog from airborne infections.

The surgical area on your dog is shaved and disinfected, and the vet or oncologist measures and marks exactly where the scalpel will make the incision into the skin. Your vet administers anesthesia intravenously and through a tube down your dog's throat, so that your dog remains asleep during the rest of the preparation and the actual surgery. Most of the time, anesthesia is maintained using a tube secured within your dog's windpipe (an endotracheal tube). Your dog's vital signs, such as breathing, blood pressure and heart rate, are monitored throughout surgery. Antibiotics and pain medications are administered directly into the blood by an intravenous port (called a catheter) or by injection directly into the body.

Surgery is inherently bloody, and it's important to make sure the bleeding ends with the surgery. To see if your dog's blood is clotting normally, a blood test, called a complete blood count (CBC), will be done before surgery (often before the dog goes into the operating room). The CBC will show if the blood cells, called platelets, are present in normal amounts.

Another blood test, called a coagulation panel or profile, can measure the levels of proteins that clot blood. Some vets do not routinely run coagulation panels. In that case, I recommend doing a simple test, called a bleeding test, to make sure that the blood is clotting normally, as it is difficult to know exactly how cancer affects an individual dog's body. Bleeding tests take a little time, but they are inexpensive and can be run after anesthesia is started while the rest of the preparatory work is done. The procedure is very simple: a tiny cut is made inside the lip, or a toenail is cut short so the wound bleeds freely. As it bleeds, the vet times how long it takes to clot. The time can vary, depending upon the test used, but generally blood clots within a few minutes. Much longer than that indicates the blood doesn't coagulate well, and the dog is at risk for excessive hemorrhaging and blood loss during or after the surgery.

If platelet levels are low and/or the bleeding test shows the blood is not clotting well, your vet will have transfusions and medications handy (or, rarely, postpone the surgery). Once your dog is fully prepared for surgery, the operation begins.

Operation: The type, size, and location of the tumor will determine what type of scalpel or other tool is used to remove it.

Most curative surgery aims for what is called a **wide excision**, which is removal of the entire tumor, along with a fairly wide, two to three centimeters, if possible, margin of tissue that looks normal to the visible eye. This margin extends around the tumor in all directions, including into the muscle layer underneath. Hopefully, this wide margin prevents a local recurrence by removing tissue that could contain microscopic cancer cells.

If a tumor is benign, a **marginal excision** is often used. In this type of surgery, the margin around the tumor is narrow. This leaves as much normal flesh intact as possible. Marginal excisions may also be used for palliative surgeries, which are meant to ease suffering or reduce tumor burden, rather than cure.

Some surgeries are more radical, or extensive, than others. In the case of a very invasive tumor, your vet or oncologist may recommend removing an entire limb, an organ (such as the spleen), or an entire portion of the wall of the abdomen.

There are also newer techniques, which may be much less invasive. Endoscopy allows us to look deep into the body with a fiberoptic camera, without creating a large opening. This instrument can also conduct small surgeries, by using robotic arms to cut and suture the tissues. For eligible tumors, endos-

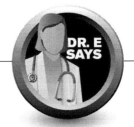

Minimally Invasive Surgery: Endoscopy

Endoscopy is becoming more and more common in veterinary medicine, and with good reason. This technique allows us to look inside organs and body cavities through a very small hole, which means the resulting scar is smaller and the recovery time is faster.

We can look inside the abdomen (laparoscopy), the chest cavity (thoracoscopy) and the bladder (cystoscopy) to get a biopsy, evaluate other organs for spread, and even remove tumors.

For example, laparoscopy enables a surgeon to biopsy a liver mass, determine if it can be removed, and evaluate the rest of the liver for metastasis. If the mass looks resectable, he can convert to a traditional abdominal surgical procedure to remove the mass. If the mass does not look resectable, or if there are other suspicious masses, he can take biopsies immediately, avoiding a large and/or unnecessary surgery.

Sometimes an entire tumor can be removed via endoscopy – for example, my surgical colleague routinely removes single lung tumors via thoracoscopy.

You may need to find a board-certified surgeon in order to take advantage of endoscopy. It may be worth checking with your vet or oncologist to see if this is an option for your dog.

copy can render larger surgeries unnecessary. Endoscopic surgery is often available at larger facilities.

Sometimes lymph nodes in the region of a tumor are suspected for spread, and are therefore removed during the surgery. There is some disagreement among oncologists about whether to do this as a default course of action. While it may initially seem logical to take out a node that seems involved in the cancer, it's not always so simple. For example, if the lymph node is biopsied and found to be cancerous, this might indicate that the cancer is metastasizing or has already metastasized. Removing that one node will not address the metastasis, and could even reduce the ability of the immune system to manage the cancer. On the other hand, if an enlarged lymph node is causing pain or interfering with normal functioning, it may be wise to remove it entirely.

After excision of the tumor and/or lymph nodes, the vet or oncologist will clean the wound and stop the bleeding. Veins and arteries may need to be sutured back together or cauterized (burned) to stop the bleeding. Muscles and other tissues may need to be sutured, as will the skin over the top of the wound.

Recovery: After the wound is sutured, a bandage may be needed to prevent infections or to provide pressure during healing. If the area must be kept still, a brace or other device may be put on your dog to keep her from moving. Then, the anesthesia is stopped, and she begins to wake up. Depending upon how extensive or intensive the surgery was, your vet may keep her for a few hours, or even overnight, to monitor her condition and administer injectable painkillers or other medications. For extensive surgeries, a few nights may be required.

If you've ever had anesthesia, you may remember feeling a little odd after you woke up. Dogs can also be a little unsteady on their feet or seem disoriented or woozy. Your dog may seem lethargic, sleep a lot, or may pant, in the hour or two immediately after surgery.

Otherwise, most dogs feel much better within three to four days, and most surgical wounds heal within ten to fourteen days.

Before then, there will likely be some at-home care you can administer. How much depends, of course, upon your dog's overall state of health and how invasive or complicated the surgery. You may have to change the bandage and clean the wound. Your dog may need an Elizabethan collar to keep her from licking the incision. Your dog may be incontinent for a while, which might mean you have to clean up after her. You might have to construct a convalescence area, where your dog can rest and not move around much while she heals. You may need to help or even carry your dog over to her food and water, or outside, when necessary. You may have to administer pain or other medications. Some dogs, particularly elderly dogs, can get depressed after surgery, so you may have to provide extra encouragement and affection.

Make sure you ask your vet to describe, in as much detail as possible, what kind of nursing responsibilities the surgery will require, once you leave the hospital. Surgery costs money, but it also costs time, both in and out of the hospital.

Follow Up

The tissues removed from any cancer surgery will be submitted for a biopsy and a comprehensive margin evaluation. If there are cancer cells along the margins, the margins are called "dirty" or "incomplete" and your vet may recommend another surgery, radiation or chemotherapy to clean them up.

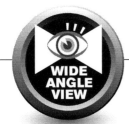

How Bad Are Side Effects?

Vets and oncologists have to walk a fine line when it comes to discussing side effects with guardians.

On the one hand, there *are* risks for every drug, surgery and radiation treatment (and many "natural" treatments as well). You, as the guardian, should be made aware of those risks, so you can make an informed decision.

On the other hand, side effects can sound so scary that they trigger fear-based thinking in guardians. Many vets are afraid that if we tell the whole story, guardians will get so scared that they'll refuse any treatment whatsoever. Immediately after vet school, I had an experience that perfectly illustrates this dilemma.

I was a brand-new vet, trying very hard to adjust quickly to my new role and responsibilities. I was working with a very nervous guardian, who felt frightened about every possible side effect for the medication I recommended.

As she asked about each side effect, I felt more and more tense. She just didn't seem to understand that I had prescribed the antibiotic because I thought its *benefits* for her dog far *outweighed* any *potential* (and *unlikely*) risk of side effects.

Finally, I couldn't take it anymore. I looked her right in the eye and said "Listen! One of the side effects is **an allergic reaction!** It's *possible* that your dog could have an allergic reaction so

Side Effects to Consider

Whether surgery removes a pea-sized lump or one the size of a grapefruit, it carries some risks and complications, which have to be proactively managed. In addition to the prolonged recovery times and intensive home care already discussed, be aware of the following risks:

- **Untreated Pain:** Most humans feel some level of pain after surgery, and it is safe to assume most dogs do, too. Often, guardians don't realize their dogs are in pain because it can be hard to pick up on canine pain signals. Your vet will probably prescribe pain medications for the days following surgery, and I recommend using them, as directed, to be on the safe side. Unmanaged pain is a stressful and horrible experience, and reducing your dog's pain is an important part of Full Spectrum cancer care (see page 229 for more details). In the unusual event that your vet doesn't bring up post-surgery pain management, make sure that you do.

How Bad Are Side Effects? *continued*

bad to this *antibiotic* that your dog could **die**!"

As you can imagine, the conversation ended rather abruptly, as did the relationship. She turned pale, called her dog, and hurried out of the office, never to return. I might as well have said to her what some parents say before spanking their children: "You want to cry about something? Cry about this!"

Losing a client, because I could not effectively communicate both the risks and benefits of a treatment (and because I was so insensitive), was a life lesson for me. It certainly inspired me to become a more supportive clinician.

I still wonder if her dog ever took an antibiotic for his infection – or did my revealing the extremely remote possibility of death, turn her away from antibiotic use forever?

The take home message is this: very few treatments are 100% safe … but there are also risks to not treating. As a vet, it is my responsibility to advocate for the health of your dog. If I think a treatment is worth the possible side effects, I will make that clear. A risk of *possible* side effects isn't the same as *probable* side effects.

Your own emotional management skills will be important as you read through this and the next few chapters, and particularly as you consult with your vet or oncologist. If you get overwhelmed, take a break and do an exercise from Chapter 2, to help you calm down and focus. Your dog will thank you for it (and so will your veterinary health professional).

- **Anesthetic Issues:** Every time we use anesthesia, there is a risk. Mild problems include stiffness from staying in one position during a surgery, throat irritation or coughing from the tube used to deliver the gas, razor burns where the shaver nicked the skin at the catheter sites, being smelly from urine that pooled underneath the body during surgery, and slightly lowered body temperatures from anesthesia. Much more serious problems include: brain damage, kidney failure, stroke, extreme hypotension (low blood pressure) during surgery, allergic reactions to medications or anesthetics, severe heart rate and rhythm problems, and death.

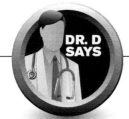

Why Be Afraid of Anesthesia?

It's a fact that anesthesia carries risks, including serious ones like kidney damage, brain damage, and death. Even mild affects, such as stiffness, nicks, and getting cold, make it unattractive. On an instinctive level, it can just seem wrong to let someone put your dog "to sleep." No wonder so many guardians are afraid of anesthesia.

To put these risks in perspective, I invite you to compare anesthesia to driving a car. If you get into a car with a very bad driver, you are more likely to experience "driving side effects" than you would be with an excellent driver. Side effects could include mild ones like an accelerated heart beat from driving too fast and a headache from loud music, and serious ones, such as broken bones, glass embedded in the skin, or even death.

There are a few studies that look at the risk of anesthesia-induced death. In one, of the 6,026 dogs who went to a specialty center (which means they were sick enough to need specialist care) over a three-year period, 20 died because of anesthesia-related accidents – or 0.33%. In another, the risk of death was less than 1% or one in 173 dogs.

Those were public studies. One private, confidential study looked at private practice vets treating dogs, cats and rabbits. In this study, the number of dogs who died due to anesthetic accidents was one in seventy-five, or 1.33%, which is higher than at the specialty centers.

The more experienced the anesthesia administrator is, the better your dog's chances of experiencing no or mild side effects. His general health is also a factor. In my experience, elderly dogs have a harder time with anesthesia than younger dogs do, and savvy clinicians will often use lower doses and gentler drugs because of this. If your dog has a known issue related to anesthesia,

Why Be Afraid of Anesthesia?
continued

the protocols will be modified accordingly.

Depending upon your budget or your location, you may or may not be able to choose your surgeon. Even so, it's worth finding out whether your vet is a "good driver" or a "bad driver" when it comes to anesthesia. You can do this by asking how many dogs have died in surgery in his practice, and how often he has seen serious side effects as a result of anesthesia. Measure his answers against the general statistics listed above and your own intuition, while you gently remind him how important it is to you for your dog to come out of the surgery with as few complications as possible.

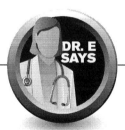

Board-certified Surgeons

If you are really worried about anesthetic accidents, seek out a board-certified surgeon. Published studies show that patients tend to have better outcomes when surgeries are performed by surgeons who have advanced training and experience.

- **Bleeding Problems:** If your dog's blood does not clot well on its own, he is at increased risk for excess bleeding on the table (hemorrhaging) or bleeding later, after the surgery is over. Ask your vet if he runs coagulation panels or does a bleeding test before he begins the actual surgery, in addition to the standard CBC.

- **Infections:** Both friendly and unfriendly bacteria can be found on the skin, and if unfriendly bacteria get into the surgical site, they can cause painful and dangerous infections. Since your dog's immune system is likely already suppressed, due to the cancer, preventing infections is particularly important. With the rise in drug-resistant bacteria, this problem is only growing. Impeccable sterile techniques are very important. Interestingly, however, the two things that most affect whether an infection occurs – especially a MRSA infection – are the length of time spent in the hospital and whether the surgical team wears masks. Humans carry germs with them all the time, and MRSA and other equally dangerous germs tend to lurk in our sinus cavities. They can be there whether we feel sick or not – and when we breathe out, they can leave our bodies and infect others. Wearing a mask, which filters the vet's breath and traps germs, is the best way to minimize surgery-related infections in your dog. If an

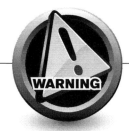

Ketamine Should Not Be Used as an Anesthetic

Ketamine has been shown to increase the odds of tumor metastasis, when it's used as an anesthetic. In a study done with rats as subjects, ketamine seemed to suppress the activity of natural killer cells, which probably made tumors more likely to metastasize, in the weeks after the anesthesia was administered. For this reason, I do not recommend using ketamine as an anesthetic when a dog has cancer.

Some vets, myself included, use very small doses of ketamine for pain control; at those low doses, it is safe for cancer patients.

In the same study, thiopental and halothane also increased metastasis, although not nearly as much as ketamine did. Although these agents are not usually used in veterinary medicine anymore, check with your surgeon to be sure. Propofol was also assessed during this study, and it was the only anesthetic not associated with suppressed natural killer cell activity.

infection does develop, a culture can be taken to find the right antibiotic to kill it. As the ten days necessary to do this can be a very long time for a dog with cancer – here in Hawaii, where MRSA is epidemic, I often give a double-dose of Clavamox immediately, when I suspect the culture will come back positive. That particular antibiotic is often effective with MRSA bacterial infections; other possibilities your vet may consider are doxycycline and clindamycin.

These risks are serious, and you want to be aware of them – but do not take my warnings as evidence to avoid surgery. Just because these side effects are possible, does not mean that they are probable. After all, cancer is serious, too. Use this information to have an open, informed dialogue with your vet or oncologist, so you can make the best decision for your dog and her particular cancer diagnosis.

Choosing a Surgeon

Most veterinarians – especially those in rural areas – are general practitioners. Because they see a wide range of problems, they often have a wide base of experience. There is still a spectrum of skill levels. Depending upon their training, whether they have supervision from another, more experienced vet, and their opportunity to practice certain surgeries, some may be more experienced – and therefore more confident – than others.

Just like human physicians, veterinarians have personal preferences about how they practice medicine. Especially in urban areas, where vets can refer out to other vets or specialists, some vets may not do certain surgeries. I know one vet who refuses amputations, because he is uncomfortable with them. He hasn't done enough to feel confident in his skills, and he's willing to refer those surgeries to other vets.

It's not rude to ask your vet whether he is comfortable with the surgery he's proposing, and it's important that you know the answer. Ask how common the surgery is, and how often he's done it. If he's not comfortable with the surgery, he will likely give you a referral.

I've been asked how many surgeries a vet needs to have done in order to be considered experienced, so I'll share with you my very general rule of thumb: fifty. Once a vet has performed the same surgery fifty times, he is probably very comfortable with the procedure. Of course, if a surgery or technique is new, or if that surgery just hasn't shown up in his practice, your vet may not have this level of experience.

Some guardians prefer to go to a specialist for surgery. If a board-certified surgeon is available in your area, at least consider consulting with her. After all, she spends every day in the operating room and will be more comfortable with complicated surgeries. There is some evidence that board-certified surgeons generally remove more tissue during surgeries, which results in cleaner margins. A few board-certified surgeons have also trained separately and are board-certified in oncological surgery. Whether you have the resources to hire "the best" surgeon or not, it's important that you have a frank and open discussion with your vet about the proposed surgery, and that you listen to your gut when it's time to make a choice.

Radiation

Radiation therapy beams a large amount of energy (which is invisible to our eyes) into one area of the body. The energy is called "ionizing radiation" and usually consists of photons or electrons. This energy is strong enough to enter cells and affect their molecules. The radiation tears electrons out of their orbits, creating those unpredictable free radicals discussed in Chapter 8. These new free radicals damage the cell's structure, most commonly by damaging its DNA.

As a result of this damage, the cell dies when it tries to divide and proliferate. Only the cells, which are dividing at the time of the treatment, will die immediately – others will die days or even weeks later, after they start to divide. This is why it can take a while – months, sometimes – for tumors to shrink, as a result of radiation therapy.

Radiation doesn't just kill cancer cells. It can damage or kill any normal cells that get in the way, such as skin, mucous membranes, eyes, and any other organs that are in the path of the radiation beam.

The resulting side effects can be quite serious. For this reason, radiation is not used in all cancer cases, and when it is used, great care must be taken to spare as many normal cells as possible. The radiation oncologist carefully considers the field of treatment, noting any particularly sensitive areas or organs, like the lungs and the intestines. The total dose of radiation is determined by how much the most sensitive areas can handle with relative safety. To minimize damage even further, the dose is divided up into many small treatments (typically fifteen to twenty). These sessions, called fractions, are helpful, because normal cells can repair themselves more efficiently after smaller, multiple doses.

The need for a radiation oncologist, several treatments and anesthetic make radiation therapy very expensive.

When to Choose Radiation

The most common time to use radiation is after surgery, in an attempt to damage irreparably and kill any microscopic cells left in or around the surgical site.

Radiation may also be considered when there is a discrete tumor, large enough to be seen with the naked eye: especially a tumor that has not metastasized or is not prone to metastasize. It's also considered for tumors that cannot be removed with surgery (inoperable or non-resectable tumors).

Some cancers respond well to radiation, including lymphoma (a lymphoma tumor can shrink to half its size after just one treatment), perianal adenoma and perianal adenocarcinoma, plasmacytoma (plasma cell tumor) and transmissible venereal tumors.

Other cancers are less responsive to radiation, but can be good candidates, depending upon the case: nasal tumors, mast cell tumors, squamous cell carcinoma, fibrosarcomas and nerve sheath tumors (hemangiopericytomas). Depending upon the individual tumor and the intent of the radiation treatments, these cancers might be reduced a moderate amount or slowed in their growth. In other cases, they may respond well, but the effect might be temporary (weeks' or months' duration).

Another use for radiation is as palliative therapy. In these cases, the goal of radiation is not to destroy the cancer completely, but to reduce the size of the tumor(s). If the tumor is pressing on nerves, organs or bones, shrinking it can reduce pain. Tumors that are obstructing important areas, like the urinary tract or prostate, may also be candidates for radiation therapy.

Radiation therapy seems to have a pain-relieving effect. For example, dogs who receive palliative therapy for osteosarcoma usually experience a lessening of pain within seven days of treatment, and that affect lasts four to six months. We're not entirely sure why their pain lessens, but we speculate that neurotransmitters (called endorphins) are released by the procedure. Endorphins are the body's natural opiates, or pain relievers. Dogs who receive palliative radiation may need less pain medication.

Palliative radiation therapy uses far fewer sessions, usually one to five, which means there is less risk of an anesthetic accident. These sessions are also less complicated and less demanding on your time for after-session care. There is also, of course, less expense, because there are fewer sessions and a shorter stay in the vet hospital.

Because radiation equipment is so expensive to purchase and maintain, radiation oncologists usually practice in large urban centers or veterinary medical schools.

What Happens in a Radiation Session

Generally, it is easier for normal tissues to repair from small doses of radiation than from larger doses. For this reason, radiation oncologists typically split up the total radiation dose into several small treatments. These small treatments are called fractions, and they ensure that cancer cells are killed and normal tissues have a chance to repair themselves. Most curative radiation protocols recommend fifteen to twenty daily treatments, over the course of three to four weeks, while most palliative protocols call for somewhere between one to five treatments (depending upon the tumor type and case), usually once a week.

Radiation therapy is usually given on a daily basis, Monday through Friday, requiring daily trips to the hospital. For convenience, some guardians choose to board their dogs in the hospital during treatment days and take them home for weekend breaks.

Dogs must be anesthetized every time they get a treatment. This is to make sure they are completely still and do not move a healthy body part into the damaging radiation beam. The repeated, daily use of anesthesia is a very important factor for guardians to consider.

(As we can sit still on our own, humans usually do not get anesthesia during radiation.)

The most common radiation machine in veterinary use is the linear accelerator, or LINAC. The linear accelerator is a large machine that produces short, rapid bursts of radiation. The dog is laid on a treatment table, which stays completely still, while the linear accelerator revolves around it, in a full 360° circle, to administer the radiation. This machine can treat from any angle around that axis, but not from any other angle, which means the radiation may fall on normal tissues. Typically, 25-50% of the total dose of radiation is delivered to normal tissues, which could cause life threatening side effects. The problem radiation oncologists have is this: how do we deliver the entire dose without causing life threatening side effects to the normal tissues in the treatment area? The solution is to break up that total dose into fifteen to twenty (or more) doses (called fractional treatments), given over the course of three to four weeks, all of which call for anesthesia.

Medical researchers have long been looking for a way to deliver radiation with more precision and less risk to the patient, and recent advances have made progress. For example, a technique called "radiosurgery" aims at getting the radiation energy directly to the tumor – even inoperable tumors – while avoiding healthy body parts that might be damaged by the beam. First, a CT (computed tomography) scan or MRI is run, to get a very detailed three-dimensional image of the tumor. Then, a computer program helps the oncologist and/or radiation oncologist to plan precise co-ordinates for the radiation beam. New, modified linear accelerators can generate very controlled, narrow beams that deliver radiation only to those exact coordinates. By the way, there is no actual cutting during radiosurgery – the name is meant to imply that radiation is accomplishing what surgery would do, if it could actually get to the tumor.

At the time of writing, this type of radio-surgery is only practiced at the University of Florida, Colorado State University, and the Animal Specialty Center in New York (Dr. Ettinger's practice). Dr. Ettinger's practice owns a particularly advanced radiosurgery machine called the CyberKnife. The machine has five "arms" and rotates around several axes. It can approach a tumor from almost any angle selected by the radiation oncologist and, while a traditional linear accelerator has two to four ports (holes where the radiation exits), the CyberKnife has hundreds. This allows for very narrow beams of energy that can be precisely directed to the tumor. Using this machine, normal tissue receives 1/100 or even just 1/200 of the total dose (instead of 25-50%). The entire dose can be given in one to

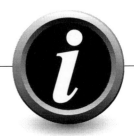

Brachytherapy

There is a relatively new radiation therapy called "brachytherapy" (which translates to "short therapy").

Instead of using a machine to beam radiation into tumors, therapeutic radio-active materials are sealed inside small bundles, shaped like seeds, needles or tubes. These bundles are then surgically implanted in the tumor itself or right next to it. The surgical site is closed up and, after a period of time, a second surgery removes the bundle. This allows the radiation direct contact with the tumor, causing much less effect on normal tissues. If you're interested in brachytherapy, ask your oncologist whether it could help your dog. To find a radiation facility near you that offers brachytherapy, check www.VetCancerSociety.org.

three treatments (instead of fifteen to twenty) and, in Dr. Ettinger's experience, acute, or immediate, side effects are greatly reduced. Dr. Ettinger's radiation oncologist colleague uses this machine to treat otherwise inoperable tumors including brain tumors, nasal tumors, spinal tumors, osteosarcoma, prostate tumors, and some oral tumors. On the other hand, radiosurgery is not recommended for microscopic cancer cells, like those left after a surgery, mast cell tumors (even non-resectable mast cell tumors) or soft tissue sarcomas (except in a few non-resectable cases).

Follow Up

Most dogs can go home right after their last radiation treatment, whether it's traditional radiation, palliative radiation, or radiosurgery. There is some recovery time involved, depending upon how intensive the therapy was and where the radiation was applied. Depending upon the case, some dogs might develop skin burns that need topical treatments (like aloe), or bandaging. If the mouth was irradiated, the tissue might be quite sore, in which case only soft food would be given. Some dogs might require antibiotics and/or anti-inflammatory medications. If the skin over a joint is burned, its movement might need to be limited and an Elizabethan collar might be necessary to keep the wound from being licked.

Side Effects to Consider

One of the main things to consider when evaluating radiation therapy is how often your dog will need to be treated. As you'll remember from the sidebar on page 118, there are inherent risks every time your dog undergoes anesthesia, and those risks apply to every radiation treatment, including all twenty rounds experienced in many traditional radiation protocols.

There are also side effects from the radiation itself, which oncologists group into early (acute) reactions and late reactions.

Acute reactions usually happen during or soon after treatment, and are very common. Most of them have to do with what is called "die off," or the death of rapidly dividing normal tissues within the path of the radiation beam. About 80% of dogs will experience some degree of the following **acute reactions** immediately after or within days of receiving traditional radiation therapy:

- **Skin conditions:** The skin is made up of several layers of rapidly dividing cells. As these cells die off or try to repair themselves, you may see redness, flaking, or blistering (like severe sunburn). Hair may fall out and, in extreme cases, the skin may even suffer necrosis (death and sloughing), leaving a hole (ulcer) that will need to be filled in by the body's natural repair processes (if possible). Sometimes dogs lose their fur or hair, or it changes color.

- **Mouth sores:** When they fall in the path of the radiation, the mucous membranes in the mouth can swell or develop sores, making eating painful. If the sores get infected, antibiotics may be required.

- **Dry Eye, Corneal Ulcers:** When radiation treatments occur near the eyes, the lachrymal gland or tear ducts can be damaged. If this happens, a condition called *keratoconjunctivitis sicca* (dry eye) may occur. In this condition, the eyeball does not receive enough natural tears or lubrication. This leads to extreme inflammation and a thick greenish discharge. As you can imagine, chronically dry and swollen eyes are very uncomfortable. To keep your dog's eyes healthy, you will need to apply lubricating ointment twice a day for the rest of his life. If the eyeball itself is in the radiation field, corneal ulcers (holes or craters) are likely to develop, causing pain and squinting. Ulcers may require ointments or antibiotics until the ulcer heals.

About 5% of dogs experience **late reactions**, which show up one month, three months, six months, and even a year or two after radiation treatments. Which effects show up will depend upon what areas of the body were treated, usually involving cells that grow more slowly. If your dog is older, you may never see any of these effects – but if your dog is young, they may pop up later in her lifetime. Here are some late side effects:

- **Bone and ligament damage,** due to the necrosis, or death, of cells in these areas. This can result in limping or other painful movements.

- **Nerve or spinal cord injury,** which can cause instability or wobbliness while walking, difficulty getting up, weakness, or difficulty moving around.

- **Other cancers,** which can arise from the damaged DNA in cells that manage to survive and replicate. For example, 3-5% of dogs whose bones are exposed to radiation develop osteosarcoma three to five years later.

- **Brain infarction,** which is a sudden loss of blood flow to the brain. Depending upon which area of the brain is affected, some signs of an infarct are: drifting to the side while walking, holding the head sideways, or having a facial droop on one side. These can be permanent changes, but sometimes dogs can make a recovery.

- **Blindness:** if the eyes were within the field of treatment, within a year or two, cataracts or retina problems inevitably show up, which could lead to permanent blindness.

- **Kidney injury,** which can cause weight loss, decreased appetite, vomiting, decreased energy, and increased thirst and urination (the kidneys are rarely included in the field of treatment for this reason).

Radiation therapy is incredibly powerful and increasingly more precise, and in the right case, its use can make sense. However, it is very expensive and carries high risks. I approach its use with caution, especially in younger dogs, and I am very concerned about minimizing risks and side effects. Make sure to weigh all these factors with your veterinarian and oncologist.

Chemotherapy

Historically, the word chemotherapy referred to the medical use of any drug. Today, we use it to mean the use of drugs in cancer treatment. Dr. Ettinger discusses the most common drugs in Part V, "From the Oncologist."

There are many chemotherapy drugs, which are usually combined with each other and administered in a series of treatments, called protocols. Like radiation therapy, chemotherapy targets rapidly dividing cells. All cancer cells divide rapidly, but so do some normal body cells (for example, those in the skin, lining the digestive tract and the bone marrow). For this reason, side effects are possible and even probable, in some cases.

Some human cancers can be cured with chemotherapy, but not in dogs. Instead, it is used to prolong life and increase quality of life by shrinking tumors and/or suppressing their growth and spread. This emphasis on life quality and extension is why I consider chemotherapy a palliative cancer treatment, not a curative one (although most oncologists wouldn't think of it this way).

Some guardians wonder why chemotherapy can't cure dog cancer, and the reason is really very simple: curative doses of chemotherapy typically come with high levels of toxic side effects. These side effects may feel awful to humans, but they can be tolerated because we understand why they must be endured. It is impossible to give dogs the same understanding, and most guardians and vets would find the severe side effects, typical in human treatments, unacceptable for dogs.

The goal of chemotherapy is to put cancer into remission, which is a reduction (not necessarily elimination) of the signs and symptoms of illness. During a remission, you may see your dog's tumor shrink (visibly or on images) or disappear, which is commonly referred to as a "reduced tumor burden." Her energy and appetite may return, and she may be in less pain, eating and drinking normally, sleeping regularly, playing, wanting to go for walks and being more engaged with you.

Veterinary oncologists consider chemotherapy a success if tumors stop growing or shrink or if they continue to grow at a much slower rate. The length of time a remission lasts varies widely, depending upon the tumor type, the stage and grade of the cancer, and many other factors. For example, Dr. Ettinger's preferred lymphoma protocol can extend life by thirteen to fourteen months, while other cancers may allow a dog just a few extra months. Remissions that last two weeks or more are considered stable and called "durable."

Researchers know chemotherapy must be as strong as possible to slow cancer – but, with stronger treatments, the side effects increase. So, what is an acceptable level of side effects? To induce remission in the majority of dogs, researchers have a set of guidelines; to be effective, any given chemotherapy protocol will not cause death in more than 1% of treated dogs, and hospitalization in no more than 5%. These results must be achieved with as few side effects as possible, most of which will be manageable at home, with over-the-counter medications.

From my perspective, chemotherapy can be a tough sell for certain cancers. Because I treat many other conditions in addition to cancer, a 5% hospitalization rate – one in twenty dogs – seems really high, in comparison to treatments used for other diseases. Many of the guardians I see in private practice feel this way, too – for some, the knowledge that their dogs have a one in one hundred chance of dying as a result of chemotherapy will cause them to walk right out the door. For others, the expense, the concerns about toxicity, the possible side effects, and the realization that there is no sure outcome, make chemotherapy a less attractive option than surgery, for example (at least surgery is guaranteed to get some cancer out of the body). Of course, there are certainly guardians who feel chemotherapy is an attractive option for their dogs. Chemotherapy certainly has its place, and should be used in the appropriate circumstances, but there are many factors involved.

In addition to the inherent risks, relapses or recurrences of the cancer are not only possible, but also, very probable. After a remission, the cancer comes back, and usually stronger. At this point, it will be your choice whether you use a "rescue protocol" to attempt a second remission. Depending upon the type of tumor and how long the first remission lasted, rescue protocols may entail the same drugs administered in the same doses, or a completely different protocol.

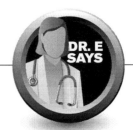

While I understand Dr. Dressler's perspective, as a chemotherapy specialist, I must respectfully disagree with him. A 5% hospitalization rate seems reasonable when I consider the benefits chemotherapy can offer dogs who are good candidates. A one in twenty risk of hospitalization seems well worth the pay-off for another year with your dog, in the case of the best lymphoma protocol, for example. Chemotherapy does not work for every cancer (please see my section for more information). When it does, you, the dog owner, ultimately have to decide for yourself: what's your risk tolerance? As a medical oncologist, I am very proactive about managing side effects, and I have rarely hospitalized chemotherapy patients. The majority of them are treated as outpatients, and they are happy dogs. Please read my section of this book for more of my advice and another perspective.

If your dog achieves a second remission, it may not seem very long before another relapse occurs.

Dr. Ettinger is in the trenches of chemotherapy, and these rates seem normal to her (although of course she wishes they were better). She takes care to inform guardians of the real odds, and her clients can afford and are willing to take the chance chemotherapy offers them, hoping that their dog will achieve some length of remission. There are many chemotherapy drugs; not all of them are useful for each cancer. There is a lot to understand, which is why Dr. Ettinger, the expert in chemotherapy, has written about these drugs, in addition to other conventional advice. Her section begins on page 289, so please make a point of using it for your research.

When to Choose Chemotherapy

Unlike radiation and surgery, which treat specific, localized areas, chemotherapy agents can circulate throughout the body, via the bloodstream. For this reason, chemotherapy can be useful when the cancer has become systemic, by spreading into the surrounding tissues (local invasion) or into the lymphatic system, bloodstream, or distant sites in the body (metastasis). For cancer types that have a high risk of future metastasis, chemotherapy may also be used as a preventive measure.

Chemotherapy is often used as a follow up to surgery. If there is micrometastasis – invisible spread – it will sometimes undergo a growth spurt immediately after surgery. Using chemotherapy five to seven days post-surgery can stunt some of that growth and make recurrence less likely. However, using chemotherapy during this time can also affect the body's ability to heal from the surgery, and for some cancers (osteosarcoma, specifically), waiting for fourteen days may not affect the ultimate outcome. For these reasons, Dr. Ettinger recommends waiting at least ten to fourteen days after surgery to start chemotherapy for most patients.

There are published chemotherapy protocols for most of the common dog cancers, which oncologists use as guidelines, not recipes. For most cancers, there is no one "standard" protocol acknowledged as "the best." Oncologists make their plans based on their observations of the particular dog, their experience with that particular cancer type, stage, and grade, and their personal preferences.

Because there are so many variables – and so many drugs – I strongly recommend reading Dr. Ettinger's advice and consulting with an oncologist, if you are considering chemotherapy. If you don't have a veterinary oncologist in your area, your vet can contact one of the commercial laboratories, which often have oncologists on staff.

What Happens in a Chemotherapy Session

The goal of most chemotherapy protocols is to give a series of the highest, most potent dose possible – otherwise known as the **maximum tolerated dose.** The shorter the time is between doses, the more effective the therapy. This intense schedule kills the maximum number of cancer cells. The trick, for oncologists, is to minimize (and manage) the possible side effects, while the chemotherapy has a chance to work.

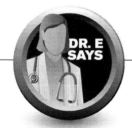

Multi–Drug Resistance

As powerful as chemotherapy agents are, some cancer cells almost always survive the treatment. Why? It could be because some cancer cells just did not come in contact with an effective dose of the chemotherapy agents. If a tumor is very large, or very dense, the agents might kill the cells on the margins, but not penetrate into the very center, especially if the blood supply to the cancer is inadequate. Sometimes it's more complicated. Some tumor cells activate a structure in the cell membrane, called a p–glycoprotein pump, to literally pump out certain chemotherapy drugs.

(P–glycoprotein pumps can be present in normal cells, too, but in those cells the pumps are used to remove toxins.)

The p–glycoprotein pump is encoded in the multi–drug resistance (MDR) gene. When it's turned on, this pump can eliminate specific chemotherapy drugs from the cell. It can eliminate many other drugs, also, even those with completely different chemical structures. This is called multi–drug resistance, and in these cases it is very hard to find a chemotherapy protocol that will be able to shrink or slow the cancer. (This is why dogs with lymphoma with multi–drug resistance have a worse prognosis.) This is an interesting area for researchers, some of whom are developing drugs that might affect multi–drug resistance and help future patients respond to chemotherapy.

While MDR is a real phenomenon for some dogs, others have the opposite problem: they carry a genetic mutation in the MDR gene, which actually makes them more susceptible to chemotherapy and other drugs. While these dogs are more likely to suffer severe side effects from chemotherapy, they also could become critically ill or even die from the use of some common parasite–control products, antibiotics, sedatives and pain medications.

Luckily, we can now test for this mutated gene through Washington State University College of Veterinary Medicine. If the results are positive for the mutation, we can significantly lower the dose of chemotherapy drugs to avoid severe toxicity. There are certain breeds at risk for this genetic mutation, so if your dog is an Australian Shepherd, Collie, Long–haired Whippet or Silken Windhound, I recommend getting her tested for this mutation, before starting chemotherapy. For more information, you can go online to www.vetmed.wsu.edu/depts-VCPL.

Most chemotherapy agents must be administered directly into the vein at the clinic, requiring a trip to the office for each dose. Depending upon the protocol, this could mean anywhere from six to twenty trips (or more). Chemotherapy treatments rarely require hospitalization overnight and most office visits last about 60 to 90 minutes. There are even some drugs in pill form, which can be given at home.

Chemotherapy doses are based on surface area, which is calculated using weight, so your dog will be weighed at each appointment. The oncologist will also do a complete physical exam, including a complete blood count (CBC). This blood test reveals, among other things, how many and what kind of white blood cells are in your dog's blood. Immune suppression is an inherent side effect of cancer, but it is also a side effect of chemotherapy (see below); monitoring your dog's white blood cell count at every appointment can help the oncologist see if the immune system is holding up under the strain.

The oncologist will ask you how your dog is feeling and what side effects may have occurred since your last appointment. Your answers, along with your dog's weight, her CBC results, and her other medical problems, if any, will be factored into the oncologist's decision about that day's dose of chemotherapy. The dose may be different from that on the last visit, for example, if the dog's weight has changed. In other cases, if there were a lot of side effects (vomiting, diarrhea, etc.) after the last treatment, the dose may be lowered.

This decision is never taken lightly, however, because lower doses can radically alter the treatment's effectiveness. For example, studies in people have shown that a 20% dose reduction can make the treatment 50% less effective: a huge drop in efficacy, compared to the drop in dosage.

There is another recent study that showed chemotherapy doses high enough to cause low white blood cell levels (neutropenia, see below) – which we typically try to avoid – were associated with longer remissions. This outcome makes oncologists even more inclined to keep doses as high as possible, while using antibiotics and other medications to keep the immune system stimulated.

Chemotherapy agents are, in general, extremely toxic, so, oncologists make safe handling a high priority. For this reason, you will likely not be allowed into the treatment rooms. Your dog will sit or lie down to receive her treatment, which is usually given intravenously, through a catheter in her forearm, or rarely into the chest or abdomen cavities. Most dogs do not need sedation to receive treatments and there is often a chemotherapy nurse and an assistant present during the entire time. Several chemotherapy agents must be delivered directly into the vein – if not, they can severely injure tissues. This is why I so strongly recommend using an experienced practitioner, or an oncologist, if you are considering chemotherapy for your dog.

Once the treatment is complete, most dogs can go home right away. Because anesthetics are not used during chemotherapy, there is usually no need to stay in the hospital for observation.

Some chemotherapy drugs are given by mouth at the hospital, or even at home. If your oncologist prescribes a home-based protocol, it's important to remember to report all the side effects, so that she isn't flying blind. To protect yourself and keep your family safe from the chemotherapy drugs, make sure to wear gloves while handling them. Keep them on until you are sure that your dog has swallowed the pill – that way if she spits it out, you can pick it up quickly and safely. When you're finished, dispose of those gloves and wash your hands well.

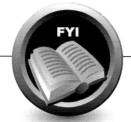

How to Give Pills to Your Dog

If the pill can be given with a small amount of food, many dogs will happily swallow pills disguised in a piece of cheese, a scoop of peanut butter or a pill pocket (a treat designed with a hollow middle, available in most pet stores, at most vet offices, and at www.DogCancerShop. com). Some dogs become suspicious of these foods, so you might give a piece without medication, before you give the loaded version.

If the pill can be given with food, you can also try hiding it in your dog's dinner. If you do this, make absolutely sure that the pill is gone, after your dog has finished eating.

If your dog is on to these tricks, or if the pill has to be given on an empty stomach, you'll need to get him to swallow the pill whole. This can get a little tricky, and it is easiest if you have an assistant. Here's how I approach it:

1. Get the pill ready.
2. Call your dog, with a super happy voice, so that he won't be suspicious. It sometimes seems like dogs can read our minds, so you might try thinking about something he likes – throwing a ball, eating dinner, taking a walk – rather than the pill, when you call him.
3. Once your dog is present, you'll need to find a way to hold him still. If he's small enough and you have an assistant, you can put him up on a counter or a couch. If he's larger, lead him to a corner or some other place where you can put his hind end against something firm, so he can't back away. You can also have your assistant hold him from behind, with her hands and arms firmly holding his shoulders and chest.
4. If you're right-handed, hold the pill between your thumb and index finger in your right hand (in your left, if you're a southpaw).

How to Give Pills to Your Dog, *continued*

5. Use your other hand to gently hold your dog's muzzle from above, with your thumb on one side and your fingers on the other.

6. Squeeze just behind the upper canine teeth and tilt your dog's head back over his shoulders. As he looks at the ceiling, his jaw will drop open a bit.

7. Lower the bottom jaw even further by hooking a finger of your hand with the pill in it between the lower canine teeth (the long front teeth), and pushing gently down.

8. Place the pill as far back in your dog's mouth as possible, and certainly over the hump of the tongue, right in the center. Do this quickly, and don't go so far in that your dog starts to gag.

9. Remove your finger and press your dog's mouth closed. Hold it and lower his head to a normal position to make swallowing easier. Gently rubbing or blowing on your dog's nose sometimes stimulates the swallow reflex.

10. Give your dog lots of praise, and a treat if you can, to make the next time easier.

11. Watch him to be sure that he doesn't hack the pill back up.

The key is calm confidence and efficiency. The more practiced and quicker you are at this, the easier it is on both of you.

If you are really having trouble, you can try filling a turkey baster or needle-less syringe with water and squirting it into your dog's mouth after you place the pill. This can "chase the pill down" and make it easier to swallow.

If you have never seen this done, you might want to ask your vet if you can have a lesson or demonstration. Personal instruction is a good way to learn this important guardian skill.

Never break chemotherapy pills into pieces, because the medication may not be dispersed evenly throughout the entire tablet. Also, breaking a pill in two creates a puff of powder, which you could inhale (the exceptions to this rule are prednisone and prednisolone). If the label on your dog's chemotherapy drugs instructs you to break the tablets, double check with your vet about the dosage.

Keep the medication in its original safety vial and do not store it near food or other medications (to avoid mix-ups). It's best to avoid having any open food or drink near you when you give your dog her medication – otherwise, you might accidentally contaminate your food supply. Be sure your dog has completely swallowed the pill, if you're hiding it in food.

If you are pregnant, nursing, or planning to become pregnant, be very, very careful when you administer chemotherapy. These drugs target rapidly dividing cells, so fetuses and babies are particularly vulnerable to their toxic effects.

Follow Up

Depending upon how chemotherapy was administered you may need to care for your dog at home. For example, there may be a pressure bandage on the leg where the chemotherapy was given. Remove this about an hour after you arrive home or circulation could be impaired and the paw might swell up. Once the bandage is off, check the injection site to make sure it looks normal. If your dog starts licking it excessively, contact your vet or oncologist, right away.

Rarely, chemotherapy drugs, that are intended to go directly into the vein, come in contact with other tissues, which can cause irritation, sloughing (skin falling off) or swelling. This is another reason why we recommend treatments be performed with an experienced team. The oncologist will tell you if the treatment accidentally contaminated the skin or other tissues, explain what to look for and give you medications or instructions for treating home care. Please follow this advice closely and keep an eye on the injection site.

In between appointments, monitor your dog for changes in the injection site and the side effects listed below. Be sure to record as much as you can, to report back at your next appointment. Contact your vet if severe symptoms develop as outlined below.

Safe Handling of Chemotherapy

Drugs often continue working after the treatment is over, and residues and by-products can come out in urine, feces vomit and, potentially, even saliva. For this reason, it's really important to take some safety precautions around these bodily fluids. I don't want you to be scared to touch your dog – normal play and cuddling is safe and good for your dog's mental and emotional health – but you should definitely take the following common-sense precautions:

- Avoid direct contact with urine, feces, vomit and saliva for at least five days. Wear gloves to pick up and dispose of wastes, gloves, paper towels and rags used to clean up messes, placing them in a tightly sealed plastic trash bag. If your dog goes outside, it's wise to pick up and dispose of feces in tightly sealed plastic bags.

- If your dog has an accident on bedding (towels, blankets) or other washable items, use gloves to pick them up and wash them separately from other laundry. Make sure to clean any floors, countertops, or carpets with a strong detergent.

- If you accidentally touch your dog's waste products or soiled items, wash your skin thoroughly, and contact your doctor if it becomes irritated.

- Because chemotherapy targets rapidly dividing cells, avoid all contact with both drugs and dog wastes if you are pregnant, trying to become pregnant, or are breast feeding, because the majority of your baby's body cells are naturally dividing rapidly, and are therefore very sensitive to chemotherapy.

- If you have a suppressed immune system, for any reason, avoid all contact with both chemotherapy drugs and dog wastes.

- Because they are growing and many of their cells are rapidly dividing, children and teenagers should not handle either chemotherapy drugs or dog wastes.

- There is some evidence that some chemotherapy drug residues can come out in saliva. The amount from a one-time exposure is likely minuscule; still, it is wise to keep your dog from licking you or anyone else for seventy-two hours.

Side effects to Consider

There are many potential chemotherapy side effects and it's important to put them into perspective. I've never known a vet who wants to see dogs suffer needlessly, and there are ways to minimize or manage side effects (see the next section), so that therapy can continue, if you feel it is helping your dog. Remember, protocols can be changed – and are changed – depending upon how well your dog is doing, and side effects can be managed.

Cancer is so common in humans these days that most of us know someone who has gone through chemotherapy. If you do, it's important to remember that humans tend to have more dramatic and intense side effects from chemotherapy than dogs do, because we don't give dogs the curative doses we give to humans. Because of these lower doses, most dogs tolerate chemotherapy better than most humans do. Veterinary oncologists push for a fine balance between maximizing the cancer kill rate and minimizing the inevitable side effects. They are well aware that, if your dog feels sick all the time – or seems sicker from the treatment than she does from the disease – you will probably not want to continue treatments.

While most dogs do experience some side effects, they are generally mild. Most dogs will vomit or have some diarrhea, at least once or twice during the entire course of their protocol and this will often be managed by take home medications or natural products (see below).

In about 5% of cases, dogs get severe enough side effects to require hospitalization, where they are usually treated with intravenous fluids, antibiotics, and anti-nausea and anti-vomiting medications. Once they have recovered, chemotherapy doses may need to be lowered and more preventative medications may be needed.

Chemotherapy typically targets rapidly dividing cancer cells. Normal cells in the body also divide – making them vulnerable to chemotherapy's effects, too. It's the harm to these normal cells that causes side effects. Normal cells that rapidly divide carry the highest risk for side effects, and others can be affected, too.

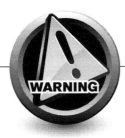

Other Health Conditions

If your dog has a history of problems with the liver, heart, kidney, blood cells, pancreas, lung, brain or any other medical condition, be sure to tell your oncologist about it. Chemotherapy drugs can have many effects in the body, and your vet or oncologist should be aware of all pre-existing problems in order to tailor your dog's treatment correctly. Make sure your oncologist has access to your dog's full medical history.

Here are the most common side effects:

• **Intestinal Symptoms:** The cells that line the digestive tract multiply very rapidly (completely replacing themselves every three days), which makes them very sensitive to chemotherapy. Nausea, vomiting, decreased appetite and diarrhea can result, and these are the most common and expected chemotherapy side effects. Symptoms usually start one to five days after a treatment and last for three days or more, while the intestines repair themselves. In most cases, the symptoms are mild and can be treated at home (see below). About 5% of dogs experience serious symptoms, such as not eating for more than twenty-four hours, vomiting three times or more in the span of a few hours or for more than twenty-four hours, a fever over 103° or severe, bloody, or black diarrhea or diarrhea for more than forty-eight hours. If your dog displays any of these symptoms, contact your vet immediately and get emergency help. In these rare cases, your dog may need to be hospitalized to receive IV fluids, anti-vomiting medications and other supportive care.

There is more information on this important topic in the section on managing side effects, below, and oncologists usually send clients home with medications and detailed instructions on how to manage side effects and what warrants emergency care. For detailed instructions on how to take your dog's temperature, please see page 267.

• **Bone Marrow Suppression:** Bone marrow is the spongy material at the core of bones, which produces red blood cells, white blood cells and platelets. Most chemotherapy drugs cause some degree of suppression of its function, which can have system-wide effects. In most cases, bone marrow suppression happens, but is mild; it shows up in blood tests, although the dog does not have any symptoms. In more severe cases, the dog may not feel sick, but is at high risk for infections and sepsis. In rare cases, your dog may experience severe suppression, and you may have to call your vet. For example, several **white blood cells** (WBC) are important components of the immune system, so, when their levels drop, immune suppression occurs. Neutrophils are one type of WBC easily affected by chemotherapy. They protect against

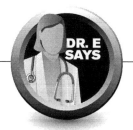

Metronomic Chemotherapy

The traditional approach to chemotherapy is oriented toward the maximum tolerated dose (MTD). The idea is to administer the highest dose possible, in the shortest amount of time, without causing severe side effects or death.

Treatments given at MTD have to be spaced out, so that normal tissues, injured during the treatment, have a chance to heal. If those tissues take a long time to recover, the next treatment is delayed - and this can allow the tumors time to recover, as well.

Recently, we have adopted a new approach, called metronomic chemotherapy. This approach doesn't attempt to kill cancer cells directly; instead, it tries to cut them off from their supply of nutrition.

In metronomic chemotherapy, low doses (sometimes only 10% of the MTD) of chemotherapy drugs are given daily (or on a regular basis), at home. At these low doses, the drugs target the lining of the blood vessels feeding the tumor. They stop new tumors from building new blood vessels (angiogenesis). As their supply lines are cut off, the tumors starve. Some tumors simply stop growing, while others actually shrink, as a result of the treatment.

The low doses mean that the normal tissues of the body are rarely affected, and side effects are greatly

continued on next page

infection, so, if their levels drop – which is called neutropenia – fevers and infections can flare up. In severe cases, sepsis (a systemic infection) can set in. Symptoms of sepsis include: severe fever, depression, lethargy, vomiting, diarrhea and/or lack of appetite. This is a life-threatening emergency that requires hospitalization, which is why your vet should carefully monitor WBC levels by drawing blood for a complete blood count every time he administers chemotherapy and, sometimes, between treatments. For this reason, it is wise to take your dog's temperature during chemotherapy (up to a week after the last treatment, especially if your dog has low white cells). Chemotherapy doses are based, in large part, on the neutrophil levels in the CBC – if levels are too low, the dose may be adjusted down. WBC usually will rebound on their own, a day or two after a session, and antibiotics can be given, along with chemotherapy, to offer protection from further drops. If antibiotics don't help, a human medication called Neupogen may be recommended. Neupogen stimulates bone marrow to make neutrophils, and, like all medications, is considered on a

Metronomic Chemotherapy,
continued

reduced.

Metronomic chemotherapy is an exciting new approach in oncology. In a recent study of dogs with soft tissue sarcomas (STS), metronomic therapy, using low doses of oral cyclophosphamide and piroxicam, was very effective at preventing tumor recurrence when used after surgery when compared with the standard post-operative radiation treatments.

I use this approach with Palladia, often combined with oral cyclophosphamide to treat dogs. I am seeing early, promising results with osteosarcoma, anal sac carcinoma and thyroid carcinoma. The effectiveness of this approach needs to be monitored in further studies.

This new approach is less expensive (because you're using less drug), easier to administer and, certainly, less toxic. However, oncologists are still learning which drugs work best with this method. There is a lot to learn about dosing, schedules and types of tumors, which respond best to metronomic chemotherapy. It's certainly worth checking with your vet about the possibilities for your own dog's case.

case-by-case basis. Although Dr. Ettinger rarely prescribes it, she feels it is worth mentioning as a possible helpful tool for cases where extremely low white blood cell counts don't improve on their own after a few days with supportive care. If **red blood cell** production goes down, anemia sets in. The cause of this is more often the cancer itself, rather than chemotherapy, but you should know about it. If it is severe, you may see low energy or lethargy, weakness, a decrease in appetite, panting and pale or white gums. (Red blood cells replenish themselves within five days, as long as the bone marrow can recover (which it usually can), and there is no cancer in the bone marrow.) If you notice symptoms like these, please call your vet or oncologist. **Platelets** help the blood to clot normally, so when platelet production drops, there is a higher risk for abnormal bleeding. Depending upon how low the platelet levels are, the symptoms can range from bruising easily, to blood in the stool, to internal hemorrhaging. If you notice symptoms like these, please call your vet or oncologist.

• **Hair Loss:** Otherwise known as alopecia, hair loss is a common side effect in humans who undergo chemotherapy. Luckily, it's less common in dogs – and just as luckily, dogs don't care about their hair like we do. If hair (or fur) loss occurs, the coat may thin out all over, or clumps of hair could fall out, exposing bald skin. Hair is usually slow to re-grow, especially in areas that have been shaved during treatments (for a catheter insertion, for example). When hair grows back, it may be of a slightly different color or texture. Many breeds do not typically experience alopecia during chemotherapy, while others are more prone to losing their hair, including Old English Sheepdogs, Poodles, Scottish Terriers, West Highland Terriers, and breeds whose hair needs a lot of clipping.

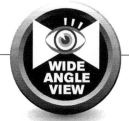

Chronotherapy and Chemotherapy Drugs

Here's something that surprised – flabbergasted – me, when I first discovered it: certain drugs are more effective and have lower toxicity at certain specific times of day.

I spoke to the American expert on chronotherapy, Dr. William Hrushesky, about the efficacy and safety of chemotherapy drugs in relation to when they are given. According to him, cisplatin, an extremely potent and sometimes extremely toxic drug, is most effective and least toxic between 4 and 6pm.

Doxorubicin (Adriamycin) – another potent drug – is best in the early morning, right after waking. It's more potent then, with fewer side effects, than if given at any other time of day.

Timing drug administration to the time of day – chronotherapy – is just about unheard of in the United States (although it's not in Europe, where it has been the subject of some intense study in French human cancer trials).

All life forms (dogs, people, worms, plants, algae) share a similar "biological clock," or circadian cycle. As the sun rises in the morning and sets in the evening, certain enzymes turn on and off at appointed times, hormones surge in and out, and organ systems accelerate or slow down.

These processes can all influence the way the body handles drugs. Perhaps, an enzyme that is very active at 10am is helpful in activating a chemotherapy drug – and helpful in suppressing nausea at the same time. Perhaps, a cocktail of hormones is released at that time, which facilitates the drug's absorption into the cancer cells (the mechanisms are not all understood or mapped out yet).

Giving a drug at a time when it is most effective and least toxic can really help us to boost a treatment's safety and efficacy. On the other hand, giving it when it is most toxic and least effective can have a serious impact on your dog's health.

continued on next page

Chronotherapy and Chemotherapy Drugs, *continued*

If the drug is more effective and less toxic, a bigger dose can be delivered – which means a bigger impact on the cancer, longer life expectancies and maybe, even a cure.

I asked Dr. Hrushesky if I could use his findings about chemotherapy drugs to help dogs in my practice, and he graciously agreed to share them with me. I am going to share them with you, too, and I want to be very clear that these results are his findings, based on studies in rats and humans (not dogs). Although these times may not yet be published in peer-reviewed journals, they represent the best, most up-to-date findings from a researcher who spends his life examining the use of circadian rhythms in administering medications.

Here are his findings:

DRUG:	BEST TIME TO ADMINISTER*:
CCNU (Lomustine)	4 pm +/- 2 hours
Doxorubicin (Adriamycin)	early morning
Platinum Drugs (Cisplatin, Carboplatin)	4-6 pm
Corticosteroids (Prednisolone, Prednisone, Dexamethasone, Triamcinolone)	early am (after waking)
5-FU	middle of the night
Cyclophosphamide	early morning (after waking)
Vinca Alkaloids (Vincristine, Vinblastine)	mid-day

*based on human and rodent studies.

Managing Side effects from Conventional Therapies

No matter which conventional treatment you use – surgery, radiation, or chemotherapy – managing side effects will be your first priority. Symptoms like nausea, vomiting, diarrhea, decrease in appetite, weight loss, anemia and immune suppression can cause a downturn in your dog's quality of life – whether they are caused by the cancer or by the treatments. Managing these side effects can help to keep your dog's spirits high, which is one of the most loving (and therapeutic) things you can do for your dog. We'll talk about both conventional and alternative treatments in this section.

Managing Nausea

If your dog refuses food completely (anorexia), drools or approaches food, but doesn't eat it, he may be nauseous. If you've ever been nauseous (and who hasn't?), you know just how uncomfortable it can be. Most vets will give you some instructions on how to manage nausea at home; here are some tips:

- Withhold food completely when you first notice the symptoms of nausea.

- Most vets or oncologists will prescribe "just in case" medication to take home after surgery, chemotherapy or radiation. Start the anti-nausea medication as prescribed. Common prescriptions include Cerenia (maropitant, a once-per-day pill that Dr. Ettinger feels is very effective, both at home and as a preventative during treatments, if necessary) and metoclopramide (brand name Reglan).

- Every few hours, offer ice cubes to keep him hydrated, and see if he's interested in putting anything in his mouth.

- After twelve hours, feed a series of very small meals (instead of one large one), and use the bland diet recommended for vomiting, below.

In addition to these measures, you can also use ginger and cimetidine, an "old-fashioned" conventional nausea medication, which has evidence for helping to slow cancer spread. These are discussed below.

Managing Vomiting

Vomiting is one of the most distressing symptoms guardians confront. Most of us are familiar with how painful throwing up can be; seeing a sick dog vomit is just plain awful. Most vets will give you detailed instructions on how to handle vomiting, and here are some tips:

- First, withhold all food and water for 12 to 24 hours. Most guardians hate doing this and find it very stressful, but it is important for your dog's wellbeing.

- If the vomiting is mild (a small amount or just one or two episodes), start the anti-vomiting or anti-nausea medication from your vet. The two most common, again, are Cerenia and metoclopramide (brand name Reglan).

- If there is no more vomiting for 12 to 24 hours, offer small amounts of water, or ice cubes, to test for nausea.

- If she does not vomit, after drinking water or eating ice cubes within the first 24 hours, offer a small amount of a very bland diet. You could offer her protein in the form of boiled chicken, boiled ground beef that has been strained of fat, or cottage cheese, mixed with a little white rice. Another option is a commercial diet such as Eukanuba Low Residue or Hill's ID. Chapter 14 lists diet recommendations and my strong opinions about not feeding white rice to cancer patients. The exception is in the case of vomiting or diarrhea. If your dog is experiencing these symptoms, she is feeling really badly, and that is our top priority. A little white rice to stop the rollercoaster in her intestines is perfectly fine.

- If the first small meal does not trigger vomiting, continue to feed the bland food in small meals every few hours and gradually mix in her regular diet until she is eating her normal food in normal amounts again.

- If the vomiting is severe (three or more episodes, large amounts, or blood in the vomit), if it persists for more than 24 hours, or if it is accompanied by a fever of 103° or higher, bring her in for emergency care immediately.

Ginger and Cimetidine can also both help with vomiting, as discussed below.

Managing Diarrhea

Diarrhea is both messy and irritating – both for you and your dog. If your dog's feces are runny and smelly, and he can't seem to control when or where he goes, here are some tips:

- Offer your dog the bland diet described above at his next meal. Also make sure to offer him fresh water in a clean bowl. As his feces return to normal, you can gradually add his normal food to the bland diet, until he's eating his regular food in regular amounts with no diarrhea.

- If you were sent home with an anti-diarrheal medication, start the medication, as prescribed. Common choices include metronidazole (brand name Flagyl), sulfasalazine and tylosin (brand name Tylan).

- If that doesn't work, or if you don't have a prescription anti-diarrheal, you could use the over-the-counter medication, bismuth subsalicylate (brand name Pepto-Bismol) every six hours. Give 2 to 2.5 ml of the liquid version for every ten pounds of body weight (there are 5 ml in a teaspoon). Some dogs dislike the taste of Pepto-Bismol; refrigeration can help to dull the flavor. Pepto-Bismol turns stools a gray-black or

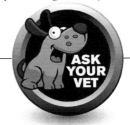

Managing side effects is an important issue. While the advice in this section is general, please keep in mind that we feel you should always contact your vet directly if your dog is having a medical issue. Most vets will give you instructions for managing side effects, including just-in-case medications and instructions on how and when to contact them; you should also make a point of asking for them.

greenish color, which can make it hard to see blood in the stool. A possible cause of vomiting is a bleeding ulcer, which would turn the stool bright red or black and tarry, depending upon where the ulcer is in the digestive tract. To make sure you can evaluate the poop for blood, you may want to use Imodium (see below).

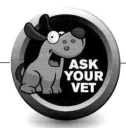

Your vet or oncologist is the best person to advise you on managing side effects in your dog's case, so don't forget to ask for his advice and guidance.

- In any case, do not use Pepto-Bismol for longer than five days. Pepto-Bismol rarely causes any other side effect.

- An alternative to Pepto-Bismol is another over-the-counter medication, loperamide, brand name Imodium. It uses a different mechanism to relieve diarrhea, and is an opiate, so it has more side effects than Pepto-Bismol. If your dog becomes constipated (strains or cannot eliminate), seems depressed or has slowed heart or breathing rates, contact your vet immediately. Collies and related breeds are particularly sensitive to Imodium. Check with your veterinarian before using Imodium, because certain health conditions can make it harmful, including respiratory diseases, severe kidney disease, hypothyroidism, and Addison's disease. The dosage for dogs is 0.2 mg/ml per pound by mouth every eight to twelve hours. It comes in either liquid or capsule form; the dosages are the same for each. Stop using Imodium if your dog is still experiencing diarrhea 48 hours after starting the medication.

- If diarrhea is severe, bloody, or black, or if it persists for more than 48 hours, or if it your dog has a fever of 103° or higher, bring your pet in for emergency care, immediately. See how to take your dog's temperature on page 267.

Full Spectrum Ideas for Managing Side effects

Some natural foods and supplements can help manage side effects. Keep in mind that "natural" does not mean "totally safe for all dogs to use in large amounts." Follow the dosing guidelines carefully and consult with your vet before using these supplements – they can be quite potent and may need to be lowered in dose or avoided altogether, depending upon your dog's other health conditions.

Ginger is a simple food that has few to no side effects, is a very good general tonic, and can help with nausea and vomiting.

Ginger

Mothers across the world give their children ginger to help tummies feel better, and there is a good reason for this. The active ingredients in ginger, called gingerols, have long been known to relieve queasiness, and Germany's version of the FDA (called Commission E) has officially approved fresh ginger root as a nausea treatment. Ginger is an excellent natural nausea remedy and I also recommend it for its other benefits.

Research has shown that gingerols have some antimicrobial effects, which can be helpful for a suppressed immune system. Gingerols also help block a chemical signal called substance P, which is often released when there is inflammation; there is some evidence that ginger may reduce pain resulting from inflammation (cancer thrives on inflammation and promotes it in tumors and surrounding tissues). Ginger may also reduce anxiety, because some of its constituents mimic the neurotransmitter, serotonin. Serotonin also soothes nausea and stimulates the appetite. Boosting serotonin activity in your dog's body is an important part of Full Spectrum cancer care.

As you can see, ginger is much more than an old-fashioned home remedy. If the conventional anti-nausea and anti-vomiting medications don't appeal to you, you can try adding ginger to your dog's diet.

Even if nausea is not a problem, I recommend ginger for its overall health benefits. Use the fresh root, which is likely to have more active gingerols

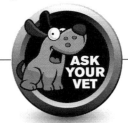

Managing side effects is an important issue. While the advice in this section is general, please keep in mind that we feel you should always contact your vet directly if your dog is having a medical issue. Most vets will give you instructions for managing side effects, including just-in-case medications and instructions on how and when to contact them; you should also make a point of asking for them.

than the powdered version. You can find ginger root in the produce section of most grocery stores and at your local health food store. Buy ginger with smooth skin and a heavy, firm feel in the hand. It will smell fresh and spicy. If it doesn't, or if the skin is wrinkled or cracked, or if the root feels light or is soft to the touch, it is too old to use.

HOW TO GIVE GINGER TO YOUR DOG

Remove the brown skin with a knife or vegetable peeler (fresh skin will be tender enough to gently scrape off with a spoon). The inside will be yellow and smell sharp. Use a heavy, sharp knife to finely mince the yellow portion of the root, or grate it with a fine-toothed grater or micro plane.

Freshly chopped ginger can be stored for up to four days in a sealed container in the refrigerator. The aroma (and possibly the effects) will decrease as it ages.

Ginger has a pungent bite, so it is best to give it with food. Mixing it with soft food or chopped, lean meat, such as chicken or turkey breast, may work, or you can add ginger to a full meal.

Dogs 10 pounds and under: give ¼ teaspoon, ideally three times per day

Dogs 10.1-35 pounds: give ½ teaspoon, ideally three times per day

Dogs 35.1 pounds and over: give ¾ teaspoon, ideally three times per day

---

PRECAUTIONS

Ginger could act as a mild blood thinner because it can affect the platelets, which are partly responsible for clotting the blood. The evidence for this is contradictory and debated; to be safe, I stop ginger intake one full week before any surgery. It can be resumed after the sutures are removed.

If your dog is on anticoagulant therapy (drugs designed to stop blood clotting), ginger should probably not be used because of its possible blood-thinning effects – check with your vet to be on the safe side.

Cimetidine

Cimetidine is an older antacid medication and the active ingredient in the common, over-the-counter drug Tagamet. Although it is not a supplement, I still recommend it for nausea and vomiting. In addition to its ability to decrease stomach acid, there is evidence that it has decreased cancer cell spread in humans and can alleviate some forms of immune suppression caused by histamine release. This little-known effect can be very helpful for dogs with cancer.

Histamines are often released when inflammation is present – and because cancer promotes and thrives in inflammatory environments, tumors may release histamines themselves (this is particularly true with mast cell tumors). To make things worse, histamines reduce the effectiveness of cancer-fighting immune system cells. According to several published studies in humans and horses, blocking histamines can help the already-suppressed immune system stay as active as possible, which may help to prevent or slow down metastasis.

This antihistamine effect is the basis of my recommendation to use cimetidine as supplemental over-the-counter anti-nausea and anti-vomiting medication. You can use it in addition to ginger to take a "double-barreled" approach to nausea and vomiting, or as an alternative to the newer anti-nausea and anti-vomiting medications listed above. You can find it in any pharmacy or drugstore.

HOW TO GIVE CIMETIDINE TO YOUR DOG

Give 5 mg per pound of your dog's body weight three times daily (for example, if your dog weighs 50 pounds, give 250 mg of cimetidine, three times per day). Give cimetidine half an hour before meals, to reduce stomach acid production.

PRECAUTIONS

For most dogs, cimetidine is a very safe drug. However, it should not be used late in pregnancy. Cimetidine may also affect the metabolism of certain drugs, including two chemotherapy drugs (5-FU and melphalan). It may increase the blood concentrations of the following drugs: diazepam, verapamil, propranolol, chloramphenicol, lidocaine, metronidazole, phenytoin, procainamide, theophylline, triamterene, warfarin, and tricyclic antidepressants. Very rarely, cimetidine may cause bone marrow suppression (2.3 per 100,000 patients). Please check with your vet or oncologist before using cimetidine with your dog.

Glutamine

If you've ever vomited or had diarrhea, you probably remember how irritated the tender tissues lining the gastrointestinal tract can feel. The feeling of soreness and raw skin can be painful and add to the inherent misery of your dog's condition.

Luckily, these tissues, called mucous membranes, regenerate themselves within three days, under normal circumstances. If your dog has cancer, she may be low on the nutrients needed to rebuild those tissues. To correct possible deficiencies and ensure she heals as quickly as possible, I recommend giving her glutamine, during and after chemotherapy and radiation treatments.

Glutamine is an amino acid, found in meat and other protein-rich foods. It fuels many body cells, especially the lining of the mouth, stomach and intestines. Supplementing with glutamine ensures that your dog has adequate fuel to rebuild those tissues, damaged by vomiting or diarrhea.

As a bonus, glutamine also feeds the cells of the immune system – which is good for immune-suppressed dogs.

Another bonus: Muscle tissue loves glutamine, preferring it to other sources for high-quality fuel. Cancer and some conventional treatments can cause cachexia, or cancer-related weight loss; glutamine feeds starving muscles, so they can rebuild and put weight back on.

Ironically, cancer cells also love gobbling up glutamine. Still, studies confirm that supplementing at the levels outlined below feeds normal body tissues before cancer tumors, so, the overall effect is good for your dog. The only exception to this is brain cancers (astroglioma, glioma and others). If your dog has brain cancer, do not use glutamine, because it can feed brain cancer cell growth before it ever gets to your dog's normal tissues.

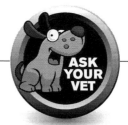

Managing side effects is an important issue. While the advice in this section is general, please keep in mind that we feel you should always contact your vet directly if your dog is having a medical issue. Most vets will give you instructions for managing side effects, including just-in-case medications and instructions on how and when to contact them; you should also make a point of asking for them.

You may see glutamine listed as its slightly different form, l-glutamine. Glutamine is not glu-

HOW TO GIVE GLUTAMINE TO YOUR DOG

Although glutamine is best absorbed on a completely empty stomach, this can cause vomiting or diarrhea in dogs with cancer. To avoid stomach upset, while maintaining optimal absorption, give glutamine with a small amount of food (not a full meal).

Give glutamine once a day at these doses:

Dogs 10 pounds and under: 250-500mg mixed into a small amount of food

Dogs 10.1-35 pounds: 800-1,000mg mixed into a small amount of food

Dogs 35.1-60 pounds: 1,500-2,000mg mixed into a small amount of food

Dogs 60 pounds and over: 2,500-3,000mg mixed into a small amount of food

Give glutamine during chemotherapy and radiation treatments and for the week following, especially if your dog is underweight due to cancer.

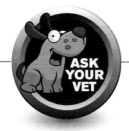

Managing side effects is an important issue. While the advice in this section is general, please keep in mind that we feel you should always contact your vet directly if your dog is having a medical issue. Most vets will give you instructions for managing side effects, including just-in-case medications and instructions on how and when to contact them; you should also make a point of asking for them.

tamate, the salty chemical used as food seasoning and commonly found in mono-sodium glutamate (MSG).

Glutamine is marketed to weightlifters and serious athletes, which makes it easy to find in health and fitness stores, and even at bulk discount stores. It comes in a powder form and is easily mixed into food.

PRECAUTIONS

Check with your vet before starting your dog on glutamine, because it is a potent supplement and not safe for all dogs. It's been shown to elevate blood sugar levels in humans, and it could do the same in diabetic dogs, which would mean that insulin needs would rise. Do not use glutamine or l-glutamine if your dog has a seizure disorder, or is on anti-seizure medications such as potassium bromide, phenobarbital or gabapentin. Do not use it if your dog has brain cancer, because it can feed its growth. Do not use it if your dog is on lactulose for severe liver disease. Your vet will be able to look at your dog's entire health profile and help you decide whether glutamine will have any unwanted side effects. He can also adjust doses of other medications, if necessary.

Cordyceps

Cordyceps is a tiny mushroom that has been in medicinal use for a very long time (some say two thousand years), in China and Tibet. It is fairly particular about its growing environment, and used to be found only in very high elevations. This made it relatively hard to find and expensive, until modern growing techniques made it more plentiful and much less expensive.

Chapter 13 explains how medicinal mushrooms like cordyceps can help many dogs with cancer, due to their anti-cancer and immune-boosting properties. Cordyceps, specifically, is important if your dog is at risk for kidney damage from certain chemotherapy drugs.

Cordyceps has anti-microbial properties and can also help restore white blood cells, which makes it good for overall immune system support during bone-marrow-suppressing chemotherapy treatments. Cordyceps has also been shown to help fatigue and support the kidneys during drug toxicity, such as that commonly experienced with cisplatin and other platinum-based compounds. It has shown similar effects in the liver and can, therefore, help support these organs when lomustine (CCNU) is used.

Cordyceps has some antioxidant effects, and some warn against using it at the same time as pro-oxidant therapies such as: busulfan, carmustine, lomustine, chlorambucil, cyclophosphamide, cisplatin, carboplatin, ifosfamide, mechlorethamine, melphalan, thiotepa, dacarbazine, procarbazine, bleomycin, dactinomycin, daunorubicin, doxorubicin, idarubicin, mitomycin, mitoxantrone, plicamycin, etoposide, teniposide and radiation therapy. While I understand this theoretical concern, the positive benefits of immune and organ support that cordyceps and other mushroom-derived polysaccharides (see page 181) offer dogs with cancer, far outweigh it.

Cordyceps is usually dried and comes in capsules. You can buy it at health food stores or at online retailers.

HOW TO GIVE CORDYCEPS TO YOUR DOG

Give 150-300 mg per pound of body weight, two or three times daily (for example, if your dog weighs 50 pounds, give 7,500 to 15,000 mg or 7.5-15 grams).

It is easiest to open the capsules and mix the dried powder into food.

Give cordyceps during chemotherapy and radiation treatments and for the week following the last dose. If desired, continue as needed, as a general cancer supplement.

PRECAUTIONS

Check with your vet before using cordyceps, because it can have several effects on the body, which may affect other treatments. For example, it can increase the body's natural cortisone production. If your dog is on other drugs that are related to cortisone – prednisone, prednisolone or dexamethasone – adjust the doses accordingly. In general, I recommend reducing cordyceps to one-third the doses above; ask your vet's advice. If your dog has Cushing's disease, do not give him cordyceps.

Cordyceps decreases blood sugar, so it should be used with caution in diabetic dogs, and possibly avoided altogether. Humans with high blood triglycerides (blood fats) can experience dry mouth, rash and stomach upset on cordyceps, so, if your dog has high triglyceride levels, you may want to avoid it.

Coenzyme Q10

You may have heard that coenzyme Q10 (also called Co-Q, CoE-Q, CoQ10 and ubiquinone) is a good supplement for cardiac problems. I recommend it for dogs who are on chemotherapy drugs, which are known for their toxicity to the heart (such as doxorubicin).

CoQ10 is a naturally-occurring antioxidant, produced in the body and taken in through the diet by eating red meat and organ meat (livers, hearts, etc.). Dog species in the wild probably get a lot of CoQ10 from their diet, because they eat the organs first, before turning to other parts of their prey.

Studies have shown that humans with a wide range of different cancers tend to have low CoQ10 levels, and supplementing with this potent antioxidant improves their survival times. In addition, there is some very interesting evidence that CoQ10 may help alleviate depression, which makes it very useful in addressing that facet of cancer care.

While I do like CoQ10 for patients at risk for heart toxicity, it has some bioavailability issues, so I do not recommend it for most dogs. If your dog is on doxorubicin and at risk for cardiac side effects, it's a good addition to your cancer care plan (to get the most benefit, start CoQ10 before doxorubicin treatments begin). CoQ10 comes in softgels or capsules, which can be purchased in health food stores or from online retailers. Some vet clinics also sell CoQ10.

HOW TO GIVE CO-Q 10 TO YOUR DOG

CoQ10 is a fat-soluble supplement, which means that it does not get absorbed without some fat present. Mixing it into food, along with some krill oil or other omega-3 fatty acid (see the anti-cancer diet in Chapter 14), will help your dog's body absorb the antioxidant.

Start giving your dog CoQ10 about a week before the use of doxorubicin or other drugs, which cause heart toxicity. Give roughly 1 mg of CoQ10 per pound of dog's body weight, once daily (for example, if your dog weighs 50 pounds, give 50 mg). Depending upon your dog's weight and the size of the capsule, you may have to split up capsules (if you can't be exact in your dosing, get as close as you can).

Some dogs will experience an upset stomach (loss of appetite or vomiting) on a full dose of CoQ10, even if it's given with a meal. In these cases, I recommend splitting the daily dose in half and giving it twice daily, which seems to work for the majority of dogs with sensitive stomachs.

PRECAUTIONS

As this supplement has anti-oxidant effects, the argument against its use may come up when a dog is on conventional pro-oxidant therapeutics such as: busulfan, carmustine, lomustine, chlorambucil, cyclophosphamide, cisplatin, carboplatin, ifosfamide, mechlorethamine, melphalan, thiotepa, dacarbazine, procarbazine, bleomycin, dactinomycin, daunorubicin, doxorubicin, idarubicin, mitomycin, mitoxantrone, plicamycin, etoposide, teniposide and radiation therapy. In the case of doxorubicin use, however, I feel the use of CoQ10 gives a benefit that outweighs any treatment negative. In the studies available, which were in humans and rodents, there was no loss of treatment efficacy with its use, combined with doxorubicin. The use of antioxidants to protect against heart toxicity is not new; the FDA approved the commercial antioxidant called dexrazoxane for this use in humans. (You can also read more about doxorubicin on page 400.)

CoQ10 can affect blood sugar regulation, so check with your vet about using it if your dog is diabetic.

CoQ10 safety studies have not evaluated its effects on infants, pregnant mothers or nursing mothers, so consult with your vet before using it, if your dog is pregnant or nursing.

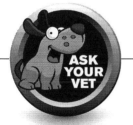

Managing side effects is an important issue. While the advice in this section is general, please keep in mind that we feel you should always contact your vet directly if your dog is having a medical issue. Most vets will give you instructions for managing side effects, including just-in-case medications and instructions on how and when to contact them; you should also make a point of asking for them.

Caught Up in the Insanity

"It was easy to get caught up in the insanity of trying to decipher what the vets were saying, looking for additional information to help with decisions, searching for others with similar experiences, and those things associated with such a horrible diagnosis that took away from the bond with the dog, the very thing we were scrambling around trying to figure out how to help. Doing the emotional management exercises, while a little underwhelming at first, were very valuable and reminded me"

- Brad Burkholder, Galt, California

Chapter 12: Step Two, Nutraceuticals

The cutting edge nutraceuticals discussed in this chapter are being investigated for use in human cancer treatments because they are apoptogens: they trigger apoptosis in cancer cells. Each has been evaluated with placebo-controlled, double-blind studies and shown to kill cancer cells in test tubes and (in some cases) shrink tumors in laboratory animals – but they have not yet been developed commercially for medical use. I've used them and seen good results in dogs – results that, many times, replicate those published studies.

These apoptogens are studied in both U.S. and international laboratories – but they are not drugs. They are plant extracts (many of which contain bioflavonoids) and some of them come from food that you may eat on a regular basis. In addition to their impact on cancer, these agents create fewer and less intense – if any – side effects than most conventional cancer treatments. (I don't think of natural-sourced apoptogens as a substitute for conventional treatments; in fact, some seem to work well when used at the same time.) As we continue to learn more about how these brand-new tools work, we may find that what we know today is only the tip of the iceberg.

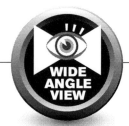

WIDE ANGLE VIEW

There's an odd circular nature to cancer research that I'm leveraging to help your dog.

Typically, cancer treatments for humans are developed by doing ten to fifteen years and millions of dollars' worth of research. A rough sketch of the process is as follows:

1. Test the treatment on cancer cells in a petri dish or in a test tube (in vitro). If the results show that the treatment works (shows efficacy) …

2. Test the treatment for efficacy and safety in live animals in laboratories. The typical test animals are mice, rats, primates and dogs. If the results are promising, then…

3. Start clinical trials in human patients. If the results are promising…

continued on next page

4. Apply for FDA approval, which takes years to get. After reviewing the data, if the FDA feels the treatment is both safe and effective, it gives approval. Once that happens…

5. The treatment can be finalized and developed for commercial application. The FDA continues to monitor the new drug; after approval, any doctor can prescribe the treatment.

Once the treatment has gone through this entire process, vets prescribe the FDA-approved treatment for species other than humans.

(There are now two chemotherapy drugs approved specifically for use in canine cancer. Palladia is one, and Kinavet CA-1 is the other. I have personally had good successes with Kinavet CA-1 when I used it as part of the FDA's compassionate use program prior to U.S. approval. You can read more about both of these drugs in chapter 41.)

Ironically, even though a treatment may be tested on dogs during the research process, it may be years before we actually start to use the treatment in veterinary clinics.

An example of what I'm talking about is included in the chapter on melanoma, where you can read about Dr. Ettinger's experience with the clinical trials in dogs for the melanoma vaccine.

Here's what Dr. George Demetri, director of the Ludwig Center at the Dana-Farber/Harvard Cancer Center in Boston, said about the vaccine, in an article entitled, *From Pets, Clues to Human Cancer,* which was published in the *Los Angeles Times,* "Now we know it's really possible. If we can do it in dogs, just give us time, and we can do it in people."

By taking human cancer research into apoptogens and using these agents in dogs, now, today, rather than waiting several more years, we're simply applying treatments to animals earlier than we normally would in veterinary medicine. That is why I recommend them for your consideration.

These agents do not need to be injected, beamed into your dog, or administered by IV. They can be given by mouth, at home. That's not to say that these are not powerful agents … in fact, in some cases, they can be quite potent.

Nutraceuticals

As you'll remember from our vocabulary chapter, a nutraceutical is any purified substance from a natural, usually dietary, source that can yield health benefits. Nutraceuticals are almost always a more concentrated and potent form of the active agent than is found in nature. In general, they are not as strong as a pharmaceutical drug and not as weak as a supplement. For example, it is assumed that a pharmaceutical will act fast once it is in the body, but nutraceuticals may need a little time (a full week or more) to build up in the system and produce their full effect.

Some nutraceuticals (including some in this chapter) are potent in vitro, or in test tubes, but diminish in potency after they enter the body and are broken down and eliminated by the liver, kidneys and digestive system (those organs are pretty good at breaking down agents, which are close to – or actually are – dietary substances).

This reduction in potency in vivo (in life or in the body) is a real problem, because if the nutraceutical is not absorbed well, is broken down, or is passed out as bodily waste before it gets to the cancer cells, it may not work as well, or at all. The challenge is to get the nutraceuticals to work in vivo as well as or nearly as well as, they work in vitro.

In the first edition of this book, the long and detailed explanations of how to prepare and administer these nutraceuticals so that they remained bioavailable daunted some readers, including guardians in my practice.

I am the first to admit that following my advice – from doing the "oxygen mask exercises" in Chapter 2, to consulting with your vet, to administering nutraceuticals, to cooking for your dog – takes time and commitment.

It's expensive and, frankly, unrealistic,

Given Three Months: Three Years Later Still "Doing Great"

"Our lab mix Buddy was diagnosed about three years ago with cancer of the spleen and liver. Dr. Dressler personally did the surgery to remove his spleen, but couldn't get all of the cancer, which had spread to his liver. We chose not to have any chemo treatment, because we didn't want to put Buddy through it. At that time, Dr. D recommended a high-protein diet of lean ground beef and chicken, mixed with vegetables, and told us he was researching cancer in dogs and was working on an all-natural treatment. He also recommended krill oil and K–9 Immunity. He asked us if we wanted to participate in helping test his new product (Apocaps). Feeling we had nothing to lose, we agreed. At that time, Dr. D told us that most dogs with Buddy's type of cancer live about three months after surgery with no chemo and about six months with chemo. March 10th of this year made three years since his surgery and he is doing great! He's been on Apocaps since his surgery and we strongly feel that Apocaps, along with Dr. D's other recommendations, have helped Buddy to live this long. He's slowed down a little since his surgery, but he still gets up every morning and plays with us and our other dogs. Apocaps is an amazing product that has allowed us to enjoy Buddy's company for a lot longer than we expected. We would like to personally thank Dr. D for his dedication and hard work in making Apocaps a reality. It really works. Our Buddy is living proof."

– *Cheryl Molina, 5-star review on Amazon. com posted April 15, 2010* to assume that everyone who reads this book can afford dozens of bottles of supplements per month, any more than they can afford thousands of dollars for radiation treatments.

Those guardians who committed the time and money to follow my method liked their results, but I was nagged by the idea that others read this book and feel they are out of reach. Eventually, in response to the obvious need for an apoptogen formula, I developed my own: a nutraceutical that combines as many of these agents as possible into a single pill, that is easier and cheaper to give to the dog. We will discuss my patent-pending pill, Apocaps, as well as the other nutraceuticals artemisinin and Neoplasene, in this chapter.

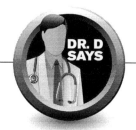

My Agenda

It's impossible for me to write this chapter without sounding like I'm promoting Apocaps. Even so, I expect you to evaluate it the same way you would evaluate any other recommendation I make. If you think it might help your dog, add it to your Full Spectrum cancer care plan and then ask your vet or oncologist for her supervision.

Apocaps

When I first formulated Apocaps, I thought I was designing a pill that would make dogs feel better, but not necessarily extend their lives. From my perspective as a conventional vet, botanical sources like luteolin, curcumin and apigenin (the main ingredients) could do little more than provide some palliative support for dogs with cancer. When I conducted the pilot study, I was hoping to see dogs perk up and feel better. I got what I had hoped for, and in some cases, even more.

We modeled the pilot study after the National Institute of Health's Best Case Series, which means that strict standards were used. I ran tests (CBCs, chemistry profiles and thyroid profiles) and I took photographs or other diagnostic images before the start of the trial, at ten days, at thirty-one days, and at sixty-six days of Apocaps use. Thirty-one dogs were included. These dogs did not receive conventional treatments (no surgery, chemotherapy or radiation), either because of the cost of those treatments or because their guardians did not wish to pursue conventional treatments. During the trial, we tracked tumor size and several factors that affect life quality, including measuring the dog's discomfort.

If you're wondering if these were placebo-controlled, double-blind trials, the answer is no. Instead, these were historically controlled trials. In this method of control, we measure the dog's progress against his own history. How did he do before he took Apocaps, and how did he do with Apocaps?

The saying, "experience is the best teacher," was demonstrated during the trials. I knew from my research that luteolin, curcumin and apigenin were apoptogens – substances that can turn on apoptosis in cancer cells. In fact, a third of the dogs in the study experienced an objective response to the treatment, which means that some positive change occurred in their tumors. Some tumors shrank. Some other tumors did not reduce their size, but their growth was stopped. Some tumors disappeared completely. I was impressed that about a third of the tumors responded; relative to what I expected, it gave me great hope for Apocaps. It also caught the interest of other vets.

From "Just One Hour to Live" to "No Longer In Danger"

"We used Artemisinin, and one of our vets wanted to use Neoplasene ... I'm not sure what worked best or if it was a combination of everything that we were doing but her cardiac hemangiosarcoma that had ruptured, did solidify and start to shrink, and over three months went from she only had an hour to live to she was no longer in danger of having that hemangiosarcoma rupture."

– *Chris Shoulet, Bethesda, Maryland*

The palliative effects were also obvious. During the trial, we measured dogs' pain responses in a series of sessions, and the results were excellent. For 78% of the dogs who showed measurable signs of discomfort at the start of the trial, there was better mobility, more energy, more tails wagged, and more playtimes requested. Pain responses during physical examination went down, and guardians confirmed their dogs seemed to suffer less pain at home.

Side effects were very rare, similar to what I see in practice when people change their dog's diet. Two dogs, or about 6%, experienced digestive upset (nausea, diarrhea or vomiting). No other adverse effects were found, after four rounds of testing on internal organ function. I could relate many stories from this exciting time, but I'm going to focus on the one that made the biggest impression on me, and convinced me that Apocaps was worth the time and effort.

Lassie[5], a pit bull mix, had a history of skin hemangiosarcoma. A single tumor had been surgically removed from her belly a year earlier, but she was back with what turned out to be a tumor regrowth, or recurrence, in the the exact same spot. There was subcutaneous involvement; the tumor was rooted into the layers beneath the skin and was palpated as a stage two hemangiosarcoma. If she had surgery, followed by chemotherapy, her life expectancy was estimated to be eight to ten months. Her guardians didn't want to use surgery again unless I could guarantee the tumor would not return, which, of course, I couldn't. Other conventional options were also declined. I offered the Apocaps trial, and they

---

[5] Lassie is not her real name, but the details of her case are all true. Every case I write about in this chapter is an accurate description of what happened during the pilot trial, according to transcripts of interviews with the vets involved. I have only changed the dog names and a few identifying factors, for privacy reasons.

agreed. I videotaped Lassie's tumor and sent them home with the pills and the instructions.

When Lassie came in for a follow up appointment, six weeks later, her guardians reported she was feeling great: eating well, moving well, wagging her tail and playing. I felt her belly for the tumor, but couldn't find it. I checked the chart in her files. *Maybe I charted this wrong*, I thought. *Maybe it is on the other side.* I felt the opposite side; still, no tumor. I reached for my video camera and found the tape from six weeks earlier. There was Lassie, with a 3.5 centimeter-wide tumor on the right side of her belly, and here, in front of me, was Lassie, with no visible tumor.

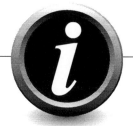

Could Apocaps Make Chemotherapy and Radiation More Effective?

The heavy hitting apoptogens in Apocaps have all been shown to be chemotherapy and radiation therapy sensitizers, or make cancer cells more sensitive to radiation therapy and chemotherapy. In some combinations, those therapies may actually work better when luteolin, curcumin or apigenin is given at the same time.

There is so much evidence for this that Functional Nutriments, which makes Apocaps, won a quarter-million-dollar grant from the U.S. government in late 2010, to study the use of Apocaps in human cancer treatments. As of this writing, we're planning on conducting trials to find out if Apocaps can help human patients, undergoing chemotherapy and radiation, get more effect from their treatments. If the planned research bears good results, Apocaps may eventually help chemotherapy and radiation treatments to kill more cancer cells in people.

In the meantime, if you choose to include chemotherapy and/or radiation treatments in your dog's Full Spectrum cancer care plan, you can often use Apocaps at the same time. The initial published evidence from research labs shows that the components in Apocaps may boost the efficacy of these conventional treatments, particularly for radiation and the chemotherapy drugs cisplatin, 5 FU, gemcitabine, capecitabine taxane, mitoxantrone and doxorubicin. (As with most topics in this book, additional citations, reading and references for the use of apoptogens as chemosensitizers and radiosensitizers are included in Appendix E.)

As always, make sure that your vet or oncologist is supervising your use of Apocaps for interactions with other drugs and supplements.

Kept My Promise and Raised My Rating from Four to Five Stars

My eight-year-old Staffordshire Bull Terrier has had frequently recurring Mast Cell Tumors. I have been giving Apocaps to my dog now for several months, along with the lifestyle and dietary recommendations I received from the Dr. Dressler's Dog Cancer Survival Guide. I have noticed significant improvements in his overall health and he has not been diagnosed with a mast cell tumor for almost six months. If he continues to stay free from tumors, I will come back and change this to a five star review. I started using Apocaps a month or so after beginning the lifestyle and dietary changes. Because I did a lot of things near the same time I can't say for sure exactly how much of his improvement is due specifically to Apocaps, but I suspect much of it is. At any rate, I continue to purchase them. **Update:** It has now been over a year since my dog has had any tumors. Considering his lifelong history of recurrent tumors, I have to assume that the Apocaps have been doing the job. I believe this is the longest he has been without any tumors since he was very young, and it is not what my Vet expected to happen. I was told the frequency would only increase. Because of this I am keeping my promise to change this review from four to five stars. The other day someone asked me how old my dog was. I said "nine". He said "months?" When I said "years", he didn't believe me at first. I think if you take the time to do the all the things Dr. Dressler has recommended, you will give your dog a much better chance at a longer, healthier life. A year later I continue to purchase Apocaps."

— *M. Hall, five-star Amazon.com review dated June 9, 2010*

I could not believe it. I actually double-checked her file and her identification tags to make sure she was the same dog. She was. I took another video to record the session — and the lack of a hemangiosarcoma — and I recommended to the guardians that they continue using Apocaps. That night, I watched the before and after videos with my wife, Allison. Over and over, Lassie's tumor appeared, and then disappeared. It was one of the best days of my life. Ten months later, several weeks past the point at which the most optimistic conventional expectations predicted her death, Lassie was still happy, waggy-tailed and tumor-free.

Other vets wanted to try my new formula with their patients and I was happy to oblige. Dr. Mark Thomas, DVM, a vet in upstate New York, gave Apocaps to a nine-year-old dog named Sherman, who had an osteosarcoma in his mouth. The tumor had started invading the teeth and the jawbone, and Sherman was facing a surgery to remove the front portion of his jaw. You can probably imagine how losing the entire front part of your lower jaw would affect life quality. Avoiding that surgery, especially in this older dog, was his guardian's priority. Sherman was a giant breed, and he had already lived past his predicted life expectancy. Without surgery, there was little that could be done for Sherman, so Dr. Thomas recommended Apocaps as a palliative treatment. At least Sherman would likely be more comfortable, even if the tumor progressed.

Sherman's guardian reported that within a few days of starting Apocaps, Sherman had more energy and a better appetite. Six weeks later, the tumor had regressed – shrunk – significantly. For example, an incisor (front tooth) was now visible, when before it had been engulfed by the tumor and completely invisible. Sherman's guardian was very happy to see the tumor shrink at all – especially with no surgery or chemotherapy. Sherman hadn't been on any other drugs or supplements, except for soy lecithin. Dr. Thomas now sells Apocaps in his clinic and recommends their use to other veterinarians.

Another veterinarian who took an interest in Apocaps is Dr. Cathy Johnson-Delaney. She is respected internationally for her work with exotic pets and is a contributing author on several veterinary textbooks. Her background in pharmaceutical testing makes her a recognized expert on veterinary drugs and nutraceuticals, and she lectures to other vets about this subject. She used Apocaps in ferrets, hedgehogs, guinea pigs and pet rats.

The first patient was a three-year-old hedgehog with a squamous cell carcinoma in her mouth, a

It's Been Eleven Months and Counting With No Obvious Signs of Cancer

"I have used Apocaps since (I think) May or June of 2010. Our dog, Maya, was diagnosed with Renal cancer April 15, 2010. We thought she had a urinary infection and following an X-ray (which showed a massive tumor instead of a kidney) we were sent to the specialty clinic for an ultrasound and to meet with an oncologist. She had her kidney removed on April 20th. We received the following as part of the histology report: "Diagnosis: Left Kidney: High-grade malignant neoplasm with multifocal to coalescing necrosis, mineralization and vascular invasion. Comment: The differential diagnosis this neoplasm includes high-grade renal cell carcinoma and nephroblastoma. Regardless of the histogenesis, this is a malignant neoplasm that has largely effaced the kidney and has metastatic potential. Although the tumor appears completely excised, moderate atypia, frequent mitosis, tissue invasion and vascular invasion warranted a guarded to poor prognosis. Close clinical follow-up for possible recurrence and/or metastasis is recommended." We were advised to expect life span of 6–8 months with the shorter span more likely. The oncologist recommended that she be placed on Palladia and low dose Cytoxan. We sought a second opinion at another clinic - same prognosis provided and same recommendation. Because we were not able to find anything that assured us that Palladia was going to be effective, we chose not to go that route. At this point we located Dr. Dressler's book and decided to follow his recommendations and commenced using Apocaps. On March 15, 2011 Maya will have survived 11 months following her diagnosis. She is showing signs of age (she is now 10+ years old), but is not currently showing any obvious signs of cancer."

– Valerie Sachs, Pepper Pike, OH

common tumor in hedgehogs. In Dr. Johnson-Delaney's experience, these tumors progress rapidly, bleed, and distort the shape of the skull. The tumors prevent hedgies from eating, and most patients die within a month of diagnosis. According to Dr. Johnson-Delaney, chemotherapy doesn't really work, and even debulking surgery can't keep pace with the tumor's fast growth. In this case, Dr. Johnson-Delaney found the tumor at the end of October and started Apocaps right away. Thirty days later, when she would have expected to hear the hedgehog had succumbed to the disease, she instead found the tumor regressed significantly, the gums and teeth firmed up, the bleeding stopped, and the pain was seemingly gone. Christmas came and went, and the hedgehog was still alive, happy, and eating normally. The hedgie lived another eight months before dying of heart failure. Dr. Johnson-Delaney could not find any apparent squamous cell carcinoma in the hedgie's jaw when she performed a necropsy (also known as an autopsy).

> ## Cancer Cells: Take a Long Hike!
>
> "I used Apocaps as soon as I could get my hands on them. Our first dog, Shadow, was diagnosed with cancer and given 2-3 weeks to live. We changed his diet to the highest degree according to Dr. D's advice, and he went on Apocaps as soon as possible. Shadow was with us for seven quality months, before he passed on in his own time. I am absolutely positive that Apocaps was an essential ingredient to this longevity. Our second dog was diagnosed with an aggressive cancer a year ago. He went immediately onto Apocaps, and we have celebrated his one-year anniversary from a cancer that has a best-prognosis of 3 months. He is fitter and healthier than ever. I am convinced that Apocaps gave both my boys the ingredients their bodies needed to support their health while telling cancer cells to take a long hike."
>
> – *Susan Harper, High Wycombe, England*

Dr. Johnson-Delaney was "very pleased" with the results of this first experience with Apocaps. She confided that she has lost her own hedgehogs to this same cancer, and has tried every tool available. Apocaps was the first thing to enhance the hedgehog's quality of life and even help with tumor regression.

Based on these results, Dr. Johnson-Delaney decided to expand her test and try Apocaps with ferrets, which, according to her "have the highest tumor rate of just about any mammal on the planet."

Ferrets often can't receive conventional treatments due to their size (less than one kilogram, or 2 pounds), and because they tend to suffer toxic side effects from chemotherapy. A common cancer in ferrets is lymphoma, and she found that using Apocaps seemed to hold these tumors in check if solid masses were detected. They didn't grow, and most ferrets had a decrease in clinical symptoms – in other words, felt better than they had. One ferret in particular, did really well. His tumor was so large

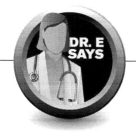

Consider Everything, Including Apocaps

As you'll see in the introductory chapter in my From the Oncologist section, my mantra in cancer care is Consider Everything. As an oncologist and chemotherapy specialist, I do not turn to alternative medicine first, but I do work closely with holistic vets who do. As long as a non–pharmaceutical supplement is safe and may help the dog, I do not object to its use.

From a conventional oncological perspective, we have a lot to learn about Apocaps, especially about how they interact with chemotherapy and radiation. I am certainly impressed with the science behind Apocaps, and their promise as a sensitizer for chemotherapy and radiation.

You may or may not be considering conventional treatments, but Apocaps is worthy of careful consideration for use in conventional protocols and/or as a stand–alone supplement.

it was keeping him from breathing fully, and normally she would have suggested immediate euthanasia. Instead, she offered Apocaps, and based on her recent experience, the guardians agreed to try it. The tumor shrank enough so that he could breathe again, and he lived another four months.

Her experience with lymphoma led her to try Apocaps with other tumors, and the results were even better. A ferret had a fibrosarcoma over his eye. These tumors usually grow so fast in ferrets that they take over the entire skull within two or three months, killing the animal. Dr. Johnson–Delaney reported that Apocaps slowed the fibrosarcoma's growth tremendously. The tumor didn't invade the bone, and she was still treating him six months later. He lived over ten months past the initial debulking surgery with Apocaps treatment.

These successes led Dr. Johnson–Delaney to try Apocaps in other species. For example, guinea pigs with inoperable mammary tumors and lymph node masses near the genitals are poor candidates for surgery, and there aren't many other options for treatment. She put two guinea pigs with this same disease on Apocaps and saw significant decrease in the masses for each. One patient saw no growth or change in the masses even after six months. In another example, she used Apocaps in combination with debulking surgery and carbergoline (an anti–prolactin medication), and saw large mammary fibromas in rats reduce significantly, fail to regrow, or grow no larger. She's even just starting Apocaps for birds with "benign" masses that are technically not malignant, but are inhibiting breathing, flying, or quality of life.

Overall, Dr. Johnson–Delaney reported, Apocaps

Once We Started, He Was His Old Self

"We used Apocaps and our dog Tyler has more energy and was his old self once we started using them. When we first learned of them we bought four bottles and then for a while they were not available. A short while later they were reintroduced to the market and we bought them and the improvement in Tyler was incredible."

— *John Arquette, Fayetteville, New York*

gave comfort time and a good quality of life to her patients. They felt better, they played more, and her clients felt it was giving them more time with their pets. She hears from her clients that they are happy to have an alternative, particularly in older animals.

When asked point-blank if she was comfortable with the plant-based supplement from a veterinary pharmaceutical standpoint, Dr. Johnson-Delaney's response was unequivocal: yes. There are a lot of chemicals in natural, plant-based sources that have real, documented, physiological actions in the body, she pointed out. Vets routinely use glucosamine chondroitin, for example, and vitamin complexes. She also said some natural substances are just as effective as pharmaceuticals, but they are not patentable, so they slip through the cracks and "don't make the evening news." Dr. Johnson-Delaney went on to say that some other countries regulate natural substances and officially approve their use for diseases, because they are potent and viable therapeutics. Our own FDA only just recently began a process for regulating botanicals, and lags behind other countries in this regard. She further noted that nutraceuticals operate according to the laws of chemistry, just like pharmaceuticals do. When you look at these substances from a chemistry viewpoint and study their actions in the body, she said, it quickly becomes obvious what is therapeutic, and what is not.

Even though I designed Apocaps for use in dogs, Dr. Johnson-Delaney clearly finds it beneficial for her exotic patients, and continues to offer Apocaps. She made a point of reminding me that Apocaps, like anything else, is not appropriate for every case (for example, it is not as effective in ferret lymphoma as it is in other tumors). She always discusses the pros and cons of different treatments, and makes sure the client understand everything, even asking them to sign a consent form for non-traditional therapies. She is comfortable offering Apocaps not just because they seem to have helped these exotic pets, but also because she has not seen any toxic or adverse side effects as of this writing. Owners tell her Apocaps is palatable (the animals take it without a problem), and they see their animal's general attitude, activity, and appetite pick up while on Apocaps.

Let's look at some of the therapeutic agents in Apocaps, including three of the heavy-hitting supplements I have recommended for years: luteolin, curcumin and apigenin.

Luteolin

There are literally dozens of *in vitro* studies demonstrating luteolin's Terminator-like apoptogen effect on cancer cells. It's very impressive to see what this bioflavonoid – a plant pigment found in celery, green peppers, artichokes, peanut hulls, and chrysanthemums – can do to cancer cells in test tubes. The challenge for me was to make it more bioavailable, so that it would work *in vivo*, in living bodies. According to published *in vitro* studies, here is what luteolin is capable of:

- Luteolin induces apoptosis in cancer cells in vitro. Through multiple mechanisms, luteolin turns on natural cell death in cancer cells, causing them to commit suicide.

- Luteolin starves cancer cells by interfering with glycolysis (the breakdown of sugars). If cancer cells can't break down sugar, they can't absorb it and they go hungry.

- Luteolin shuts down fatty acid synthase, a system of enzymes that are involved in metabolizing fatty acids for energy. When this system is tuned down, cancer cells lose energy and starve.

- Luteolin sabotages the ability of a cancer cell to replicate its DNA, making it unable to multiply.

- Luteolin cuts cancer cells off from the blood supply by blocking angiogenesis (the making of new blood vessels), which makes it harder for them to feed themselves or metastasize.

- Luteolin shuts down "self-stimulating"

More Energy, Happier After Mammary Cancer

"I started one of my older girls on Apocaps after a diagnosis of mammary cancer. She had the tumor removed and I had purchased Dr. Dressler's Cancer Survival Book (which is excellent). I was already using many of the natural products he suggested at the time. When Apocaps became available I was able to stop many of them and just give her the Apocaps. That was about a year ago. Besides still being cancer free at over eight years of age, I noticed that she started having more energy, was happier, was picking up toys and running around the house with them, was able to frolic with our youngest Leonberger and had an overall better and happier attitude toward life. Apocaps was the only change. When I got a diagnosis of osteosarcoma on a couple littermates of one of my other girls, I chatted with Dr. Dressler and he recommended that I start my girl on a lower dosage of Apocaps and I have seen a similar, although not such a drastic change, in her. However, we have been able to get weight off her because she is exercising well and has more energy. I have just started an older male on the product as well - too soon to see any change in him, but will keep you up to date!! To date, I am overall pleased with the product. Wish it could come down in price and come in larger bottles."

– *Beverly J. Travis posted this story on Amazon.com on February 23, 2011* communication in cancer cells. One of the first steps a cancer cell takes when it wants to multiply is to manufacture chemical messengers called autocrine agents. The production of these agents stimulates the cell and/or its neighbors to multiply faster. Luteolin slows the autocrine process, rendering the cancer less capable of multiplying itself.

- Luteolin decreases inflammation, which, as we have learned, is a central mechanism in cancer development and progression.
- Luteolin boosts the effects of both chemotherapy (cisplatin and doxorubicin) and radiation therapy.

As you can tell, luteolin is a very potent anti-cancer agent on its own, and it can help both radiation and chemotherapy do their jobs more effectively. So why isn't luteolin widely used? There are a few reasons.

Everything to Induce Apoptosis

"We've used about everything Dr. D recommends to induce apoptosis. Along with a lot of other supplements, we give Angus three Apocaps at mid-day and we cycle Artemisinin 4 days a week, giving Essiac & Transfer Factor on the other three nights at bedtime. Along with breakfast, he gets K-9 Immunity (medical mushrooms), Colostrum Plus, Krill Oil, IP-6, Indol-3-Carbinol, Beta Glucans, Probiotic Complex and a couple Veggies for Life tablets. Along with dinner, he gets Turmeric, a Quercetin/Bromelain capsule, a Carnitine/Co-Q 10 mix, Milk Thistle, D-3, Red Clover, Astralagus, Alpha Lipoic Acid. Other things that have been mixed in from time to time include garlic, green tea extract, digestive enzymes, pine bark capsules, etc."

– *Al Marzetti, Raleigh, North Carolina*

One is that it is not easy to find luteolin. It's a tiny chemical compound found in parts of plants (peanut hulls, artichokes, and chrysanthemums). It is just not a common supplement.

Another reason is that it's a naturally occurring substance, which makes it hard for pharmaceutical companies to patent. If they can't patent it, they can't make as much money off of its use as they can other drugs.

On top of this, there is little research on luteolin in the United States, although there is a firestorm of luteolin research in China.

The fourth reason it's not commonly used is: while it kills cancer cells *in vitro*, it can't do it so as effectively *in vivo* (in the body) when given by mouth. Luteolin is broken down in the intestines and in the liver and often doesn't even reach the cancer cells.

This lack of bioavailability is a major challenge I had to overcome when I designed Apocaps. Eventually I found the right combination of techniques to boost luteolin's bioavailability. I call it the Trojan Horse, because the combination distracts the body while sneaking luteolin into the blood-stream – and soon thereafter into cancer cells.

Luteolin is a powerful apoptogen, but it's not the only player in Apocaps. Another agent I've recommended for years, that made it into the pill, is familiar to anyone who loves Indian food: curcumin.

Curcumin

Turmeric is a popular Indian spice, closely related to ginger. Anyone who's ever had a bowl of yellow curry is familiar with its earthy, spicy flavor, but few realize that one of its bioflavonoids – curcumin – is an apoptogen.

Researchers recognize curcumin's potential for safe and potent cancer treatments. As I write this, curcumin is undergoing several clinical trials, aimed at creating new human cancer therapeutics; at just one research center, The Ohio State University, curcumin is the blueprint for forty different synthetic anti-cancer drugs. Here's what curcumin does *in vitro*:

- Curcumin helps increase apoptosis, natural cell suicide, in cancer cells

- Curcumin is an antioxidant when taken in low doses, but when it is used in higher doses it has a pro-oxidant effect. As you'll remember, pro-oxidants cause free radicals to form, which can damage and even outright destroy cancer cells (leaving normal cells untouched).

- Curcumin slows angiogenesis (the making of new blood vessels) in cancer cells, making it harder for them to feed themselves or metastasize.

- Curcumin decreases the activity of the enzyme COX-2, an enzyme associated with inflammation. COX-2 inhibitors have been shown to be beneficial in cancer cases.

- Curcumin blocks the topoisomerase enzymes, which are critical to the DNA replication process. As topoisomerase enzymes are disrupted, new cancer cells have diminished ability to "turn on" their growth genes.

In vitro and some *in vivo* studies have shown that curcumin sensitizes cancer cells to the effects of radiation therapy and chemotherapy (specific drugs studied were cisplatin, gemcitabine and capecitabine). Its ability to help induce apoptosis, help kill cancer cells directly with free radicals, impede angiogenesis, slow or in some cases stop cancer cell division, and reduce metastasis with few to no side effects made it an obvious choice for inclusion in Apocaps.

T-cell Lymphoma Responds

"My mixed breed/pitt was diagnosed with t-cell lymphoma in October, 2009 when she was nine and half years old. At that time I found The Dog Cancer Survival Guide on the internet and have used it as my guide to Full Spectrum treatment. That has included a full course of chemo (Wisconsin Protocol, and recently a modified second course). As soon as our vet was sure she was able to handle the chemo with little side effects, I added a number of complimentary protocols based on Dr. Dressler's book: we switched to grain free dog food (a mix of wet and dry) and ordered Apocaps (at that time it was still distributed in powder form). I also incorporated K-9 Immunity caps and Salmon Oil into her food. As it is difficult to get a dog to take the caps- I open them and add to her food. In the case of the Apocaps- which she gets twice a day half hour before meals- she gets the cap contents mixed with small bits of boiled chicken in the chicken broth- and loves it. Everything else (we have recently added liver and joint support meds proscribed by our vet) is crushed and added with the K-9 Immunity to her dried food, which is then pre-bagged for an entire week's servings and added to her wet food. Although this seems complicated, we have it quite organized, and she has been thriving so far. I think it is necessary to mention that there is a significant financial cost to taking this path. In our case, I believe the complimentary protocols- particularly Apocaps and the K-9 Immunity caps- are what kept Honey's immune system strong enough to hit the lymphoma hard (we were told t-cell was an aggressive form), and we have had the resources (and ongoing results) to make that decision an easy one. Our primary vet told us that Honey only had a few months without treatment, and our oncologist was wary because it was the t-cell, not b-cell variety. It's now a full year and a half since her initial diagnosis and I'm hoping she can make it through at least one more summer so she can go up to our lake and muck around with the frogs and chase chipmunks again."

— *Lyn Pentecost, New York City, New York*

In addition to its anti-cancer effects, curcumin has some other benefits. Like its cousin ginger, it has been approved for use in treating nausea and stomach upset by Germany's version of the FDA, Commission E. Like luteolin, curcumin has anti-inflammatory effects in the body. And finally, rodent studies have shown curcumin provides some protection for the kidneys during doxorubicin treatments.

Curcumin comes from a spice, so the body has evolved to excrete it in the waste easily, which is probably why isn't well absorbed when taken by mouth. However, I found other evidence that it still helped, even when taken by mouth: in early clinical trials involving mice, for example, curcumin shrank prostate cancer cells. In other trials involving humans, participants showed chemical marker changes in their bloodstreams after taking curcumin.

My concern about curcumin's bioavailability was the reason I created the Trojan horse, which boosts curcumin's blood levels in the Apocaps formula in several different ways.

Let's look at the third major apoptogen found in Apocaps: apigenin.

Apigenin

If you have ever eaten a sprig of parsley, you've eaten the apoptogen apigenin. This bio-flavonoid, commonly found in edible plants (artichokes, basil, celery and others), has many of the same effects as luteolin and curcumin do on cancer.

After you read through its actions in the list below, you'll understand why api-genin is the subject of so much study in

It's Almost As If He Doesn't Have Cancer

"I am still using Apocaps and have just picked up the K-9 immunity. I'm not sure if it is the Apocaps, or the diet ... but Charlie has shown an increase in energy over the past two weeks. It's almost as if he doesn't have cancer at all."

– Audry Arnall, Kelowna, British Columbia

cancer research. There are several impressive studies, but the one that jumps out for me was published in the journal of the Federation of American Societies for Experimental Biology (FASEB). In this study, apigenin, fed to mice by mouth, shrank prostate tumors to one-third or one-half of their original sizes. Here is what apigenin can do:

- Apigenin helps turn on apoptosis genes in cancer cells.

- Apigenin increases cell cycle arrest in many different kinds of cancer cells. Although the mechanism or mechanisms are not all understood yet, it's clear that it may stop cancer cells from multiplying by literally stopping their replication process.

- Apigenin slows angiogenesis (the making of new blood cells), making it harder for cancer cells to feed themselves or metastasize.

- Apigenin helps block COX-2, an enzyme cancer cells use to "self-stimulate" replication and inflammation.

- Apigenin helps block gap junctions, impeding cell-to-cell communication. When cancer cells can't talk to other cancer cells, they can't coordinate many different activities.

Like luteolin and curcumin, in vitro studies have shown apigenin decreases inflammation and sensitizes cancer cells to the effects of chemotherapy (the specific drugs studied were cisplatin, 5-Flu-orouracil and gemcitabine) and radiation therapy. Some oncologists are not sure about the use of apigenin as a radiation and chemotherapy sensitizer. The controversy is complex and deals with several different molecular compounds that can be extracted from apigenin. For our purposes in this book, I will simply say that I have taken these factors into account, and am confident that the way that apigenin is extracted and compounded for use in Apocaps preserves its chemo- and radiosen-sitizing properties. If your vet or your oncologist has any concerns about this, please direct them to www.Apocaps.com, where I have presented my thoughts and the relative issues in some detail.

Other Ingredients

Although apigenin, curcumin and luteolin work well together and are the most promising apoptogens I've found, they're not the only ingredients in the patent-pending Apocaps formulation. Some ingredients are part of the Trojan Horse formula, used to boost bioavailability, while others stimulate the immune system. Some have evidence of being chemotherapy sensitizers or radiation therapy sensitizers. Others provide support for the internal organs, offer nutritional support, or have evidence for reducing side effects from radiation and common chemotherapy drugs.

Apocaps took years to research, develop and refine, and I'm really proud that it has safely helped so many dogs. It's my number one supplement recommendation for any dog with any type of cancer, including dogs undergoing conventional treatments. If you or your vet or oncologist need or want more information, including the product label and frequently asked questions, go to www.Apocaps. com. You can also find Apocaps on www.Amazon.com and at many veterinary clinics, as well as at www.DogCancerShop.com. If your vet or oncologist has any questions about its use in your dog's specific case, they can contact Functional Nutriments and get the information they need (see Appendix C).

HOW TO GIVE APOCAPS TO YOUR DOG

Bioavailability is highest when Apocaps are given on an empty stomach, so I recommend giving Apocaps between meals. Waiting at least one hour before or after a meal is sufficient; ideally, administration will occur four hours before or after a meal. There is also some justification for giving Apocaps late in the morning (around 11am) and/or late at night (around 11pm). It is not mandatory to give Apocaps at this time, but if you can, it might be helpful.

Taking a pill (any pill) on a completely empty stomach can cause tummy upset in humans and in dogs, so I recommend giving Apocaps with a small amount of food (not much, just one or two tablespoons). If your dog gets an upset stomach, even with food, you can give Apocaps with a full meal. The bioavailability will go down, but it's better to give some Apocaps than none.

The exact dosing instructions will always be on the label, and here is a general schedule for giving Apocaps to your dog:

5-10 lbs.: one capsule in the morning and one in the evening

10.1-20 lbs.: two capsules in the morning and two in the evening

20.1-40 lbs.: three capsules in the morning and two in the evening

40.1-60 lbs.: three capsules in the morning and three in the evening

60.1 lbs. & over: three capsules in the morning, three in the afternoon, and three in the evening

---

Precautions

As with any change in your dog's care, your vet or oncologist should supervise the use of Apocaps, including the management of side effects, if there are any.

Apocaps rarely cause stomach upset (nausea, vomiting or diarrhea). If this happens to your dog, stop giving Apocaps until these symptoms clear up, use the strategies in Chapter 11 to relieve the symptoms and consult your veterinarian or oncologist. Once your dog is feeling better, your vet or oncologist may suggest trying Apocaps with a full meal, to prevent stomach upset.

Most veterinary medications are safe to use with Apocaps, but there is a possible exception in the case of anti-inflammatory medications. Doubling up anti-inflammatories can cause stomach upset; because Apocaps has an anti-inflammatory effect, adjustments need to be made if your dog is on anti-inflammatory medication. Common examples of NSAIDs (non-steroidal anti-inflammatory drugs) include aspirin, piroxicam, Rimadyl, Metacam or the generic meloxicam, Deramaxx, Previcox and Etogesic. If a dog in my practice is on an anti-inflammatory, I drop the dose of either the NSAID or the Apocaps down to one quarter or one half of the full strength dose. The choice of which and how much to reduce depends upon the specifics of the case, so rely on your veterinarian or oncologist for advice. I also advise giving Apocaps with a full meal if anti-inflammatories are used simultaneously.

The same advice applies to dogs on corticosteroids, such as prednisone, prednisolone, methyl-prednisolone, Vetalog, budesonide, and dexamethasone, for the same reasons.

Because NSAIDs may also have a mild "blood-thinning" effect, Apocaps may, too (I have never seen this, but, theoretically, it's possible). To be safe, if your dog has blood-clotting problems, make sure your vet or oncologist knows this, so she can advise you about how to proceed with your dog.

If your dog has liver or kidney problems, you already know that NSAIDs should be avoided. Because Apocaps share some similarity with NSAIDs, I recommend avoiding Apocaps in these cases, as a precaution. To be clear, I did not see Apocaps affect liver or kidney markers in the pilot trial, and I have never heard of this problem from guardians or other vets. However, because the components in

Combination Works for Sienna

TRUE TAILS

"We've used Apocaps, in rotation with other anti-cancer supplements, since Apocaps first became available [March 2010] after Sienna's cancer diagnosis. Sienna's cancer hasn't returned to date. We believe the combination of changes we made to her diet, as well as cancer-fighting supplements we've introduced along with positive life changes have all come together in bringing her back to health. We can't pinpoint exactly which supplements are helping her most, but we do believe Apocaps has something to do with her continued health!"

— *Tammy McCarley, Sacramento, California*

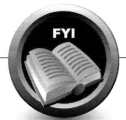

Antioxidants and Apocaps

Apocaps has a pro-oxidant effect, so, theoretically, antioxidants (or compounds with an antioxidant effect) can interfere with Apocaps, if they are given at the same time.

Give these supplements separately, ideally 4-6 hours apart from administration of Apocaps. Most of these supplements are best given with meals, so this is rarely (if ever) a problem for guardians. Here is a list of common supplements with antioxidant effects (some of these aren't recommended for dogs with cancer, but I include them because they are so common):

- Multivitamin supplements (see page 186)
- High potency antioxidant supplements (Max GL and Poly MVA for example)
- Supplements with the phrase "anti-oxidant" on the label
- K-9 Immunity (see page 182)
- Fatty acid supplements (including fish and krill oils, page 202)
- Oral algae supplements (see page 417)
- Most herbal supplements
- Most immune-boosting supplements
- Coenzyme Q-10 (CoQ10, see page 149)
- IP-3 and IP-6 (see page 421)
- Cordyceps (see page 148)

An ideal schedule would look like this:

1. Give supplements other than Apocaps with morning and evening meals.
2. Give Apocaps with a small snack in late morning (11am) and at night (11pm). Some dogs may require an additional mid-day dose, which can be given in the late afternoon with a small snack.

If this is not possible, here is an alternative schedule:

1. Early morning snack with Apocaps
2. Wait one hour, then feed meal with other supplements
3. If your dog requires a mid-day dose, give it in the late afternoon, with a small snack.
4. Evening meal with other supplements
5. Late night snack with Apocaps dose.

Antioxidants and Apocaps, *continued*

Very few dogs get stomach upset when they take Apocaps with a small amount of food; if your dog does, you can give Apocaps with a full meal. The bioavailability will go down, but it's better to give some Apocaps than none. If forced to make this choice, I recommend eliminating the use of other the supplements in favor of the use of Apocaps.

NOTE: This advice and schedule also applies if you choose to use the apoptogen artemisinin.

Apocaps share some similarities to NSAIDs, I am cautious. Your own veterinarian or oncologist may or may not share my concern, and can help advise you on the specifics of your dog's care.

Safety has not been evaluated in dogs who are pregnant, nursing, breeding, diabetic or less than six months old, so I do not recommend using Apocaps in these cases.

Using Apocaps with Surgery, Chemotherapy and Radiation

Anti-inflammatory medications, like NSAIDs, may have mild "blood thinning" effects and, because Apocaps has NSAID-like effects, I exercise caution around surgeries. I have not seen Apocaps actually affect blood-clotting, but there is theoretical evidence that this could be a possibility. To be completely safe, I recommend stopping Apocaps use at least three days before surgery. You can start giving Apocaps again after healing is complete (usually ten to fourteen days after surgery).

The apoptogens in Apocaps have been shown to make some cancer cells more responsive to chemotherapy and radiation treatments in *in vitro* studies, which may make these treatments more effective. Using Apocaps as an adjunct nutraceutical for these treatments is being researched, and as of this writing, I do not have hard data to share with you about Apocaps specifically. For this reason, I recommend following your vet or oncologist's advice about using Apocaps at the same time as conventional treatments; your vet or oncologist can also call Functional Nutriments for the latest advice.

Note that rutin, which is included in Apocaps, is an extract of grapefruit, but does *not* contain the other grapefruit compounds known to alter the way the body metabolizes chemotherapy drugs.

Apocaps and Other Apoptogens

Using potent wormwood preparations such as artemisinin, Artemix or artemether (see below) at the same time as you use Apocaps, has not been evaluated for safety, so it is not recommended. If you choose to use wormwood preparations, use them in alternation with Apocaps, on a rotating schedule of five days on Apocaps (and stop artemisinin), five days on artemisinin (and stop Apocaps),

More Energy: He's Doing Great

"I used Apocaps and found them to be very helpful in helping Hydro gain his energy and not be so lethargic, he's willing to take walks and it's not such a struggle. He's not having difficulty walking anymore. He's doing great."

– Maria J. Neal, Aurora, Colorado

I Will Continue Using Them

"Since Dr. Dressler's Apocaps became available [in March of 2010] I have been using them for Lucy. It is two years now since she was diagnosed and treated for the Mast Cell, with a mitotic index of 4. I truly feel that the Apocaps have been helping her and I will continue using them."

– Shirley, Salem, Oregon

I Have Tested This ... by Running Out of Apocaps

"I use Apocaps on my dog. I do see an improvement in how she recovers from exercise, being a Tripawd. I have tested this a few times, by running out of Apocaps."

– Tracy Snow-Cormier, Portage, Maine

I Only Wish They Were Available Earlier

"I used the Apocaps and Artemisinin with Apollo. I do believe they helped. I only wish they had come out and been available when Apollo was first diagnosed."

– Sandy Miller, Palo, Iowa

five days on Apocaps (and stop artemisinin), and so on.

The use of oral Neoplasene (see page 176) with Apocaps has not been evaluated for safety, and is not recommended. If your veterinarian has prescribed the topical form of Neoplasene, for use on the skin, you may use Apocaps under veterinary or oncologist supervision.

Some vets and oncologist choose to use a combination of these apoptogens, in these cases, follow their advice.

Other Apoptogens

Readers of the first edition of this book will remember that I once recommended the apoptogens EGCG in addition to luteolin, curcumin and apigenin. Since that edition was published, I have developed Apocaps and have more experience with all of these apoptogens. I no longer recommend EGCG unequivocally (see page 419). I still recommend artemisinin, however, and I also recommend topical Neoplasene (in select cases).

Artemisinin

Artemisinin is a compound extracted from an ancient Chinese plant called Qing Hao, which has been used for centuries to treat malaria and fever. It is the focus of much current cancer research for both humans and dogs, and gets a lot of attention in online forums for its effects on osteosarcoma, lymphoma and other cancers.

Interestingly, Qing Hao is a member of the wormwood family, and wormwood is used to make the powerful and notorious alcoholic spirit, absinthe.

Artemisinin works by interacting with iron stored in cancer cells to create free radicals. Most normal body cells don't have much iron, but cancer cells have relatively large amounts, because iron favors cancer cell growth. These iron-rich stores in cancer cells make them a natural "target" for artemisinin. It enters the cancer cells relatively easily, and, once inside, uses the iron to create free radicals, which can help destroy the cancer cell from within. Artemisinin also seems to slow angiogenesis. It is a powerful apoptogen, which should be used with care.

Remarkably Healthy and Strong

"After a lot of online research, I finally found places from which to purchase Apigenin and Luteolin, both of which were used in my dog's cancer-fighting diet. My golden doodle Ellie had a very aggressive form of cancer, yet the time she had with us was remarkably healthy and strong right up until the very end. I have no doubt this is due in part to the nutraceuticals we used."

— *Sarah N. Bertsch, Hudson, Wisconsin*

You may see artemisinin, itself, or one of its two derivative compounds, artemether and artesunate. There is also a product called Artemix, which combines all three compounds. There are several researchers working closely with these, and not all of them agree yet on a standard protocol.

Herbal preparations often seem more effective if they are given for a while, then stopped, then given again, because the body seems to build up a tolerance to the herb, making it less effective as time goes on. For artemisinin specifically, the lining of the intestine literally stops absorbing it after five days. Giving the body a break every few days keeps this herb's effect more potent (see below).

Artemisinin may or may not be helpful for your dog. I use it in some advanced cancer cases, including osteosarcoma, but not as often as I use Apocaps; consult with your vet or oncologist about your dog's specific case. If you are interested in learning more, there is an artemisinin forum at http://pets. groups.yahoo.com/group/Artemisinin_and_cancer, and the main research is being conducted by Dr. Henry Lai at the University of Washington and Dr. Guillermo C. Couto at Ohio State University.

Artemisinin and Iron-Rich Foods

Artemisinin doesn't react with all forms of iron; it only reacts with the unbound ferrous ion form. If you start researching artemisinin, you will see some debate about whether to give your dog an iron-rich diet, while using this agent. Some folks advocate iron-rich diets (featuring red meat), and even supplementing with iron, supposing that cancer cells will gobble it up and become even bigger targets for artemisinin. Others wonder if the iron ever makes it to the cancer cells before the artemisinin interacts with it.

As always, this is a complicated situation and it's impossible to make blanket statements. Here's

Did the Nutraceuticals Work?

"I primarily used Luteolin, Curcumin and Artemisinin as Apocaps were not yet available. I also changed her diet to include as many naturally occurring version of each. We were also attending a clinical trial for Palladia. Did the nutraceuticals work? I can't say for certain either way, but if I had to do it again, I would definitely go the same route."

– Julian Trevino, Roseville, Michigan

what we know:

1. Artemisinin creates free radicals when and where it encounters the unbound ferrous form of iron.

2. About half of the iron in red meat is unbound, and a small portion of that unbound iron is also ferrous.

If that relatively small fraction of unbound, ferrous iron from a meal with meat is still in the digestive tract when artemisinin is administered, then yes, theoretically it could create free radicals outside of the cancer cells rather than inside of them. The active artemisinin would be consumed before it could be absorbed into the bloodstream.

This possibility is just one of the factors behind my recommendation to give artemisinin at least four hours before or after meals. I do not recommend supplementing with iron.

To read more about artemisinin and how it interacts with unbound ferrous iron, visit the following links.

http://www.irondisorders.org/iron-we-consume/

http://the-medical-dictionary.com/artemether_374_article_5.htm

http://library.med.utah.edu/WebPath/TUTORIAL/IRON/IRON.html

Precautions

Artemisinin is a powerful apoptogen, and it's important that you discuss its use with your vet. It's worth repeating that there is no standard protocol at this time, and each researcher has her own opinion about its best use. My dosing recommendation is a starting point for discussion between you and your vet. In the meantime, there are a few complicating factors to keep in mind.

Occasionally, this agent can cause excessive stomach acid production and vomiting, loss of appetite or diarrhea. Stop giving artemisinin for at least a week to get the problem under control and contact your veterinarian or oncologist. When you start giving artemisinin again (under veterinary supervision), give it with full meals.

If your dog is receiving radiation treatments, do not use artemisinin, and wait until two months after finishing radiation treatments before your resume giving the herb. Radiation treatments may

HOW TO GIVE ARTEMISININ TO YOUR DOG

Artemisinin's pro-oxidant effects are similar to Apocaps, which means its effects can be quenched by antioxidant type supplements. I recommend giving it at least four hours before or after a meal with a small amount of food. Read the sidebar about Antioxidants and Apocaps on page 170 and follow the exact same advice when giving artemisinin.

There is no agreement on a standard protocol for artemisinin use; my recommendation is to give about 10 mg of artemisinin per pound of body weight, once daily, between meals or right before bed-time, and always at least four hours before or after food. To disguise the pill and mask its bitter taste, you can use a small amount of food, and preferably one that contains some fat (fish or krill oil, peanut butter, milk, coconut milk, or cream cheese). The fat in these foods helps boost blood levels of artemisinin. If your dog's stomach is sensitive to fat or if he has a digestive problem, like pancreatitis, which could flare up with fat, instead choose a protein snack like lean meat.

As mentioned, artemisinin may stop being absorbed if used continuously, so use a five-days-on, five-days-off cycle for administration. To keep your dog's body pumped full of apoptogens, I recommend using Apocaps on the days that you are not using artemisinin. Give in five-day cycles: five days on artemisinin (stop Apocaps), five days on Apocaps (stop artemisinin), and so on.

There some is evidence that artemisinin, like Apocaps, may be best given at 11am or 11pm or as close to that time as possible. Again, this is not a mandatory rule, only a suggestion.

Most dogs can tolerate the dose I recommend, although some may experience nausea. If this happens to your dog, you could try splitting the single dose into two half doses, given at the same times of day as Apocaps is given (but not on the same days as Apocaps, of course).

To get the best protocol for your own dog, consult with your veterinarian or oncologist, because there is no agreement at this time on a standard protocol. I've seen protocols for as low as 2 mg of artemisinin per pound of body weight given continuously with no breaks, and others as high as 16 mg per pound of body weight. Some vets prefer just artemisinin, while others like a combined approach. Some favor injections over oral methods, in certain cases. What works for your dog may not work for another, so be sure to consult with your veterinary professional and monitor your dog.

cause dying cancer cells to release iron into the surrounding tissues, including normal tissue. If there is a lot of free iron in the radiated area or in the body, artemisinin may react with some of this free iron to form damaging free radicals, and these may harm normal body cells.

A few humans have experienced elevated kidney markers and suppressed white blood cell counts while on artemisinin. As a precaution, it is wise to monitor these levels in your dog, while he's on artemisinin.

There are also scattered reports of rare brainstem toxicity with this compound. For this reason, in dogs with seizure disorders or brain tumors, artemisinin is not recommended.

Artemisinin has been tested in vitro with many chemotherapy agents. As all interactions have not yet been assessed, consult closely with your vet and/or oncologist before using artemisinin with chemotherapy agents.

Most dogs do not experience any toxic side effects on artemisinin at the doses recommended above (2-16 mg per pound of body weight). However, some humans have experienced cramping, stomach upset and fevers on artemisinin.

Neoplasene

Neoplasene is what I call a "salvage technique" – something to use when nothing else is working. I did not include it in the first edition, because it's a tough protocol for the average dog-lover. Enough people have asked me about it, however, that I decided to include it in this edition.

You may have heard of "black salve," a Native American remedy, used for centuries, which contains the herb, bloodroot. Neoplasene contains some of the components present in bloodroot, as well as other proprietary components. It comes in three forms: salve, pill and injection.

Neoplasene is a powerful apoptogen, and may be useful for tumors of the skin such as fibrosarcomas, mast cell tumors, and mammary tumors. It is not available for home use because it is such a potent substance with possible toxicity for some dogs. Buck Mountain Botanicals, the manufacturer, will only sell Neoplasene to veterinarians, never to consumers.

Here's why they're so resistant: Neoplasene applied to a tumor on the skin typically induces apoptosis relatively quickly (usually within ten days) and causes the tumor to die and slough off (fall out) of the body, leaving a hole where it was. In addition, any invisible cancer cells around the tumor may also die, leaving an even larger hole than the size of the visible tumor. This can be scary. It can also be medically dangerous, if a veterinarian does not supervise the process. Tumors which have spread deep into body tissues can leave a hole large enough that you can actually see the underlying bone. Clearly, large holes require quick and immediate medical attention, which is why vets should supervise this process.

Meanwhile, NSAIDs, prednisone and other anti-inflammatory agents may reduce the efficacy of Neoplasene. This is a problem, because Neoplasene can cause pain and swelling in both the tumor and the surrounding tissue. Depending upon the case, this may make Neoplasene a rather uncomfortable agent.

(Note that, even though Apocaps has an anti-inflammatory effect, I use it along with topical Neoplasene because the apoptogens in Apocaps offer so many other benefits that outweigh the possible decrease in efficacy for Neoplasene. I do not combine Apocaps with the liquid oral or injectable forms of Neoplasene.)

Using Neoplasene is not a decision to make lightly. The application of the salve is not straight-forward, and is best done under veterinary supervision. The injections for tumors deeper in the body must be performed at the hospital, and the liquid oral version can cause such severe vomiting that I don't recommend it at all.

Another consideration, when using Neoplasene, is that you cannot biopsy the treated site later. Some guardians may want to use Neoplasene without getting a biopsy, and then, if other health issues or tumors occur later on, wish they had more information about the treated tumor (type or grade, for example).

I use Neoplasene in special cases on inoperable tumors, especially nasal tumors that are ineli-gible for conventional approaches. I think of Neoplasene as a last-ditch effort or salvage procedure. In essence, it's a plant-based form of surgery that, in most cases, does not require anesthesia, is cheap, and requires no cutting. In addition to killing the primary tumor, Neoplasene can also help destroy the microscopic cells that have invaded tissues around the tumor – the ones surgery typically misses. This may sound like a good thing; the problem is that you can't predict ahead of time how much tissue will actually fall out during the treatment. Consider, for a moment, the case of a nasal tumor that looks like it is just on the bridge of the nose, but actually extends into the sinuses, through the skull, and into the brain. The removal of a tumor that large and complicated is not something most guardians can handle, at least not in the home environment. It requires medical attention and intense follow up.

HOW TO GIVE NEOPLASENE TO YOUR DOG

Do not use Neoplasene on your own; get your vet to apply it. Your vet will apply Neoplasene according to the very detailed instructions Dr. Fox provides. If you are using topical Neoplasene, the wound must be kept from drying out by applying a salve over it. Use the products Dr. Fox recom-mends. If your dog is receiving the Neoplasene injection, your vet must follow Dr. Fox's protocols closely.

Because of the potential for vomiting, nausea and loss of appetite, I do not use the liquid oral form of Neoplasene (not every vet or guardian agrees with me). If you choose to use the oral liquid, your vet can get protocols from Dr. Fox. To avoid stomach upset, you can try giving the liquid with food, and milk may enhance its absorption.

Make sure you follow up with your vet for proper and quick attention to any wounds left by the treatment. Some may need surgery to close. Pain medication may be needed during and after Neoplasene treatments.

As I mentioned above, I use Apocaps concurrently with the topical form of Neoplasene, not with the injectable or liquid forms.

I'm being particularly graphic in my descriptions, so you understand how graphic Neoplasene treatments can be. Especially for tumors that have a high degree of local invasion, otherwise invisible to the naked eye, the wound that results from the tumor's dissolution may be more than anyone has bargained for. On top of this, good pain control may be difficult, without using drugs that interfere with Neoplasene. In my practice, we use medications like high dose Tramadol and gabapentin or amantadine for pain control in these patients.

In my experience, and from the anecdotal evidence that I've found, Neoplasene does make tumors go away, at least, temporarily. However, its use is not a permanent solution to cancer. Regardless of the form of Neoplasene used, cancer still may regrow locally or show up in distant sites. Also, there are no published studies on Neoplasene, other than case reports, and its safety and efficacy have not been established, as of this writing.

This is an aggressive but natural

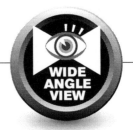

Which Nutraceuticals Should I Use?

This question used to be a lot harder to answer before I developed Apocaps, and is what led me to develop the apoptogen formula in the first place. Apocaps safely combines the most effective nutraceuticals I have found and can be used in most dogs with cancer of any type (see page 169 for precautions). It is my overall number one supplement recommendation. Depending upon the specifics of an individual case, I sometimes also add the apoptogens, artemisinin and topical Neoplasene, to a treatment plan. As always, I urge you to consult with your vet or oncologist about the specifics of your dog's case.

Also, consult the Supplement Hierarchy in Appendix A, which lists all of my supplement recommendations, in order of importance.

treatment that you may want to include in your treatment plan, if your dog has a tumor that cannot be removed surgically and is not responding to any other treatment. At the very least, you may be able to debulk it (reduce its size and impact on other body parts) and reduce the overall tumor burden in your dog. This can be a risky strategy, and those risks must be weighed carefully.

Your vet can get Neoplasene from Dr. Terrence S. Fox. Ph.D. at Buck Mountain Botanicals, www.BuckMountainBotanicals.net. There is a lot of information on his website about the use of Neoplasene, including many before and after pictures.

Precautions

Your vet must be consulted in order to use Neoplasene. I do not recommend contacting Buck Mountain Botanicals directly.

Your dog must be kept from licking the salve and the resulting wound, so an Elizabethan collar may be needed.

As mentioned above, the use of anti-inflammatories may interfere with Neoplasene efficacy, including Apocaps, prednisone and all other corticosteroids, and NSAIDS, such as aspirin and piroxicam. I use Apocaps with topical (not oral or injectable) Neoplasene because I feel its benefits outweigh the possible negative effects. The use of any other supplements is not well evaluated with Neoplasene and cannot be advised at this time.

The intravenous injections of Neoplasene trigger high rates of allergic reactions in dogs, so be sure that your vet is monitoring your dog for symptoms and using preventative medications, if he can.

It takes about ten days for Neoplasene to act on cancer cells, during which time dead tissue may slough off the site. Changing the bandages and keeping the wound from drying out are very important to keep the area safe from infections, so follow Dr. Fox's maintenance protocols carefully.

Chapter 13: Step Three, Immune System Boosters and Anti-Metastatics

"Look deep into nature,
and then you will understand everything better."

–Albert Einstein

When I take Einstein's advice and look deep into nature, I am often in awe of what I find. A rainstorm darkens the sky and floods the ground, but once it is gone plants are greener and everything looks brighter. If I cut my finger, my body immediately takes steps to clean and heal the wound, and a few days later the skin is whole and clean.

The ointment and bandage I put on the wound did not actually cause this healing. They gave extra shelter and protection to the wound, while the body healed itself.

In these moments of introspection, it is clear that nature is capable of solving many problems, when given enough time, shelter and support.

Cancer is a big problem, one the body is (theoretically) equipped to handle. A normal immune system has tools it can put to use to identify cancerous cells and eliminate them from the body.

As we've seen, the consequences of our daily life can overwhelm the im-

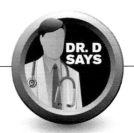

Good Advice

I am a veterinarian, not a medical doctor, and this book is about dog cancer, not human cancer. Regardless, research shows that the ideas in this chapter may have application for humans. It's my hope that this book inspires all of us to take excellent care of ourselves, as well as our dogs. We all deserve it.

mune system. On top of that, cancer can actively suppress the immune system, and even use it to nurture developing cancers. When this happens, there are ways to offer the immune system shelter and support. The strategies and supplements in this chapter are like ointments and bandages for your dog's immune system. They offer support, shelter and, hopefully, time, as they attempt to correct some of the common effects of our modern lifestyles.

Some of the advice in this and the next two chapters may remind you of your mother's. Most mothers I've met advise their children to eat well, get enough sleep, relax and exercise regularly. Most of the children of mothers I know end up ignoring this advice at least once in a while. Ignoring it may be leading us to epidemics of "diseases of civilization," including cancer.

Taking good care of your dog's basic bodily needs is not just helpful; many of these supplements and lifestyle choices have published evidence supporting their benefits for cancer patients. I recommend using at least some of these in your Full Spectrum cancer care plan.

Mushroom-Derived Polysaccharides

When I first came across the scientific literature about how effective mushrooms are at stimulating the immune system, I was very skeptical. But as I read, my skepticism softened. I remembered that penicillin – perhaps the greatest advance in medicinal history – was created from fungus. Maybe the use of mushrooms isn't such a weird idea, after all.

Mushrooms contain natural compounds, called polysaccharides (simple sugars which are strung together), and the most important polysaccharides for cancer patients are called beta-glucans. Beta-glucans have a wide variety of effects in the body, a couple of which are of particular interest to us. Beta-glucans can bind to the outside of natural killer (NK) cells and other immune system cells, responsible for destroying cancers, and help "turn them on" and increase their activity. Beta-glucans may also be able to increase overall white blood cell activity in the body. Beta-glucans and other mushroom-derived polysaccharides can harm cancer cells in several other ways, too. They can increase cell cycle arrest (which slows down replication), help induce apoptosis, and interfere with angiogenesis.

There are many studies that look at medicinal mushrooms and cancer. There is some evidence for direct anti-cancer actions in the body when they are given by mouth, but even stronger evidence that they boost the immune response and increase life quality for cancer patients.

He Puts Himself to Bed!

"I have made sure the room is totally dark now for sleeping. He actually puts himself to bed at 10:00 every night, even if we're still downstairs watching TV!"

– Vicki Hagopian,
Hudson, Massachusetts

There has been discussion that mushroom-derived polysaccharides cannot be absorbed into the bloodstream when taken by mouth, and instead should be injected into the body to achieve reasonable blood levels. Rodent studies show that this is not the case and that these substances are indeed active when taken by mouth, making them ideal candidates for inclusion in Full Spectrum cancer care.

Many mushrooms contain beta-glucans and other polysaccharides; the main species that have been shown to be effective for cancer are Cordyceps sinesis, maitake (Grifola frondosa), shiitake (Lentinula edodes), Phellinus linteus, Coriolus versicolor and Agaricus blazei. While shiitake mushrooms can be found in the produce section of your local grocery store, it is difficult to determine how much of any given mushroom to give your dog, because individual mushrooms may vary greatly. A beta-glucans supplement is a better choice.

I like beta-glucans so much that I included them in Apocaps as an immune booster. If you would like to further boost your dog's immune system, I recommend you also give a separate beta-glucans supplement. There are several medicinal mushroom supplements on the market. I have used and recommend K-9 Immunity from Aloha Medicinals[6], for a couple of reasons. It's engineered specifically for dogs, they include a wide variety of potentially beneficial mushrooms, the enzyme bromelain is added (which helps the polysaccharides get absorbed and into circulation even more quickly and efficiently), and they also sell a companion product, called K-9 Transfer Factor, which seems to support the activity of the beta-glucans.

There is also an all-in-one formulation, called K-9 Immunity Plus, which includes both K-9 Transfer Factor and fish oil. Unfortunately, it is formulated with cane sugar and corn syrup as binders and taste enhancers. While I understand they want to make it more palatable for dogs, I do not recommend feeding sugar to dogs with cancer, even in this small amount. In addition, the dose of fish oil is far too low to have significant anti-cancer benefits. As you'll see in the next chapter, I highly recommend supplementing with fish oils in higher doses. For these two reasons, I prefer using the separate K-9 Immunity and K-9 Transfer Factor supplements over the newer all-in-one K-9 Immunity Plus formulation.

The Bottom Line on Mushroom-Derived Polysaccharides

Supplementing with beta-glucans may help boost your dog's immune system. There are some beta-glucans in Apocaps and, if your budget allows for it, further supplementation may be helpful.

How to Give Mushroom-Derived Polysaccharides

The dosing for Apocaps is on the product label and also discussed on page 168. K-9 Immunity

---

[6] Knowing I'm from Hawaii, and seeing the name Aloha Medicinals, you may wonder if I have ever been connected with or a ever had financial interest in this company. The answer is no – it is pure coincidence. By the way, Aloha Medicinals is headquartered in Nevada.

has specific dosing instructions on their label, and I also recommend using the product called K-9 Transfer Factor. For all other formulations, follow the labeled dosing.

The easiest ways to give these supplements is to empty capsules and/or grind tablets into a powder, then mix them into your dog's food. These products can both be used concurrently with Apocaps; please read the sidebar on page 170 for timing recommendations.

Precautions

If your dog has a disease caused by an over-active immune system (an immune-mediated disease), medicinal mushrooms could theoretically exacerbate the condition. Please check with your vet or oncologist, if you are unsure about this.

Mushrooms can stabilize blood sugar, and diabetic dogs may need less insulin when they're on mushroom-derived polysaccharides. If your dog is diabetic, your vet will need to monitor his blood sugar levels and adjust insulin doses, as needed.

Mushroom-derived polysaccharides can occasionally cause digestive upset, such as nausea, vomiting or diarrhea.

Melatonin and High Quality Sleep

If you're like most guardians, you probably remember your mother's advice to go to bed early, especially when you were sick. This is excellent advice for you, and for your dog, espe-

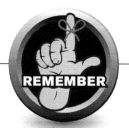

Possible Side Effects

In general, the supplements I recommend are safe for most dogs. Any new supplement or change in diet may cause temporary digestive upset (nausea, vomiting or diarrhea). If you notice these symptoms in your dog, discontinue the new supplement or food and take steps to address the symptoms under veterinary supervision. You can find detailed conventional and alternative methods in the side effects discussion that starts on page 140. Once stomach upset resolves, you can assess whether you want to continue giving the supplement. Some dogs need to start with smaller doses and work up to full doses. Others may need a smaller dose on an ongoing basis. You may want to eliminate that supplement from their Full Spectrum cancer care plan. Your veterinarian or oncologist will be able to help you decide what is right for your dog.

Be sure to review the listed precautions for each supplement and treatment in this book, and weigh those precautions carefully, as you work with your vet or oncologist.

cially if he has cancer. With artificial lights, over one thousand television channels, twenty-four hour news cycles, computers and unlimited long distance phone plans, we're more likely to "stay productive" long into the night and skimp on sleep. These extended hours are not nearly as productive as we'd like to think they are. They can lead to insomnia and rob our bodies of their natural rhythms. Our dogs – our closest companions – are right there with us. They need quiet rest in the dark, just like we do.

As we discussed on page 86, there is a powerful hormone called melatonin that boosts the immune system and also has a direct anti-cancer effect on the body. According to studies in lab animals and humans, melatonin has been shown to limit metastasis, reduce tumors, extend survival times and restore body weight, lost to cancer cachexia.

In one study, melatonin more than doubled the survival time of human cancer patients receiving chemotherapy (cisplatin and etoposide) for advanced non-small-cell lung cancer. It's also been shown to benefit humans with cancers of the breast, metastatic renal cell carcinoma, hepatocellular carcinoma and brain metastases from solid tumors.

There is evidence that melatonin may decrease side effects related to chemotherapy. Patients in studies experienced better platelet counts and less irritation of the mouth (stomatitis). There was also less nerve damage and heart toxicity for patients on melatonin.

Melatonin is secreted by the pineal gland – the tiny gland nestled in the center of the brain – but not unless there is complete darkness. The light from television screens, computer monitors, overhead lights, lamps and streetlights may reduce melatonin levels.

It may not feel like it, but creating a "den" atmosphere for your dog at night could be considered a cancer treatment. Whether you put a thick cover over her crate or install light-blocking shades in the bedroom and turn off the TV, you'll be doing your dog a huge favor by keeping her in complete darkness for at least nine hours every day. This can encourage the pineal gland to accelerate its production of that cancer-fighting melatonin.

Melatonin is also available in supplement form, online and at health food stores. I do not generally recommend this, because some dogs seem to suffer from grogginess on the oral supplement.

The Bottom Line on Melatonin

I recommend every guardian try to boost melatonin levels through natural methods. The easiest and most comfortable way to do this is to make the sleeping environment completely dark, and to make sure that your dog sleeps for at least nine hours at night, if possible. I do not usually recommend oral melatonin supplements for dogs because of their side effects. However, if you choose to try them for your dog, I have included the doses.

HOW TO GIVE MELATONIN

Always give melatonin late at night. Natural melatonin peaks, in human studies, at around 1:30-2:00 am, and it is wise to try to mimic the natural circadian cycle of melatonin in the body. If you give melatonin during daylight hours, your dog's circadian rhythms will be altered and she may suffer from excessive sedation. If you've ever taken melatonin for insomnia or to recover from jet lag, you'll remember that it can make you feel very sleepy, and it is very uncomfortable to take it when you can't go to sleep.

The more advanced your dog's cancer is, the more melatonin I recommend. For cancers caught relatively early, use 1-2 mg of melatonin per 40 pounds of body weight. For more advanced cancers, use about 5 mg of melatonin per 40 pounds of body weight.

Some dogs will develop unacceptable sluggishness the day after receiving melatonin. This has prompted me to be selective with my use of this supplement in dogs with cancer. This often goes away within three days or so, but many guardians find this side effect unacceptable.

Precautions

Side effects like nausea, vomiting and diarrhea are rare when taking melatonin, but any new supplement or change in diet can trigger these symptoms.

Diabetic dogs may need their insulin adjusted if they take oral melatonin. Dogs on calcium channel blockers (which are in some types of heart and blood pressure medications), fluoxetine (Prozac), and epileptic dogs should not take melatonin. Melatonin may also interfere with fertility.

In the past, there was some concern about the use of melatonin with immune-mediated disease. I believe this concern was likely unfounded, because melatonin is used to treat some of the common immune-mediated diseases.

Sunlight

The idea that sun is bad for cancer has been proven to be a myth in all but two dog cancers: squamous cell carcinoma and hemangiosarcoma of the skin or the eyelid. For all other cancers, getting some sun is good for dogs.

Sunlight stimulates the body to make high levels of vitamin D, which has a much stronger effect in the body than the vitamin D found in fortified milk or vitamin supplements. Hormonal vitamin D attaches to the outside of cancer cells and may slow angiogenesis, cancer cell division and metastasis. In human studies, sun exposure resulted in less cancer in thirteen different types of cancer.

The current recommendation for humans with light skin is 10-30 minutes of sun every day, while those with dark skin may need several hours. It is logical to apply the same recommendations for dogs, who also have different skin colors (dogs with light coats usually have light skin, while dogs with dark coats usually have darker skin).

While natural sunlight is best, it is important to take some precautions. Your dog should not be allowed to overheat, for example. Hair needs to be clipped short, if your dog is outside in the sun for more than thirty minutes at 75°F or higher. Dogs with short muzzles (Boxers, Pugs and Bulldogs) are particularly susceptible to heat stroke. To be safe, I do not recommend being in direct sun for more than a few minutes, if the temperature is above 85°F, regardless of breed.

If natural sunlight is not available or if the heat is preventing your dog from enjoying it, you can use a UVB light therapy lamp. These lamps have been used with great success to treat depression in countries without a lot of sunlight, and I recommend getting one, if your dog can't get direct sunshine. (Hint: the most beneficial wavelengths of light may burn out before the bulb dies, so change bulbs when recommended, regardless of whether it still lights up.)

I do not recommend supplementing with oral vitamin D, because not enough reaches the bloodstream to be effective as a cancer treatment, and the levels that do reach the bloodstream create toxicity.

The Bottom Line on Sunlight

The bottom line on sunlight is this: unless your dog has squamous cell carcinoma or the hemangiosarcoma mentioned, get your dog out into the sun for some time each day. The hormonal vitamin D manufactured in the body when exposed to sunlight is a good addition to your Full Spectrum cancer care plan.

Multivitamin Supplements

We've already covered the pros and cons of antioxidant supplementation in some detail; let's summarize again.

Vet Was Amazed at Blood Results

"During Lucy's chemotherapy she was on Aloha Medicinals' K-9 Immunity and K-9 Transfer Factor. Her doctor had warned us that she would probably develop lower white cell levels and maybe even stop eating, but during the entire four months of chemotherapy her blood levels were always well in the normal ranges. Her food intake was good, and she remained a joyful Golden. Her doctor was always amazed at each week's blood results and I attribute this to the K-9 Immunity and K-9 Transfer Factor she was on."

– *Shirley, Salem, Oregon*

Vitamins and minerals are vital for health. They are absolutely necessary, in order to make tens of thousands of normal body processes occur, including nerve communication, muscle movement, growth and development, hormone production and a wide range of other necessary functions.

Some vitamins also have antioxidant properties: they scavenge for and neutralize free radicals.

You'll remember that some researchers believe that excessive free radicals are one of the causes of cancer. But it's not as simple as "free radicals are bad for dogs with cancer." In fact, some cancer treatments actually use free radicals to kill cancer cells (certain chemotherapy drugs, radiation, Apocaps, and artemisinin, to name a few).

Since antioxidants neutralize free radicals, I do not recommend massive doses of antioxidant vitamins, when you are using free radicals to treat cancer. If you're going to give your dog a multi-vitamin, I recommend one that provides maintenance doses – just enough to satisfy the dog's basic needs.

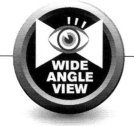

It Can Be Safe to Use Antioxidants with Chemotherapy and Radiation

Conventional and alternative veterinarians sometimes argue about whether or not to use antioxidants for dogs on chemotherapy or radiation treatments. As you know by now, there are many factors to consider and there is no black and white answer. Each dog, each cancer and each treatment is unique and must be evaluated on a case-by-case basis.

Some cancer treatments are pro-oxidant; they kill cancer cells by generating free radicals. These include: busulfan, carmustine, lomustine, chlorambucil, cyclophosphamide, cisplatin, carboplatin, ifosfamide, mechlorethamine, melphalan, thiotepa, dacarbazine, procarbazine, bleomycin, dactinomycin, daunorubicin, doxorubicin, idarubicin, mitomycin, mitoxantrone, plicamycin, etoposide, teniposide and radiation therapy.

If your dog is on one of these, there is a risk that you could suppress the drug's free radical mechanism by giving a potent antioxidant formula (for example, Max GL, Poly MVA, or any other formula advertised as a potent antioxidant). I would also be careful about using herbs known to have potent antioxidant effects.

I would, however, recommend giving a dog on these drugs maintenance (low) levels of

It Can Be Safe to Use Antioxidants, *continued*

antioxidants, because there is enough evidence to show that human cancer patients on chemotherapy and radiation actually benefit from receiving low, dietary levels of maintenance vitamins and antioxidants. They experience shorter hospital stays and fewer side effects, for example.

Some supplements with antioxidant properties also have other beneficial properties that may outweigh the theoretical impact on pro-oxidant therapies. These supplements and foods, in my opinion, are beneficial for cancer patients enough to use:

- A general multivitamin with low maintenance levels of antioxidants
- Cordyceps and other mushroom-derived polysaccharides, like those found in K-9 Immunity and K-9 Transfer Factor
- Fresh garlic (found in the dog cancer diet)
- Fresh ginger root (used for stomach upset and also in the dog cancer diet)
- Coenzyme Q-10 (if indicated, see page 149)
- Fatty acid supplements (krill and fish oils, found in the dog cancer diet)
- Melatonin

Of course, each guardian must weigh the decision to use any supplement, including these, with her veterinary professional. The Supplement Hierarchy in Appendix A will also provide more food for thought.

I'm afraid that vitamin manufacturers have convinced us that we humans all need a "daily multivitamin." Some guardians may generalize this belief and think their dog also needs a multi-vitamin.

Your dog needs vitamins and minerals to maintain normal bodily processes, but how much of each can vary widely from dog to dog. The need for different vitamins and minerals varies based on the dog's state of health, weight, age and even stress levels. There are so many factors at play, that it is nearly impossible to make a general recommendation about what to take every day for most dogs.

Instead of trying to find a one-size-fits-all multi-vitamin, it may be better and more accurate to realize that the vitamins and minerals found in natural food sources are easier for your dog to absorb than the ones found in pills.

Studies clearly show that there is a link between eating lots of vegetables and lower cancer rates.

We used to think this was because vegetables have a lot of antioxidants; current studies show that it may be the other substances in vegetables – enzymes, bioflavonoids, apoptogens and others – that do the heavy lifting.

Switching to the dog cancer diet in the next chapter helps provide good levels of the following from natural sources:

- Vitamin A (found in liver)
- Vitamin C (found in red meat, fish, poultry and fruits and vegetables)
- Vitamin E (found in broccoli)
- Lutein (found in leafy greens, such as spinach and kale)
- Carotenoids (found in leafy greens, such as spinach and kale and colored vegetables, such as red and yellow peppers)
- Selenium (found in both vegetables and meat)

These agents, along with the anti-inflammatory compounds and natural apoptogens found in the foods I recommend, will give your dog a valuable baseline of support.

Supplementing this diet with a general multivitamin could be a good idea, as long as it is not a mega-dose of antioxidants. A general multivitamin that supplies maintenance levels of vitamins and minerals may have an overall good effect for your dog and help ensure that he is getting everything he needs for optimum nutrition. Recommended Daily Allowance (RDA) levels for dogs are set by the Association of American Feed Control Officials (AAFCO), which controls all animal food and supplements. Multivitamin manufacturers marketing to pet owners are following AAFCO's guidelines on normal, dietary levels of vitamins and minerals. As long as it's a general multi-vitamin designed for dogs, you can assume the amounts listed on the label are in accordance with their guidelines.

Despite what's on the label, some supplements may not be all they claim. They may contain fillers, be contaminated with substances such as lead, or not actually contain as much of a given substance as they claim. If you are concerned about this, you can

We Were Very Afraid of Recurrence ... But It Has Been Over Two Years

"My Boxer had mast cell tumors. We had them removed but were very afraid of recurrence. I have used several immune boosting strategies that Dr. Dressler recommends. I feed the highest grade food along with his recommended immune boosting food. I also use Birkdale K9 Immunity daily; give a good sleep environment and plenty of exercise and activities. She is doing great and it has been two years."

– Jon Marshall, Norman, Oklahoma

call the vitamin manufacturer directly and ask for the Certificate of Analysis or equivalent paperwork. They will be able to give you the breakdown of their supplements, in terms of purity and contaminants.

Your vet's own experience with multi-vitamins and his knowledge of your dog's general health and other disease conditions will provide the best guidance in this matter.

You can buy multi-vitamins through your vet's office, online or in a pet store.

The Bottom Line on Multivitamins

My bottom line on a general multivitamin that supplies maintenance levels of nutritional support is that it is a good idea, to help meet the nutritional guidelines set by AAFCO. However, it's probably more important to feed the excellent "dog cancer diet" – which is packed with vitamins and minerals, good fats, and naturally occurring anti-inflammatories – and use other supplements, such as Apocaps and mushroom-derived polysaccharides. If you feed a completely home-cooked meal for your dog, a general multi-vitamin that provides maintenance levels, not mega-doses, of antioxidants is a good idea.

HOW TO GIVE MULTIVITAMINS

Follow the dosing instructions on the label or follow your vet's recommendations. Some vitamins like A, D, E and K, are oil-soluble, which means that absorption is lower without some fat present. For this reason, I recommend giving multivitamins with food that contains some fat. Good fat choices include krill and fish oil (see the dog cancer diet in the next chapter). Please note that high fat diets are not appropriate for dogs with pancreatitis, so your vet may not want you to take this step. Always remember to consult with your vet about treatment steps.

Precautions

Any change in diet, new supplement, or new multivitamin can cause stomach upset (nausea, vomiting or diarrhea).

Modified Citrus Pectin

You may have heard of pectin, a natural compound found in plants like apples, plums and the peels of citrus fruits. Pectin has been powdered and used for centuries as a thickening agent in food, as a natural stabilizer in beverages and as a supplemental source of dietary fiber.

In its original form, pectin cannot be absorbed by the body. When it is slightly altered into what is called modified citrus pectin, it can enter the blood stream, bind the outside of spreading cells, and help keep them from attaching to the walls of blood vessels.

Studies have shown that modified citrus pectin can help block cancer cells from binding to their targets and keep them from metastasizing. It can also reduce angiogenesis, which may stop tumors from creating new blood vessels. In a study published in the Journal of the National Cancer Institute, mice with cancer experienced reduced tumor growth, less metastasis and less angiogenesis when they were given modified citrus pectin (MCP).

You can get MCP, in either powder or capsules, at health food stores or online at www.Dog-CancerShop.com.

The Bottom Line on Modified Citrus Pectin

While not as important as some other supplements, modified citrus pectin is a nice addition to your dog's diet because of its demonstrated anti-cancer effects.

HOW TO GIVE MODIFIED CITRUS PECTIN

Open the capsule(s) and mix the powder or gel into your dog's meal. If you are using powder, keep in mind that it is still a natural thickening agent, so it will turn into a gel as it gets wet. This is completely normal.

Capsules:

Note: If your dog is less than 35 pounds, you may have to open and divide capsule contents.

Under 10 lbs.: 200 mg per day, mixed into food, once daily

10.1-35 lbs.: 400 mg per day, mixed into food, once daily

35.1-60 lbs.: 800 mg per day, mixed into food, once daily

60 lbs. and over: 800 mg per day, mixed into food, twice daily (1,600 mg total)

Powder:

One heaping teaspoon is approximately 5 grams of powder. MCP is a safe supplement, so you can be approximate in your dosing.

Under 10 lbs.: ½ g powder, (just under half of a ¼ teaspoon) per day, mixed into food once daily

10.1-35 lbs.: 1 g per day, (just under ¼ teaspoon) mixed into food once daily

35.1-60 lbs.: 2 g per day, (just under a ½ teaspoon) mixed into food once daily

60 lbs. and over: 4 g per day, (just under a teaspoon) mixed into food twice daily

---

Precautions

Modified citrus pectin is a food product, included in many common foods, so side effects are very rare; even so, any dietary supplement or change in food can trigger upset stomach (nausea, vomiting and diarrhea).

Doxycycline

Doxycycline is a well-known antibiotic, which is why some vets scratch their heads when guardians mention it as a cancer treatment. It has been the subject of several cancer studies over the last decade. In addition to helping the immune system fight infections, doxycycline has been shown to block the activity of matrix metalloproteinases (MMPs). These enzymes are used by cancer cells to break down normal body tissue and make room for growth, so limiting their activity may help limit tumor growth. In fact, studies using mice show their tumors were reduced by about one-third when they were given doxycycline. Doxycycline has also been shown to help induce apoptosis in cancer cells.

Based on the available literature, doxycycline also may be most useful in helping to slow metastasis, particularly if there is bone involvement. Doxycycline can slow angiogenesis, which makes it harder for tumors to feed themselves or metastasize to distant locations.

There is an in vitro study, showing that doxycycline decreased sensitivity of breast cancer cells to chemotherapy, so be sure to discuss the pros and cons of its use with your veterinarian or oncologist. Doxycycline is a prescription drug, so you have to get it through your vet.

The Bottom Line on Doxycycline

Doxycycline is a nice addition to your Full Spectrum cancer care plan, particularly if there is bone involvement.

HOW TO GIVE DOXYCYCLINE

To give doxycycline as a cancer treatment, give 5 mg per kilogram of body weight, which is roughly 25 mg per 10 pounds of body weight, daily. I recommend giving it with food, to avoid stomach upset.

Using any antibiotic for a long period of time can cause complications later, because while it does kill bad bacteria, survivors can breed more germs resistant to the drug. For this reason, I suggest using doxycycline for no longer than two weeks at a time, with at least two weeks as a break in between cycles.

Precautions

The most common side effect is digestive upset (nausea, vomiting and diarrhea), especially when given on an empty stomach. See page 140 for detailed instructions on managing these side effects.

If your dog is on antacids, including Pepto Bismol, famotidine or cimetidine, do not give them at the same time as doxycycline, because they may decrease its absorption. Give doxycycline at least two hours before or after antacids.

Calcium can block the absorption of doxycycline, so I recommend avoiding cottage cheese, bones, calcium supplements or any other calcium-rich food when giving doxycycline.

Never give doxycycline to nursing or pregnant dogs. It can retard the development of the fetus' skeleton, and can be passed in the mother's milk. Young dogs given doxycycline sometimes experience yellowed teeth.

Chapter 14: Step Four, Diet

When cancer strikes, it can bring with it weight loss, muscle weakness and depression, all of which can lower your dog's quality of life. Luckily, there is a cancer treatment that can help improve all of these factors: eating good food.

Most dogs like food, and many crave a good diet – what I call a Wild Diet – as much as they crave sunshine and a walk outside. A good cancer diet, like the one described in this chapter, can accomplish several important tasks:

- Feed your dog's healthy cells foods dense with nutrition to keep them strong.
- Help restore weight and muscle mass.
- Eliminate foods that do not help your dog – or worse, may help the cancer.

In Chapter 8 we enumerated some of the carcinogens found in some commercially prepared dog foods, but carcinogens aren't the only problem. For example, protein that has been processed loses some bioavailability in the body. The bioavailability of key minerals, such as iron, zinc and calcium, is also significantly affected by the levels of fiber, phytic acid and tannin in foods. These substances can be reduced or altered by milling, fermentation, germination, extrusion and thermal (heat) processing. Vitamins, especially ascorbic acid, thiamin and folic acid, are also highly sensitive to some processing methods.

In this chapter, we'll explore food a little bit more, including what to include in your dog's diet, some important supplements that have not been fully discussed yet, how to switch your dog to his new diet, and my step-by-step approach to making a meal for a dog with cancer.

I have two pieces of good news for you. The first is that when you feed your dog according to this recipe, you are helping him immediately. The dog cancer diet is made up exclusively of foods that encourage healthy cells and discourage cancer growth.

The second piece of good news is that your dog is likely to love switching to this diet. It's composed of hu-

When you feed your dog according to this recipe, you are helping him immediately. The dog cancer diet is made up exclusively of foods that encourage healthy cells and discourage cancer growth.

man food, and most dogs like to eat tasty, lovingly prepared human food.

Let's get a quick overview of what dogs used to eat in the wild, because this Wild Diet is the basis for our dog cancer diet.

The Wild Diet

A dog's natural diet consists of protein, fat and some vegetables (usually not grains, like corn and wheat). We know this by looking at what dogs and their relatives eat in the wild.

Dogs and their wild cousins (wolves, coyotes, foxes, etc.) eat freshly killed animals, not highly processed kibble. They typically satisfy their wild cravings by hunting prey animals, like deer and rabbits. These prey animals feed on plants and grasses, which are naturally full of vitamins and minerals.

After the wolves take the prey down, their first target is the internal organs. These rich, meaty organs are filled with nutrients, derived from plant material. After devouring the organ meat, wolves tear into the flesh and bones as a second helping.

A dog with cancer often loses weight and becomes physically weak. Feeding him a good cancer diet, based on his wild cravings, may help counter some of those side effects.

In fact, according to human cancer research, including that done by Sir Richard Doll, a British epidemiologist (awarded Knighthood and several other honors for his work with cancer), about one third of cancers can be prevented just by improving the diet.

Raw Foods and Cancer

Some dog lovers believe that feeding their dogs only raw foods – raw meat, raw bones, raw vegetables – is closer to the healthy, "wild diet" I describe above.

I have no objection to a fresh, raw diet for healthy dogs with normal, non-cancerous body cells. After all, based on human studies, cooking food can create carcinogenic compounds, which could actually set the stage for cancer development (see Chapter 8).

Given this, it might seem logical to think that feeding raw – which reduces carcinogens – is good for a dog with cancer; it's not that simple.

In general, dogs suffering from cancer have completely different body chemistry from healthy dogs. They have compromised immune systems, too, so – no matter how counter-intuitive this may sound to "raw foodies" – an all-raw diet is actually not good for dogs with cancer. There are a couple of reasons for this.

First of all, it is fairly difficult for us modern-day humans to replicate a fresh kill in our dog's food bowl. Even the highest quality meats, veggies and fruits available in the supermarket, health food stores, and farmer's markets are not as fresh as a deer that has just been brought down by the pack.

———— • ————

An all-raw diet is actually not good for dogs with cancer.

———— • ————

Let's look at meat, for example. You probably have heard of microbes like E. coli (sometimes found in ground red meat). This and other microbes grow over time on the surface of just about any red meat, chicken, pork or fish product, even when it is sealed in plastic and then refrigerated for prolonged periods. The longer the time between killing the animal and eating it, the more likely these foods are to have large populations of surface microbes.

There's a second place that germs can hide out and multiply: inside the flesh of chicken, pork and fish. Salmonella and trichinella, as well as other parasites, can be found within the flesh of these foods (interestingly, beef carries very few microbes within it).

As you probably know, if these microbes are not killed during cooking, they can make dogs very sick. In healthy dogs, the immune system might be able to fend off the microbes; infections are more likely in dogs with cancer. This is why I recommend cooking your dog's food long enough to destroy microbes and minimize carcinogens.

Cooking Meat for Your Dog

We can minimize carcinogens by cooking with low temperatures, and only long enough to kill the microbes. It's been shown that when food is boiled (which happens at 212° Fahrenheit at sea level), almost no carcinogens are created. Raise the temperature above 390° Fahrenheit or so and we see the production of carcinogenic heterocyclic amines.

(There are many probable sources of carcinogens in your dog's life – so avoiding them when you can is reasonable. Avoiding carcinogens produced while cooking is one of the few things guardians can really control – which is why I include so much information about it in this book.)

To avoid even moderate levels of carcinogens, you can simmer food. This is the simplest way to guarantee that the temperature is not too high. Another benefit to simmering is that food becomes very tender and evenly cooked.

If you love to sauté food in a pan, you can do that, of course, keeping the temperature low. Because every stovetop is different, as is every pan, it is difficult for me to tell you "how low" on your particular stovetop. A food thermometer will tell you how hot your food has become.

Poultry, pork, fish and organ meats like liver must be cooked all the way through to kill microbes both inside and on the surface of the meat. Ground red meat of any kind must also be cooked all the way through, since the surface microbes are mixed into the interior of the meat in the grinding process.

A cut of red meat – like a beefsteak, for example – is a different matter. Since red meat rarely has microbes on the interior, you only need to cook the outer shell of the meat. Cooking the outer 1/8th inch leaves the interior still very pink or red (nearly raw, like it would be in the wild) but kills the surface microbes.

Preparing Vegetables for Your Dog

In the wild, vegetables have already been broken down inside the prey animal's digestive system before the wolf eats them. The internal organs are loaded with the nutrients, vitamins and minerals derived from the vegetables, in a form that the wolf can easily absorb into his body.

If you've ever fed your dog carrots or corn, you've likely noticed they "come out the other end," looking nearly intact. This is because the dog's gut doesn't break down intact vegetables easily. So, when you feed your dog completely raw veggies, he may not be extracting as much nutrition as he could be.

Cooking vegetables helps break down the plant matter and "pre-digest" it, so that your dog is better able to absorb all those essential vitamins, minerals and nutrients. Cook vegetables until they are very soft, and then chop or process them in a food processor into very small pieces.

If you want to feed raw vegetables instead, you can process them through a food processor or blender until they are a mushy puree, which can then be mixed into the rest of the meal. This way, the blender "pre-digests" the veggies by breaking them down.

Overfeeding and Cancer

I'm probably no different from most dog lovers when it comes to the temptation to feed table scraps to my dog, Björn, or give him extra food as a special treat. The problem is, when we feed by hand, we may feed too much without realizing it.

Overfeeding is not healthy for our dogs, because it shortens life expectancy. In one study, forty-eight Labrador Retrievers from four different litters were followed. Half of the dogs were fed a lot of food – as much as they could eat with no restriction – and the other half were fed 25% less.

The lifespan of the dogs on the restricted diet was significantly longer than that of the ones who ate at will. The dogs in the restricted group lived an average of two years longer than the excessively fed dogs, which is a long time in dog years.

Another study found that half of the dogs who were fed a restricted diet lived to the age of thirteen, while only five percent of dogs who ate as much as they wanted did. That's a tenfold increase in the number of dogs who lived to thirteen!

A large excess of body fat, or obesity, is also linked to cancer in dogs (mammary tumors and transitional cell carcinoma). The precise link is not yet completely defined; new research has shown that fat cells secrete a chemical called adiponectin, which may block the development of cancer cells. You may think that more fat cells produce *more* adiponectin, but the opposite is true. According to studies in rodents and humans, fat cells secrete much *less* adiponectin when the body has excess fat in storage, while secreting more adiponectin when the fat cells are being burned for fuel (which happens in leaner bodies). This means that a lean body has more adiponectin than an obese body, so a lean body may be more able to resist cancer.

Many guardians comfort their dogs with food. Others get very concerned about their dogs' cancer weight loss, and end up overcompensating with extra food. While I certainly understand the impulse, it is best to consult with your vet or oncologist about how much to feed your dog given all of the factors in her case.

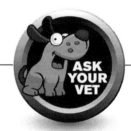

How much should you feed your dog? That's a complicated question, and there is no one-size-fits-all answer. Dogs with cancer vary so widely in their age, metabolism and stage that there is no chart or system we can turn to for feeding guidelines. If your dog has another disease or problem in addition to cancer, that may also affect how much to feed him. I offer general guidelines in the Dog Cancer Recipe section, which will give you an approximation of how much to feed your dog. If you have further questions, I recommend consulting with your vet to get an answer tailored to your dog's unique health situation.

Reduce Omega-6 Fatty Acids

Essential fatty acids, or EFAs, are molecular building blocks of fats and oils. The two main types are omega-3 fatty acids and omega-6 fatty acids. In addition to their being fuel for the body, the balance between these two fatty acids affects body functions such as inflammation, mood, behavior and intracellular communication.

According to researchers, the ideal ratio of omega-6 to omega-3 fatty acids is four to one. Our modern diets typically have ratios of ten to one, and some have ratios as high as sixteen to one.

The health consequences of this imbalance can be severe. Excessive omega-6 fatty acids have been associated with cardiovascular problems, arthritis, osteoporosis, depression, obesity and cancer, in humans. Excessive omega-6 fatty acids may result in immune suppression, and can activate several genes (up to a dozen) that create inflammation, which plays a significant role in cancer.

It's Really Quite Simple

"I now make food for both of my beautiful Black Labs. Once I got "in sync" with making the food, it is really quite simple. I make it in bulk, portion it out into containers and freeze it. I also make all of my girls' treats. I bought a $30 dehydrator and I dehydrate boneless, skinless chicken breast strips and brown rice mixed with all natural peanut butter. Feeding my pets in this fashion in something I will always do...it makes sense for all dogs!!"

– *Cynthia McKinnon, Sanford, Florida*

It's very important for your dog to eat the right balance of fatty acids. High omega-6 fatty acids are primarily found in corn and other vegetable oils and the fat of grain-fed animals. If you look at some commercial dog foods and treats, you may find these ingredients. Some of the most common ingredients are meat or meat by-product (which can include anything from bones to cartilage to entrails). The animals used in dog food are often farm-raised beef and poultry. If left to forage, cows would eat grass and chickens would eat insects, worms and seeds. Commercial operations, however, often feed these animals inexpensive grains like corn to keep expenses down, "fatten them up," and keep their flesh tender. Unfortunately for our dogs, this food increases the amount of omega-6 fatty acids in the meat.

On commercial dog food labels, fats like corn oil, vegetable oil and beef tallow are often listed. These are all rich in immunity-suppressing omega-6 fatty acids. In addition to minimizing the preservatives and carcinogens sometimes found in commercial dog food, this is one of the main reasons I urge you to cook for your dog at home.

Supplement with Omega-3 Fatty Acids

It's been shown conclusively that omega-3 fatty acids can help minimize the immune-suppressing and inflammatory effects of excess omega-6 fatty acids. Omega-3 fatty acids also protect against cancer cachexia (weight loss), been shown to help reduce depression and, in some cases, shrink tumors, in human studies.

Omega-3 fatty acids can be found in cold-water fish, such as sardines, mackerel and menhaden. They're also found in the tiny shrimp-like plankton, krill, which is an important food source for many whale species. Flax and some other seeds contain omega-3 fatty acids, although not the higher amounts of certain very beneficial types (DHA and EPA) that are found in fish and krill oils.

Deliberately reducing the presence of omega-6 fatty acids in your dog's diet, and increasing the amount of omega-3 fatty acids, is a cornerstone of the dog cancer diet. You'll find more specifics about how much and what kinds of oils to use later in this chapter.

Reduce Sugar

Cancer has a sweet tooth. Cancer cells prefer sugar to any other kind of food, including foods with a higher calorie count. Even before any actual signs of canine cancer begin, the metabolism of sugar in the body starts to change as cancer cells signal the liver to create more sugar. The increase in sugar favors the growth of developing cancers, which then send signals to release even more sugar – and so the cycle continues. Sugar both favors cancer development and continues to feed it once it has taken hold.

We've discovered that the way sugar is used by the body is a reliable indicator of the progression of cancer. Positron emission tomography (PET) scans are even used to detect human cancer in tissues by looking for sugar "hot spots."

Clearly, limiting sugar is an important step to take when your dog has cancer (I also recommend doing this for healthy dogs). Carbohydrates break down into sugars during digestion, and certain carbohydrates break down more quickly than others. Unfortunately, the first ingredient on most commercial dog food labels is often a high-carbohydrate food such as corn, corn meal, wheat or flour. These grain-based foods are cheaper than meat, which is probably the main reason they are used so often in dog food. Sadly, they don't just feed the dog; they may also feed the cancer. Some brands have recognized that high carbohydrate diets are not appropriate for dog wellness, and are producing low-carbohydrate foods.

The diet I recommend later on is a low-carbohydrate diet. The carbohydrates that are included are from low-glycemic grains that break down slowly, so there are no spikes in cancer fuel.

Weaning Your Dog to the Dog Cancer Diet

Whether your dog has cancer or not, it is advisable that any change in diet always be started slowly by gradually phasing out the old food as the new is added. Dogs can experience diarrhea, bloating, loss of appetite, vomiting, and other problems if their food is changed suddenly. Your patience will pay off.

The way to introduce these foods is over a long period, usually about two weeks. Every day, increase the amount of new food and decrease the amount of old food, tablespoon by tablespoon. If a small amount of diarrhea occurs, lessen the amount of the new food at the next meal un-

> ### Best Decision We've Made
>
> "[The dog cancer diet] has helped her tremendously. Olivia is full of life and energy. Her blood tests have come back normal. Overall it's been the best decision we've made."
>
> – *Margherita Ferlita, Surrey, England*

til the symptoms subside. Then try to increase it again in a few days. If problems still continue, or get worse, be sure to call your vet or oncologist.

After one week, your dog's ration will probably be half the dog cancer diet and half the previous food. After two weeks, your dog will probably be on the new dog cancer diet. If your dog has trouble adjusting, it might take a little longer.

The dog cancer diet is flexible, with several choices for ingredients, which can be mixed and matched according to your dog's taste. As you go, you might find your dog does not like something in particular, and you might have to try out several different combinations before you can find one your dog enjoys.

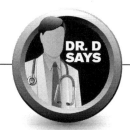

Remember the most important thing: eating something is better than not eating at all. If you have to choose between feeding your dog something less-than-healthy and starving your dog, choose the less-than-healthy food.

The Full Spectrum Dog Cancer Diet

The Full Spectrum dog cancer diet is mainly based on what dogs eat in their natural state in the wild. It also includes several foods that may help the body fight cancer or lessen the consequences of cancer in the body. You will likely recognize many of the ingredients, and, depending upon where you shop, most are relatively inexpensive. These ingredients can also be purchased in bulk or on sale, and frozen for later use.

If you already cook for yourself, shopping for and preparing your dog's food will take no more time than for any other meal. Because this recipe makes enough for two to four days' worth of food, you will not have to cook every day. If you do not cook, this may initially pose more of a challenge (well worth taking on); previous readers often report this home-cooked diet makes a big difference in the life quality and even the health of their dogs.

Mealtime is an excellent time to give your dog many of the supplements I recommend. A detailed recipe follows; before I tell you how to make your dog's meal, I want to go over the general guidelines for this diet.

Dog Cancer Diet Guidelines

Try to include at least one ingredient from each of the following categories at every meal. Don't worry about memorizing all of this information right now. I will tell you how to combine these

---

Previous readers often report this home-cooked diet makes a big difference in the life quality and even the health of their dogs.

---

ingredients, and in what amounts, in the Recipe section.

At Every Meal: High Quality Lean Protein

Protein is a very important component of your dog's cancer diet. For one thing, dogs love the flavor of most proteins, and that encourages them to eat. Protein is also a dense source of amino acids, vitamins and minerals. The following are good choices for protein: beef, chicken, fish, turkey, venison, duck, pork, goat and lamb. The exception is if your dog has mammary cancer; if this is the case do not feed her red meat, because it has been shown to be a risk factor for tumors of this type. Offer her white meats, including fish and chicken, instead.

Buy lean cuts of meat (chicken breasts instead of thighs, for example), because the fat in most animal flesh contains more omega-6 fatty acids than I recommend for a dog with cancer. Trim skin or fat off the meat before you cook it. After cooking, remove fat by pouring it out of the pan or straining.

Don't worry about losing flavor with the fat; you'll add cancer-fighting omega-3 fats later on and there are several non-carcinogenic flavor-boosters in the recipe section.

At Every Meal: Cancer-Fighting Fats and Oils

Excess omega-6 fatty acids suppress the immune system; supplementing with additional omega-3 fatty acids can offset this effect. Omega-3 fatty acids can also help to offset the effects of inflammation in your dog's body. I recommend two sources.

The two recommended sources of omega-3 fatty acids are krill oil and fish oil (my favorite picks are available at www.DogCancerShop.com). Pick one of these oils, use it for three to four weeks, and then switch to the other, alternating oils throughout the treatment. There are many brands of fish and krill oil; when choosing one, the most important factor to pay attention

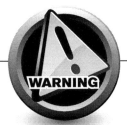

Some people suggest that tofu be used as a protein substitute. I do not recommend tofu, because most dogs do not digest it very well. When your dog is fighting cancer, anything that unnecessarily strains her system is best left off the menu. The value of tofu as a protein does not outweigh its digestive difficulties for a significant number of dogs.

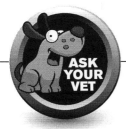

If your dog has a pancreatic disease, a "sensitive stomach," or other digestive issues, your veterinarian may alter portions of this diet, as high levels of fat in the diet may worsen such a condition.

to is the level of DHA and EPA available. For maximum benefits, try to find good concentrations of these in the formula. Formulations are constantly changing, of course, so it's hard for me to give you the "correct" concentrations, because what's on the shelf today may be reformulated tomorrow. A good guideline, however, is this: for every 1000 mg serving of oil, about 180 mg should be EPA (18%) and 120 mg should be DHA (12%). Most fish oils are in this range.

Krill oil comes from krill, the tiny shrimp that are the primary source of food for whales. I like krill oil for several reasons. Krill are near the bottom of the food chain; fish higher on the chain live longer and their fatty tissues tend to accumulate heavy metals like lead, some of which are carcinogens (most, but not all, of these are removed from fish oil). There is also evidence that krill oil, taken in high doses over time, may help with depression in humans. There is more evidence for this effect with krill oil than fish oils. We know from human studies, that depression and cancer are linked, so efforts to fight depression in dogs are logical. Finally, living on Maui makes me acutely aware that the oceans are getting overfished.

HOW TO GIVE KRILL OIL

Krill oil typically comes in 1,000 mg soft gel capsules. To feed it to your dog, just mix the whole capsule into food, or cut the capsules at one end with a pair of kitchen shears and gently squeeze the oil into the food, mixing thoroughly. If your dog can swallow softgels whole, feed your dog krill oil this way.

The sudden introduction of fatty acids can cause stomach upset and diarrhea, so work up to a full dosage over about fourteen days.

Up to 10 pounds: 1,000-2,000 mg daily

Dogs 10.1 - 35 pounds: 3,000-4,000 mg daily

Dogs 35.1-60 pounds: 6,000-9,000 mg daily

Over 60.1 pounds: 10,000-12,000 mg daily

Note that the doses are given in a range. This is because there are so many brands, which each formulate the oil in different ways. Use these doses as guidelines, rather than hard-and-fast rules. Alternate the use of krill and fish oil every month.

Precautions:

Krill oil may have some "blood thinning" effects. Stop giving krill oil ten days before any surgery and wait until ten days after surgery or after sutures are removed or dissolved, before giving it again. Also, allergic reactions to shellfish or fish are rare, but possible. Immediately stop use and consult your vet if you think your dog is having an allergic reaction.

The second oil rich in omega-3 fatty acids, which I recommend, is fish oil (from menhaden, mackerel, salmon, etc.). The effects of fish oil are generally similar to those of krill oil. It's more readily available and usually cheaper than krill oil, which may be important to some guardians. However, fish oil also shows less evidence for impact on depression. There used to be some concern about the heavy metal levels in fish oil, but today name brand fish oils have lowered these to allowable levels.

HOW TO GIVE FISH OIL

Administer fish oil in the same way you administer krill oil. For these doses, I assume each 1,000 mg soft gel contains about 180 mg of EPA and 120 mg of DHA. Check the label on your bottle to see if this is true for your brand and adjust accordingly. Remember to work your way up to these dosages over fourteen days if you are just starting your dog on a fatty acid supplement.

Up to 10 pounds: 1,000-2,000 mg daily

Dogs 10.1 - 35 pounds: 3,000-4,000 mg daily

Dogs 35.1-60 pounds: 6,000-9,000 mg daily

Over 60.1 pounds: 10,000-12,000 mg daily

Note that the doses are given in a range. This is because there are so many brands, which each formulate the oil in different ways. Use these doses as guidelines, rather than hard-and-fast rules. Alternate the use of krill and fish oil every month.

Precautions:

Fish oil may have some blood thinning effects. Stop giving fish oil ten days before any surgery and wait until ten days after surgery or after sutures are removed or dissolved before giving it again.

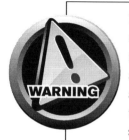

I do not recommend cod liver oil as your fish oil supplement. Cod liver oil contains high levels of fat-soluble vitamins, ingestion of which can lead to serious toxicity levels. I discourage using salmon oil from the name brand EHP, also. In an independent analysis, Consumer Labs found that EHP's salmon oil actually contains less EPA than stated on the label. Since EPA is such an important source of omega-3 fatty acid, there's no excuse to skimp. Other brands of salmon oil are fine to use.

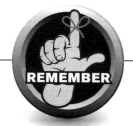

At Every Meal: Vegetables

Vegetables which are low in carbohydrates and have anti-cancer benefits are an important part of your dog's cancer diet. For example, brightly colored vegetables are important: at least one publication has shown that dogs (Scotties) that ate colored vegetables three times weekly had a lower risk of developing the most common form of bladder cancer. You can mix and match these vegetables or just include one in each meal: shiitake mushrooms, brussels sprouts, broccoli, cauliflower, cabbage, (cooked) mung beans and red or yellow bell peppers.

I prefer fresh vegetables, or you can find

REMEMBER

Stay away from high-carbohydrate vegetables like potatoes, carrots, peas and corn. These vegetables break down quickly into simple sugars in the body and may end up feeding the cancer. Also, do not feed onions, because they are toxic for dogs.

these vegetables in the frozen food section. To prepare them, steam or boil until they are very soft to make them easy for your dog to digest. Once cooked, chop or process the vegetables into fine pieces or a puree.

If you are choosing to feed your dog a partially raw diet, I advise pureeing raw veggies. Roughly chop the vegetables, place them in the bowl of a food processor, and puree them until they are mush. This will help your dog fully absorb their nutrients.

At Every Meal: Calcium

Your dog will definitely benefit from a good source of calcium, which is a vital mineral for all sorts of normal body functions. Bones and teeth need calcium, of course, and did you know that your dog's muscles can't contract without it? Similarly, muscle strength, proper blood clotting, regular heartbeats, inter-cell communication and even the transmission of signals from one nerve

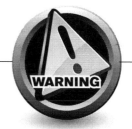

WARNING

Do not give the anti-cancer antibiotic doxycycline within two hours of a meal containing calcium. The calcium will bind the doxycycline in the stomach and block its absorption.

to another are all vital processes that require calcium. Because dogs cannot produce it in their bodies, they must get it from their diet. Good sources of calcium include cottage cheese, chicken or turkey necks and calcium citrate tablets. The necks can be simmered according to the low-temperature cooking recommendation above. Adding necks at least a few times a week is ideal, because the phosphorus found in the bones is an important nutrient.

Bone meal has a lot of calcium, but, there is evidence that the bones ground into meal have accumulated fluoride, which, as you'll remember, is something we may want to avoid in a body that is fighting cancer (based on the human studies of osteosarcoma). Additionally, I advise avoiding oyster shell calcium, which may have high lead levels (a carcinogen).

At Every Meal: Filling and Nutritious Whole Grains

Most grains, like corn and wheat, are not good for your dog with cancer because they provide too much sugar. However, brown rice and oatmeal are both healthy and filling, and there are advantages to adding small amounts to your dog's diet. The polysaccharides found in the bran in these grains may help to fight cancer. They are also much lower on the glycemic index, which means that they release lower levels of the simple sugars that cancer loves into the bloodstream.

Choose steel-cut or rolled oats over instant oats. Cook oats and brown rice according to the package instructions, until soft. Add these cooked grains individually or in combination

I Had to Keep My Human Family from Eating Her Food

"I was scared that she would get a sore tummy and have diarrhea to try differently. I tried your suggestions. Pre-packing then freezing it made it easy to heat and serve. It looked so good; I had to label the packages so my human family wouldn't eat it by mistake. Kristi never lost her appetite while on this diet and her stool would be a little softer but still formed."

– *Lois Boesing, Ewa Beach, Hawaii*

She Eats Like a Horse

"Sadie has allergies so at first I was worried about adapting it, but the book is so easy to understand and I got ideas I'd never thought of. Sadie is looking and acting so much better and loves her new diet. She had pretty much stopped eating her premium dog food (grain free fish and sweet potato) and even showed little interest in the homemade stuff I had been making, but the combination of foods in the cancer diet has her eating like a horse and I think she might even be regaining some weight."

- *Ellen Slater, Redmond, Oregon*

in the recipe that follows.

At Every Meal: A Dog Multivitamin

Even though this home-cooked diet provides well-rounded nutrition, it's a good idea to be safe and make sure that all of your dog's dietary vitamin and mineral needs are met. For this reason, I recommend giving a general multivitamin along with completely home-cooked meals. An added bonus for dogs dealing with cancer is that, based on human studies, a multivitamin may help with chemotherapy side effects and speed recovery post-treatment.

As I've made clear elsewhere, I do not recommend mega-doses of any vitamin or mineral. A general multivitamin you can get from your vet or oncologist will do just fine, and you can give it as directed.

At Every Meal: Optional Healthy Additions

These ingredients add flavor to your dog's meal, but they also pack it with cancer-fighting, immune-boosting properties.

You can add: fresh garlic cloves (peeled and minced); fresh ginger root (peeled and minced); fresh minced leafy herbs like parsley, basil and oregano; virgin coconut oil; sardines packed in oil (minced); goji (wolf) berries; fresh blueberries; fresh raspberries and fresh blackberries.

Digestive Enzymes

I strongly suggest using digestive enzymes in your dog's food. Dogs in the wild get their plant matter "pre-digested" for them by their prey. Adding digestive enzymes to your dog's food to pre-digest both mimics a wild diet and helps cancer patients in general. There are several good enzyme preparations available. Brands I particularly recommend include Dr. Goodpet and Wobenzym N, a popular European brand. Both can be found online and at www.DogCancerShop.com.

Precautions: Digestive enzymes may have "blood-thinning" effects. Stop giving digestive enzymes ten days before any surgery and wait until ten days after surgery or after sutures are removed

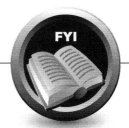

The dosing instructions on enzyme labels assume that you will use enzymes between meals. Using digestive enzymes to pre-digest food like we are doing requires many more enzymes than a regular dose. If you are using Dr. Goodpet, I recommend using three times the label's dose per meal. If you are using Wobenzym N, I recommend using two times the label's dose per meal. Dr. Goodpet comes in a powder form and Wobenzym N comes in tablets. Please grind tablets into powder before mixing into food, so that the enzymes can contact the entire mixture. If you don't have a little mortar and pestle or a pill grinder, you can use two spoons to mash the tablets.

Note: Some guardians ask about giving their dog digestive enzymes in between meals. There is fair evidence that enzymes used between meals have an anti-inflammatory effect, but the evidence that they have anti-cancer actions is not there. For this reason, using enzymes between meals is not a priority in Full Spectrum care.

Half the Food Is Cancer Diet

"I feed Orijen, some can food (Wellness and BC) I add in the diet supplement in Dr. Dressler's book along with added (Birkdale) omega-3 fatty acids. The home cooked meals in Dr. Dressler's book accounts for 1/2 of each meal. All combined I know that it has helped greatly, my boxers look great and I know they feel great."

– Jon Marshall, Norman, Oklahoma

Increased Well-Being and Life Span

"I think that Dr. Dressler's dog diet with his home cooked foods, plus the Omega-3 oils increased Thor's wellbeing and also most definitely increased his lifespan."

- Connie Almy,
San Antonio de Belen, Costa Rica

or dissolved before giving it again.

Salt Substitutes

While adding salt to food typically enhances its flavor, normal table salt (also known as sodium chloride) could theoretically promote cancer cell development by creating a slightly acid environment in the body. Instead of salt, you can use a salt substitute called potassium chloride, which you can find in most grocery stores or online. (If your dog has a disorder where there is high blood potassium such as uncontrolled Addison's disease, occasional instances of kidney disease, or other issues creating high blood potassium, do not use salt substitutes.)

Another way to add flavor is to use a splash of Bragg's Liquid Aminos (be very sparing – this is concentrated), balsamic vinegar, or watered down pan juice from the cooked meats. You could also use a little of the water that canned tuna is packed in.

The Full Spectrum Dog Cancer Diet Recipe

Now that we've gone over the ingredients for your Full Spectrum Dog Cancer Diet, let's mix and match and put them together into a meal that tastes good.

The recipe that follows provides about four days of meals for your fifty-pound dog, who eats twice a day, depending on her activity level and metabolism. If your fifty-pound dog is very active, this may only last two days. If your fifty-pound dog is not a big eater, it could last four days. You may scale this recipe up or down, depending upon your dog's weight. For example, if your dog weighs 25 pounds, cut this recipe in half; if your dog weighs 100 pounds, double it.

A small kitchen scale can be very helpful. Some of the ingredients need to be cooked before you weigh and assemble them in this recipe.

This recipe has several steps, so I recommend reading all the way through, before you start cooking. Most of the food can be prepared and combined all at once into what I call the Base Mixture. Assuming the ingredients are not close to expiring, this can be stored in the refrigerator for up to four days.

Do not chop or mix in the optional ingredients until you are actually serving the meal to your dog. This is to preserve their freshness and active ingredients. The digestive enzymes will be added last, mixed in thoroughly, and allowed to work for thirty minutes before serving.

Once you have done this a few times, a rhythm will develop and it will be easy and less time-consuming.

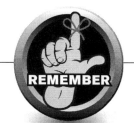

Krill oil, fish oil, garlic, ginger and digestive enzymes all have blood-thinning effects. Do not feed these foods ten days before any surgery and wait until ten days after surgery or after sutures are removed or dissolved before feeding them again.

Base Mixture Ingredients:

- 2½ to 3 pounds[7] of lean meat: beef, chicken, fish, turkey, venison, duck, pork, goat or lamb

- 1½ cups oatmeal, or 1¼ cups brown rice

- ½ – ¾ pounds of any combination: shiitake mushrooms, brussels sprouts, broccoli, cauliflower, cabbage, mung beans and red or yellow bell peppers.

- ½ – ⅔ pounds beef, chicken or pork liver

- 1 to 1½ cups cottage cheese

- 8 skinless chicken or turkey necks, or calcium citrate tablets

- (optional) ¾ teaspoon salt substitute or other flavorful addition: Bragg's Liquid Aminos, balsamic vinegar, pan juices from the meats or a little tuna water

- 16,000–18,000 mg of fatty acids in the form of krill or fish oil, depending upon the size of your dog and her activity level

Healthy Options to Add Before Serving:

These can be added as available and desired. All amounts are for one serving of food.

- 1 teaspoon minced fresh garlic[8]

- 1-2 teaspoons minced fresh ginger root

---

[7] All measurements are standard in the U.S.

[8] There is evidence that large amounts of garlic (½ teaspoon per pound body weight) causes problems in the red blood cell of dogs. I am not concerned about this for the majority of dogs, because the amount of garlic in this recipe is extremely low compared to the amounts used in the study. However, if your dog has anemia, check with your veterinary professional before giving garlic.

- 1 teaspoon minced fresh berries (goji, blueber-ries, raspberries, blackberries)
- ½ tablespoon virgin coconut oil
- 1-2 teaspoons minced fresh leafy herbs (parsley, basil and/or oregano)
- 1 oil-packed sardine, chopped
- Digestive enzyme powder (see note on page 207 for amounts)

Step One: Base Mixture

If you are using digestive enzymes to pre-digest your dog's food, you will need to add them when the food is at rool temperature or cooler. To give it time to cool down, I recommend making the Base Mixture well before you plan on feeding your dog. Until you figure out how long this takes you, I would al-low at least ninety minutes for cooking, assembling and cooling the food to room temperature.

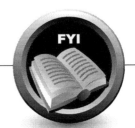

Garlic offers some evidence for anti-cancer effects, which are seen with garlic constituents found in higher amounts in the whole, fresh version. These tend to become in-activated when prepared in capsule form. I recommend adding garlic to your dog's diet, not the capsules. See page 420 for more informa-tion.

Trim your chosen meat of excess fat, and then cook it. My favorite method is to simmer meat in water or low-sodium chicken or beef broth, but you can also use a skillet on the stovetop (use very little fat and monitor the temperature – if you cover the skillet, you will cook the food more evenly). If you are using fresh red meat like beef, lamb, venison or goat, cook the outer 1/8" only to retain the benefits of the raw meat, while killing off any surface microbes. Cook pork, fish, ground meat of any kind, and poultry all the way through. Pour off or strain any fat after cooking (this is particularly important with duck). Chop or food process meat into smaller-than-bite-size pieces.

Meanwhile, cook the liver and turkey or chicken necks (if using). You may be able to cook them in the same pan as the meat, depending upon what method of cooking you are using. Chicken and turkey necks are best skinned and trimmed of fat, and then simmered and chopped or food processed. Even though the fat in liver is desirable and contains beneficial vitamins, some dogs may experience digestive upset from too much fat. For this reason, I recommend chopping the liver before you cook it, to increase surface cooking area and reduce the amount of fat it contributes to the recipe. Remem-ber to skim off excess fat or strain the meat before using it.

Meanwhile, cook oats or brown rice until soft, according to package directions.

Cook your vegetables, according to the package directions, or, if fresh, preferably by steaming

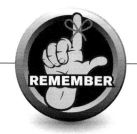

Do not add any of the fresh optional additions to this Base Mixture. Also, do not add the digestive enzymes. It is better to wait until you serve the food to chop and add these ingredients.

or simmering in water, until they are soft. After cooking, chop the vegetables into small pieces, or use a food processor or blender. If you prefer raw vegetables, puree them until mushy. Note: mung beans must always be cooked.

In a large bowl, add the meat, liver, and if used, chicken or turkey necks. Mix well with a spoon or with your clean hands. (When you put your hands in your dog's meal, you are also adding your scent and associating yourself with the food.)

Add brown rice or oatmeal. Mix well.

Add vegetables into the meat and grain mixture. Mix well.

In another large bowl, mix together the cottage cheese, salt substitute and fatty acids (krill or fish oil). Some dogs will eat the capsules of krill oil or fish oil whole, while others will need the capsules opened and emptied into the mixture.

If you are using calcium citrate instead of chicken necks, grind the tablets with a mortar and pestle, or other grinding implement. (I have calculated the correct dosage for the brand I use, Citracal Maximum, as twelve tablets). Add to the cottage cheese mixture. Mix well.

Add cottage cheese mixture to the meat/rice/vegetable mixture. Mix thoroughly.

For flavor, consider adding a splash of Bragg's Liquid Aminos, balsamic vinegar or a little of the pan juices from the cooked meats or water from canned tuna.

Store entire mix in an airtight container in the refrigerator for up to four days. Use as needed, twice a day.

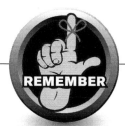

If you use a commercial dog food as part of this recipe, keep it to one quarter to one half (¼–½) of the overall portion. I particularly recommend Halo foods, although other good choices might be found in dehydrated and frozen dog foods. Add the commercial food in Step Two, when you add the supplements and the enzymes and scale down the helpings of homemade food in proportion to how much commercial food you are using.

Step Two: Healthy Options at Meal Time

Start this step about forty-five minutes before mealtime to allow for prepping and assembling ingredients and letting the digestive enzymes work.

Dish out a portion of the Base Mixture appropriate for your dog.

Depending upon which healthy options you are adding to your dog's meal, mince garlic, ginger, berries, herbs, and sardine. Add them to the serving and mix well. If using, add the coconut oil and mix well.

This is a good time to add any supplements or vitamins that can be served with meals, including the multi-vitamin. Grind tablets into powders using a mortar and pestle, and, if needed, open capsules. Add all to the serving. You can also add pills and capsules whole, if your dog will swallow them that way (just make sure they are gone at the end of the meal).

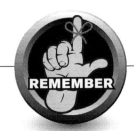

If your dog is using Apocaps, give them on an empty stomach between mealtimes (at least an hour before or after, but preferably four hours before or after), as the label recommends. The same advice applies for artemisinin. See page 170 for details on how to schedule these supplements. You can use the Base Mixture as the snack for her supplements.

Mix the digestive enzyme powder into the food, using the dosages recommended in the sidebar on page 207. Heat can inactivate the digestive enzymes, so if the food is hot, cool to room temperature or below (you can put it back in the refrigerator for a few minutes), before you stir them in. Mix very well to distribute the enzymes evenly throughout the food. Allow the food to sit for at least 30 minutes at room temperature (or slightly cooler) to let the enzymes pre-digest it.

After thirty minutes of pre-digestion, give your dog his meal.

NOTE: If you are giving Apocaps or artemisinin with the meal (for example, if your dog has a sensitive stomach), open the capsules and add the powder to the meal *after* the enzymes have worked for thirty minutes. Remember to mix well before feeding your dog.

Meal Time

When you feed your dog, make sure to take at least a moment or two to enjoy your dog while she enjoys her meal. As we've discovered, your attitude, mood and emotions may impact your dog's attitude, mood and emotions. In turn, her mood and emotions may impact her ability to heal. High quality moments like sharing an enjoyable meal cement the bond between the two of you, and feeling your love and enjoyment is very important for your dog while she deals with cancer. Leave the dishes for when she's finished.

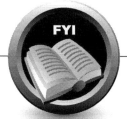

Cancer Diets for Other Health Issues

If your dog has disease or damage of the liver, kidneys, pancreas or any other organ or bodily system, the diet outlined in this chapter may need to be modified.

For example, if your dog has a liver issue, the relatively high amounts of fat in this diet may need to be reduced. If your dog is allergic to dairy, you won't be able to feed him cottage cheese. Everything depends upon your individual dog's health.

This diet is ideal for most dogs with cancer. If your dog cannot tolerate an ingredient or it isn't good for her, or if your vet tells you not to feed it, exclude it. I have included as many healthy options as possible, so that you can find a way to give your dog a balanced diet, even if you can't do absolutely everything I recommend.

I recommend you consult with your veterinarian directly. Go over the diet and get her feedback about what to include and exclude.

Chapter 15: Step Five, Brain Chemistry Modification

"I just want her to feel better," guardians tell me, "because as long as she's still happy and wags her tail, I know she's OK."

Preserving your dog's happiness – and increasing it as much as possible – is the fifth step in Full Spectrum cancer care. Once you've taken care of your dog's physical needs with conventional treatments, apoptogens, immune-boosters and an excellent diet, it's time to turn your attention to optimizing her brain chemistry.

The treatments in this chapter may seem "out there" or even a little frivolous when compared to "big gun" therapies and important supplements; they are not.

According to research conducted in humans and lab animals, stress may reduce the activity of cancer-fighting cells, such as natural killer cells and cytotoxic T-cells, not only diminishing the number of these cancer fighters, but their effectiveness at finding and killing cancer cells. Stress can also increase angiogenesis (blood vessel creation) in tumors, allowing them to grow faster. Some lab studies even show that stress hormones directly stimulate cancer cells. Reducing stress is not just a nice idea – it's crucial for cancer care.

One of the clearest studies I found in my research involved 826 women with breast cancer, each of whom was surveyed about her loneliness, marital contentment, life changes and emotional repression. The researchers then ranked each respondent, from most depressed

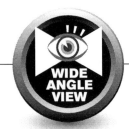

Psychoneuroimmunology

The scientific field of study called psychoneuroimmunology explores the intimate connections between brain chemistry (psychiatry and neurology), immunology and physiology. This interdisciplinary field looks at how our mental and emotional states directly impact our health. Experts in this field are currently studying many of the strategies in this chapter.

to least depressed, and compared the results with the severity of their cancers. Surprisingly (or maybe not so surprisingly), the more repressed, depressed and lonely a woman was, the more severe her cancer.

Humans are social creatures – and so are our dogs. If humans with cancer benefit from support, companionship and esteem-building exercises, dogs do, too. I consider these exercises essential. To my knowledge, this treatment has not been deliberately applied to dogs with cancer; it's time to change that, because ignoring the body-mind connection is a mistake.

To my knowledge, this treatment has not been deliberately applied to dogs with cancer; it's time to change that, because ignoring the body-mind connection is a mistake.

Based on what we know from human and lab animals, many negative mental states could weaken your dog's ability to fight cancer. Depression, loneliness, repressed emotions (or lack of an emotional outlet), low self-esteem and stress may impair your dog's body. If you can help your dog ease these emotions and replace them with ease, relaxation, connection, contentment and even joy, you may get an edge on cancer. The strategies outlined in this chapter tap into your dog's instinctive drives, which are likely connected with brain chemistry, physiology and the immune system.

When My Wife Isn't Looking …

TRUE TAILS

"Angus gets a couple of walks per day. Mostly what he looks forward to is walking by, and in, the ocean in the morning. He's got a "sister", Maggie, to hang out with during the day. We play fetch with his stuffed monkey for short periods, but don't press it for fear of an accidental injury to his remaining rear leg. He gets massages and, when my wife isn't looking, energy therapies (the few times she's seen me do this, she rolls her eyes and asks me what planet I came from)."

– *Al Marzetti, Raleigh, North Carolina*

Exercise

Daily physical movement can "burn off" stress and provide your dog with a dependable outlet for excess emotions and energy. Exercise may also help build muscles, wasted from cancer or cancer treatments, and improve the immune system's function. Exercising with your dog has the added benefit of giving him time with you, which makes it a social activity that decreases loneliness. Daily exercise helps dog to sleep better, which can increase melatonin levels, and, out in the fresh air and sunshine, your dog's body is stimulated to make the hormonal form of vitamin D.

Most dogs are used to taking walks outside, and this is a wonderful form of exercise for a dog with cancer; you don't need to create a track star. Get your dog walking; he may not be able to walk down the block, but he might be able to walk around the room.

Walking isn't the only way to move. Depending upon his physical condition, personality, and disposition, he could jog with you, run while you bike, swim, sprint, chase a ball, play with his toys, wrestle or fetch. Even yowling or barking can burn off steam. Getting dogs moving can help a lot, even if they can't do what they used to.

It may sound kind of silly, but even climbing a short flight of stairs can feel like an accomplishment. Aiming for that top stair can give a dog a sense of purpose, get his blood pumping and make him feel good about reaching the top.

No matter which form of exercise you try, the key will be to start out gradually. If your dog is a couch potato, a five-mile walk could overwhelm him. Start with a manageable amount of exercise, and then gradually increase it, a little every week. Consistency and routine is more important than the length of time you spend exercising. For example, a ten-minute walk in the morning and another ten-minute walk in the evening are better than one half-hour walk, once a day, and five minutes of exercise is better than no exercise at all.

Dogs like routine and they also like surprises. Switch exercise activities once in a while to keep mind and body stimulated.

Not every dog can handle a lot of exercise, and some dogs with cancer are truly limited in their mobility. If that applies to your dog, there are several things you can do to improve his circulation and burn off some steam (see the sidebar).

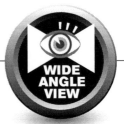

Stimulation for Dogs with Reduced Mobility

There are many ways to get your dog to move without his having to move, himself.

Assisted Movement: Help your dog along by using a harness or a towel slung under the belly. (See www.DogCancerShop.com for mobility aids.)

Physical Therapy. To increase blood flow and help with general stiffness, repeatedly and slowly flex and extend every joint in your dog's legs. Spend about three minutes on each limb before moving on to the next.

Grooming. Gentle brushing with a soft-bristled brush stimulates the skin and feels relaxing for your dog. If he doesn't like brushes, you can use your fingers to give a thorough and gentle pet.

continued on next page

Stimulation for Dogs with Reduced Mobility, *continued*

Warmth. Applying low heat can increase blood flow and relieve stiffness, and is especially useful if your dog is thin or old. Soak a washcloth in warm (not hot) water and apply it to the low back, hips, knees, shoulders and elbows. You can also use hot water bottles (make sure the water is warm, not hot). Another option is to buy a pillow designed to be heated in the microwave to gentle warmth. Always test the temperature on your own skin before you apply anything to your dog's skin or fur. If it's too hot to keep on your own skin, it's definitely too hot to keep pressed to your dog's. I do not recommend electric heating pads or blankets, because skin can burn if the elements are not padded adequately or if they get wet.

Fresh Air and Sunshine. Just getting outside in the breeze and sunshine can feel good to your dog. Take a meandering ride in the car or move his bed out onto the porch. One client bought a playpen and set it up on her back porch, then carried her dog out to rest comfortably in the fresh air. Even opening a window can help. At my hospital, I bring all my patients outdoors, regardless of their age or mobility, because I see an immediate lift in their mood.

Play Dates

We know from human studies that feelings of isolation worsen cancer outcomes, so I propose using this information to help our dogs.

Dogs can get lonely, especially when they're the only dog in the house. Most feel a natural instinct to congregate with other dogs, and satisfying this need is not only a life quality booster, it may even be considered a cancer treatment. Social connection decreases loneliness and stress, especially when it is pleasant.

Arrange play dates with other dogs you think will be compatible with your dog. For example, if you have a slow, slightly deaf, elderly lady, she might not want to deal with a bouncy, barky puppy or a large and athletic German Shepherd. Your dog should be able to hold her own with her friend, without getting intimidated, overwhelmed or physically overpowered. It is a good idea to start with one easygoing dog and invite more friends later.

If your dog does not enjoy the company of other dogs, she may enjoy meeting other people. Have your friends over, especially if they are dog lovers. Playing, walking and even cuddling with other humans can be therapeutic for a dog with cancer.

Training

Just like people, most dogs like to have jobs and tasks to complete. Training engages your dog's mind and emotions and builds self-esteem. Remember, self-esteem does not come from unearned praise – it comes from facing a challenge and overcoming it. Getting a reward, in the form of a healthy treat or lavish praise, is even better.

While a full agility training program is not appropriate for a dog with cancer, responding to simple commands like Sit, Stay, Come, Speak, Shake, Fetch, Roll Over and others, can build self-esteem and connection between the two of you. Even five minutes a day can help your dog feel productive and happy.

If it's been years since your dog went to puppy kindergarten, you might want to pick up a copy of a good book on low-key dog training. I recommend Tamar Geller's book, **The Loved Dog.**

Keep in mind that you are not training for your own benefit, but simply to give your dog a chance to manage a challenge and receive abundant, lavish praise. Your enthusiasm and excitement can make your dog feel like he has just won a gold medal, which will help elevate his life quality and may even help him fight his cancer.

It's a Shame to Assume He's Not Up for It!

"Exercise every day is a must, and enjoyed by all. If one dog doesn't have high stamina every day, he does what he can and thoroughly enjoys it. We simply roll the ball closer rather than throwing it far, and let him walk while the others run around. It's totally accepted, never seen to be a sad thing, and I can tell he enjoys it as much as ever. It would be a true shame to not go out because I assume he's not up to it. We mediate or just stay quiet together a lot. Touching, singing to him, sending boundless love and joy to him has benefitted us all."

- Susan Harper,
High Wycombe, England

Manageable Challenges

Sometimes just doing something new can make you feel good. You may remember the joy and pride you felt as a child, when you mastered tying your shoes or riding your bike. These were manageable challenges that your parents knew you could meet and overcome.

You can come up with your own list of manageable challenges for your dog, and every once in a while encourage him to master one. Walking in a new area is a manageable challenge, as is going up stairs, learning to roll over for a belly rub or learning to shake paws. When your dog overcomes a manageable challenge, give her abundant praise!

Joys of Life

Every dog is unique in her appreciation of life. Some dogs love to run fast, while others love to chase balls. Some would rather cuddle on your lap than take a walk and others love to swim. Whatever makes your dog feel uniquely happy is what I call a *joy of life*. You probably already know

Ellie Led Me to a New Healing Ability

"When we got the diagnosis of splenic hemangiosarcoma for our golden doodle Ellie, I dove into learning as much as possible about any and every treatment option. I already had experience with the power of prayer, meditation and visualization but I had never heard of Reiki (a form of light-touch/energy therapy). I was so intrigued. There was just something about it that sounded so powerfully comforting. Now, thanks to Ellie, I am a Reiki teacher and practitioner - for pets and people. All of my dogs benefit from Reiki treatments with increased relaxation and decreased pain & stress. I hear the same reports from people. My elderly arthritic dog has a way of nestling into my hands whenever he wants a Reiki session - he and Ellie used to share Reiki sessions together and their moods and bodies always seemed lighter afterward. One of the greatest gifts I received from Reiki was its calming effects when it was finally time for Ellie to cross-over. In the midst of that very difficult decision, the presence of positive Reiki energy helped me know I was doing all I could for Ellie's well-being. Reiki also helps me know that Ellie and I continue to be connected in energy and spirit."

– Sarah N. Bertsch,
Hudson, Wisconsin

what your dog's joys are, and I encourage you to view those joys as opportunities to treat her cancer. Make a list of her joys and make sure that she gets them on a regular basis.

Sometimes we can't provide a joy, the way we once could. For example, a dog who once adored running on the beach, who is no longer able to romp, may enjoy sitting on a towel and sniffing the salty breeze. Whatever your dog's joy is, indulge it as much as you can. While you do so, create some extra positive emotions in your dog by getting excited yourself. Express your own enthusiasm for her joy through your voice and gestures. For example, if you are sitting on the beach and she is sniffing the wind, sniff it yourself and rub her behind her ears. A big smile and a gentle "yay!" or "all right!" can express your pleasure at being with her and sharing this moment. This enhances your connection and can elevate her joy quotient.

Meditation

Benefits of dog meditation are not just emotional closeness, calm thinking and a relaxed mind. Meditating with your dog, being present with each other can help your dog feel calm, relaxed and connected to you. Many dogs will get a life quality boost from this practice. See page 26 for a simple dog meditation.

Visualization Exercises

Though it may sound "new age" to some, visualizing what you want to happen is not just a "far-out" concept. It's a technique used by elite athletes, NASA astronauts and other top performers, to maintain their mental muscles. A mental rehearsal can train your brain to help achieve a desired outcome in real life.

Basketball stars, like Michael Jordan, often imagine a basketball going through the hoop, even before they take the shot. Interestingly, elite coaches train their clients to use positive visuals, even in the face of failure. For example, if the basketball misses the hoop, the player re-visualizes the shot and imagines it going in the hoop. This prepares the mind for success the next time.

So what can you visualize for your dog? Pick something that feels good to you and don't limit yourself. Perhaps your desire is for your dog's pain to be eased, for a good life quality or that your dog will beat the odds. Whatever it is, spend some time imagining what your desire would look like, then see it, actually happening. Add any sounds, smells, or textures that make the visualization even more real. Remember to imagine what it feels like to actually have this.

Just like a child playing with sand, you can make this as real as possible. Allow the feelings of success, peace and joy to carry you away a little. This is how the world's top performers make their lives what they want them to be,

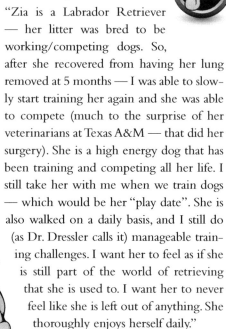

Competitive Retriever Never Left Out

"Zia is a Labrador Retriever — her litter was bred to be working/competing dogs. So, after she recovered from having her lung removed at 5 months — I was able to slowly start training her again and she was able to compete (much to the surprise of her veterinarians at Texas A&M — that did her surgery). She is a high energy dog that has been training and competing all her life. I still take her with me when we train dogs — which would be her "play date". She is also walked on a daily basis, and I still do (as Dr. Dressler calls it) manageable training challenges. I want her to feel as if she is still part of the world of retrieving that she is used to. I want her to never feel like she is left out of anything. She thoroughly enjoys herself daily."

- Sheril Allen, Austin, Texas

and it can't hurt to try. Your dog can pick up on your good feelings, even if she doesn't understand why you feel good.

Some people have trouble with this. They feel like it's fake to imagine something good. If you just can't get yourself to feel good and believe in what you want to have happen, ease up on yourself and visualize something that still feels good, but is more attainable. If imagining your dog as pain-free doesn't work, perhaps imagining his feeling more ease when he sleeps will do the trick. Being realistic is prudent and sensible; sometimes, however, we get tangled up in negatives and our dogs might pick them up. Allowing ourselves to focus on the good things can also be prudent and sensible. The point of this exercise is not to lie, just to practice feeling more positive states of emotion. If this exercise doesn't work for you, that's OK; there are plenty of other ways to get your dog and yourself to feel good.

Intercessory Prayer

If visualization seemed weird to you, then using intercessory prayer for your dog might seem really bizarre. Please, bear with me.

Whether you believe in a traditional religion or not, intercessory prayer is a direct request to a higher power to intercede in the situation and to help bring about a good outcome. After researching intercessory prayer, I am sort of intrigued with its potential as a cancer treatment.

One very important (and controversial) study published in the *British Medical Journal* particularly caught my attention. The study attempted to determine whether patients with bloodstream infections (sepsis) were helped by remote, intercessory prayer. In other words, were patients helped if people who did not know them and were not present prayed for their health and recovery?

In July of 2000, over three thousand (human) patients with sepsis were categorized into two groups: the intervention group, which was prayed for, and the control group, which was not. This was a blind, randomized study, which meant that the doctors, patients, and the people offering prayers did not know which patients were being prayed for, and which were not.

The prayer offered was for the well-being and full recovery of the intervention group. No prayers were offered for the control group.

The outcome of the study was that patients in the intervention group had statistically significant shorter hospital stays (although the difference was not large) and their fevers went away faster than those in the control group.

The other detail of that study is quite bizarre: the patients involved were hospitalized years earlier than the prayer was offered – between 1990 and 1996! In other words, intercessory prayer seemed to help the treatment group, *even though it was offered years later.* Plus, the lead scientist was a skeptic, who was actually trying to prove that prayer doesn't work at all. After analyzing the results, however, the study authors concluded that intercessory prayer "should be considered for use in clinical practice."

As you can imagine, this study received intense scrutiny and negative feedback from the academic community. Follow up reviews did not support or refute the effects, and the study's methods were attacked. The fact that it was done in the first place was roundly criticized.

Not everyone prays, and not everyone is comfortable with thinking about prayer. Praying for a different outcome, when the event has already passed, may seem positively silly to most people. I am offering this information so that you can decide for yourself whether you want to pray for your dog. Asking others who pray to do so certainly can't hurt. When your dog is coping with cancer, every little bit helps.

Massage and Touch Therapies

In addition to feeling pleasurable, massage has been shown, in humans, to elevate cancer-fighting natural killer cells, increase circulation, reduce stress, ease constipation, lower blood pressure and relax stiff muscles. In fact, massage has been shown to be so beneficial for cancer patients, that a premier human cancer treatment center, Sloan-Kettering Cancer Center in New York, has incorporated massage into its treatments. Their own trials have shown that massage decreases pain, nausea, depression, anxiety and fatigue by more than 50%. This is a great treatment to add to your Full Spectrum cancer care plan.

Some think massage is not appropriate for cancer patients, likely based on reports of bruising and muscle pain in healthy humans, following massage. Some humans are allergic to massage lubrications, and there have been reports of internal bleeding and dislodging of blood clots, which created blood flow issues. It is clear to me that these events are very rare and/or result

> ### *Interactive Toys, Reiki, Prayer All Help*
>
> "We found a toy called the Dog Brick which requires brain power, a good nose and not too much physical power and it's a great interactive game for Daisy, we would hide cookies and she figured out where they were. Great toy for a dog who can't move too much. She also loved her trips to the holistic vet too for ozone therapy, massage therapy, reiki, and all over energy healing. And lots and lots and lots of prayers. There were 100's of people praying for Daisy every day. She had touched so many people throughout her life and truly was an amazing dog who had done so much and impacted so many dogs and people during her life."
>
> *- Chris Shoulet, Bethesda, Maryland*

from excessive force during massage.

The evidence points to massage as being beneficial in reducing cancer-related symptoms in people, and we can safely use it to help our dogs. Just don't use deep and excessive force. The massage exercise on page 29 is a good place to start. You can also get professional massage for your dog from a good massage therapist in your area (some even specialize in pet massage). General massage techniques like the lighter strokes in Swedish massage are useful and there are many other types of bodywork and massage therapy that focus on healing through light touch or energy. These have not been studied as much as regular massage; they are worth mentioning because, in humans, they can provide social support, ease loneliness and reduce stress levels.

The following techniques usually involve very light touch, so they can be used in conjunction with any other treatment.

- **Tellington Touch or TTouch:** Created by Linda Tellington-Jones, a horse trainer, to calm them down, TTouch creates changes in brain patterns by lightly drawing circles all over the body. It may sound strange, but something about the repetitive motions and the attention to all body parts (even the gums) seems to relax and calm animals, including dogs. TTouch has even been shown to be helpful for humans in a controlled study, which measured anxiety, pain, heart rate and blood pressure. In the treated group, both blood pressure and heart rate dropped significantly as a result of the treatment. At the very least, trying TTouch with your dog is an excellent way to be social and loving with each other.

- **Acupressure:** Acupressure uses finger pressure to manipulate and restore balance to the Chinese acupuncture energy meridians. Skilled acupressure therapists understand the Chi-

At Least as Important as Chemotherapy

"Exercise, play, massage, and prayer really helped all of us (dogs and people) to live with and through Casper's year with lymphoma. Few doctors will go so far as to recommend these healing strategies, yet we know from ages past that they have worked for others. These therapies are at least as important as traditional chemotherapy in managing cancer in dogs."

- *Connie Hardy, Ames, Iowa*

He Dazzled My Clients

"I took Max with me everywhere I went. He came to the office and dazzled my clients with his charm and good looks. If I did errands, he came along and we went for short walks at each stop we made. We visited friends, meditated together, continued training on a low-intensity basis. I continued body work on him and did tons of praying and visualizing."

- *Judith A., Willingboro, New Jersey*

nese medical model and are familiar with the points on the body, which Traditional Chinese Medicine uses to treat everything from asthma to cancer, and it may have some benefit for your dog.

- **Reiki:** Reiki is an energy therapy from Japan that involves the laying on of hands. As the patient rests, healing energy called Reiki (which translates to "universal life energy"), is transmitted through the therapist's hands and into the body. Some patients feel tingling or warmth coming from the hands and most feel a deep peace and contentment throughout the session. Some dogs may respond to Reiki with enthusiasm, deeply relaxing and letting go of tension.

- **Healing Touch:** Nurses in human western medicine developed Healing Touch, also known as Therapeutic Touch, to counteract what some felt was the impersonal and clinical approach of modern medicine. According to practitioners, there are energetic fields within and outside of the body. These fields

carry the imprint of illnesses, and impact the physical body; by working with the energy "bio-fields," physical illness can be relieved. Recipients report that it is deeply relaxing and very restorative.

Meditation, Visualization, and Massage

"As our Jack Russell Terrier, Gorilla, starts to age and his health decline, we had to adjust his exercise, but we still insist on getting him out for some controlled exercise every day. Meditation, visualization exercises and massage are also a big part of our life. Our little "G-man" loves his Reiki sessions especially. He also gets great benefits from regular acupuncture and from the occasional hydrotherapy swim session."

- Lola Michelin, Shoreline, Washington

True Believer in Home Cooking

"I have seen a difference in my puppy's energy level and overall wellbeing. He seemed to chew at his feet a lot and he has completely stopped doing this. I am a true believer in the home-cooked meal."

- Tina Holloway Johnson, Surprise, Arizona

Just Do It!

All of these strategies engage the power of the body-mind connection to heal, reduce stress and elevate happiness. Engaging your dog in these activities might help him get an edge on cancer and it also bonds the two of you, which is guaranteed to make him feel better. I urge you to consider adding at least one to your daily routine. Now, it's time for you to take a look at yourself, your budget, and your dog's cancer case and do some serious analysis. When you're ready to start, turn to the next chapter.

Part IV:
Making Confident Choices

In this part of the book, you will begin to formulate your own Full Spectrum cancer care plan. To start, I will answer some questions that are frequently asked at this stage. We'll also discuss pain and pain management, other life quality issues, and see some statistics on life expectancy in purebreds and mixed breed dogs. You'll answer a series of questions, which will help you to identify your overall philosophy about cancer care and guide your treatment choices. We'll work through each of the five Full Spectrum steps in a treatment plan analysis, and you'll get you my best advice about how to take that plan to your veterinarian or oncologist. We'll also cover working with loved ones who may be involved in your dog's life, and you'll learn how to keep a journal to stay organized. We'll discuss outside-the-box ways to finance cancer treatments and, if you need it, there is a section dedicated to hospice care, euthanasia, and saying your final goodbyes.

Chapter 16: Dog Cancer Treatment FAQs

*I*want to take a moment now to congratulate you for getting this far. We've covered a tremendous amount of material and you've absorbed a lot of information. Even if you don't yet have a firm plan in place, your dog will benefit from your research. You can be, and should be, proud of yourself for taking this time for education.

One of the most difficult things for many guardians to accept is the fact that there is no "one right way" to treat dog cancer. Depending upon the cancer, there may be too few treatments or too many – and not knowing which one will definitely benefit your dog can be tough.

This section is designed to help you take a step back and analyze what you've learned, so you can make confident decisions about your dog's cancer. Obviously, although I cannot consult with you through the pages of a book, I can tell you how to consult yourself, and give you some advice about how to work with your vet or oncologist.

First, I'll answer two very common questions guardians ask me at this point:

How do I know whether this treatment is really worth it?

I know I would do almost anything to help my dog. How do I know if treatment is for my dog, or really, for me?

These are important questions to consider before you draft a plan for your dog, so, let's look at them now.

Is all this treatment really worth it?

Sometimes guardians ask this when they have a limited budget, limited time to devote to nursing their dog or when they feel their dog may be very near the end of his life. They often recognize that treatment might help, but they are not sure whether they can provide it.

The sad truth is that cancer far too often wins, in the end. I firmly believe in, and have personally experienced, dogs who beat the odds, sometimes by large margins. Of course, I cannot predict that your dog will be among them.

She Wanted to Eat the Delicious Food!

"Learning about canine diet was one of the most important things I took away from my experience with canine cancer .... The change in food definitely helped keep my dog strong during chemotherapy because she wanted to eat the delicious, nutritious food. Her legacy lives on in the health of my other dogs because they are benefiting from what i learned from Dr. Dressler. This dietary improvement has made a positive difference for my elderly dog who suffers from arthritis, too."

– Sarah N. Bertsch,
Hudson, Wisconsin

Answering the question "is treatment really worth it?" tears at the heartstrings, no matter who you are. Contemplating the "worth" of your dog's remaining time can seem cold and callous, and some guardians don't even want to consciously contemplate the question.

It's actually an excellent question and this section of the book will help you to answer it for yourself. No one else can do it for you. The "right" answer is as individual as your fingerprint and as unique as your dog.

The next part of this book will address all of the relevant issues, so that you can make a decision that truly is best for you and for your dog. Please read it with care.

Is this for my dog, or for me?

Some guardians worry that, because they love their dogs so much, they will proceed with treatments that are not ultimately in their best interest. It's true that some of us have a hard time differentiating between our own needs and the needs of our dogs. This is understandable, especially when there is a close and loving relationship in place. The best advice I have for you is to work the question from both angles.

I suggest writing down how your dog's cancer and possible treatment looks from your own point of view, totally excluding your dog's point of view. Get it all down. Are you worried about your dog's dying? ...that you are somehow failing your dog if he doesn't get better? ...that you won't have tried everything possible? Are you worried about the logistics of getting to the vet for multiple treatments, taking time off from work or paying the bills? What about negatives, like wasting money or that a treatment won't work? Write down everything you can.

Now, let's look at your dog's cancer from your dog's point of view. Does he worry about dying? ...about pain control? ...about you? ...about money? ...about eating well? ...about whether a treatment will work? The answer to all of these questions is: no. Dogs do not blame or judge us. Their opinion of us, their love for us, is not based on how much money is in the bank, how much we spend on their treatments or whether we make mistakes. They don't worry about the future – they have more immediate problems. When a dog is in pain from surgery, he just wants the pain to stop – he doesn't worry that it won't get better later.

Keeping this in mind can really help you to evaluate whether you are taking on a treatment or pursuing a particular course of action for yourself, or on behalf of your dog. As your dog's guardian, it is extremely important to examine your responsibility and anchor yourself to doing the best you can with what you have. Sometimes that will mean pursuing a treatment that is likely to help, and at other times it will mean stopping something that isn't working. Keeping this exercise in mind can help you a great deal as you analyze your dog's cancer case.

Seemed Labor Intensive Until We Were Fighting Cancer

""Home cooked meals seemed like a labor intensive tasks until we had a cancer diagnosis to fight. It is now so easy – all the dogs get cooked chicken or lean beef at every meal as the main ingredient, along with loads of cooked broccoli. Krill oil supplements add the highest quality omega-3s we can give. They love their diet; there is never any food left in the bowl."

- Susan Harper,
High Wycombe, England

Chapter 17: Pain and Pain Management

There is no doubt that pain feels bad and blocks your dog from experiencing many of her joys of life. Your concern about your dog's pain is real and valid, so I'm going to cover it in some detail.

My personality type makes me particularly sensitive to quality of life issues, and pain management is a top priority. Most vets and oncologists share this sensitivity, although, every once in a while, I hear about a veterinary professional who does not take pain management seriously. I recommend making a point of addressing the topic of pain with your own vet. To do that, you need to have some background information. Let's start by describing how a dog in pain behaves, as a "reality check".

A pain-free dog is generally content, relaxed, playful, affectionate and engaged in enjoyable activities. How much affection, playfulness and engagement are shown depends upon the dog – some are love bugs with lots of energy, while others are more reserved in their affection and less enthusiastically athletic. You likely know your dog well enough to know what is normal for her.

A dog in pain, on the other hand, can seem withdrawn, listless and tense when han-

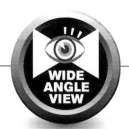

How Bad Is the Pain?

This is one of the hardest questions to answer, because it is so difficult to truly know and understand our dog's experience.

Dogs have a nervous system that works the same way ours does, so it is logical to think they feel pain.

It's not logical to assume your dog feels or thinks about his pain the same way you feel or think about your pain, however. It's also not logical to think your dog ascribes the same meaning to pain that you do.

It's hard enough for us to understand what another human is feeling, let alone our dogs. Let's take the common example of a headache. Some people can have a headache and go about their day as if nothing

dled, particularly if the pain is chronic. More sudden or acute, "sharp" pain, usually elicits the expected response: vocalization, flinching, licking or pawing at the area or limping.

The best approach is to assume that your dog has some level of pain, if there is injury or tissue irritation. Not every tumor causes pain – in fact, some cause no pain at all, especially in the early stages. Just because your dog has cancer, does not mean that he is in pain, but he could be and, if he is, you want to know it. There are several signs to look for.

Please note that while all of these signs are consistent with pain, none points to pain, specifically; other issues may also cause these signs:

How Bad Is the Pain?, *continued*

were wrong. They can sit in a meeting with a splitting headache, while no one else has a clue they are in pain. Others, with a similar pain, simply cannot ignore it: they moan, tell everyone else about it or go home, to ease the pain.

Some Guardians assume that if a dog is hurt, he will yowl or whine or yelp. This isn't true for dogs any more than it is for humans. While barking or vocalizing can be a sign of pain, it does not mean there is pain. By the same token, a lack of whining or yelping does not mean there is no pain.

- **Limping:** Dogs only limp when it hurts to bear weight on a limb. Limping is a reliable sign of pain.

- **Resistance to using the affected area:** When your dog is not using a part of her body, she may be experiencing pain. For example, if she suddenly holds her tail down, it may mean her tail is painful.

- **Bunny-hopping:** When either both hips or both knees are painful, her gait can look like a bunny hop, with both hind limbs advancing at the same time.

- **Resistance to manipulation:** When you touch the area that seems to be painful, for example by manipulating a joint, your dog may quickly look back at you or pull away. It's the same way you might react if you had sunburn on your shoulder and someone slapped you there in greeting. You might flinch, turn your head quickly or even shake them off.

- **Yelping:** When you hear your dog give a short yelp for no apparent reason – for example, while he's lying quietly – this can be a sign of a sharp, sudden pain.

- **Panting:** Some dogs will pant excessively when they are uncomfortable (during times that they would not be panting normally).

- **Trembling:** Occasionally dogs will "shiver" when they experience pain, although other conditions can also cause this. (Sometimes even non-health related conditions; I know one dog who lets her owner know she needs to go outside by trembling.)

- **Resistance to changing levels:** If your dog doesn't want to jump on or off the couch or climb stairs, this can be because of pain, especially back pain or other orthopedic pain. The same can be said if a dog does not easily rise when lying down or has difficulty sitting or lying down from a standing position.

- **Guarding:** If your dog has a "hunched" posture, where the back arches up when it did not previously, she may be experiencing abdominal discomfort. If you've ever had a stomach ache yourself, you'll recognize this posture. Occasionally dogs with back pain or neck pain will do this, as well.

- **Straining:** Both straining to urinate and urinating frequently can indicate bladder or urethra pain or discomfort. Some dogs lick or chew their genitals when they're in pain in this region, but this is not always a sign of pain. Straining to pass stool, along with soft feces and/or feces coated with mucous or blood, can indicate a colon problem, which could mean there is discomfort in the lower digestive tract.

- **Apathy:** Internal pain can cause a decrease in normal activity levels. Turning back on walks, half-hearted playing or refusing to play, and staying in one place for an extended period of time, can be a sign of pain.

- **Lack of appetite:** Sometimes pain can cause nausea or a lack of appetite. If a dog doesn't feel well, she may eat less, turn her nose away from treats or stop eating altogether.

- **Lack of engagement:** Pain, especially chronic pain, can cause isolating or withdrawn behaviors. Many times, dogs will stop playing or retreat to a private, protected area to nest under a bed or in a corner, and refuse to come out unless coaxed repeatedly. Many guardians mistakenly think their dogs' personality is changing, or that they are "getting old" when the real problem might be chronic pain.

- **Aggression:** Dogs may become aggressive when they are enduring a painful condition.

Of course, dogs differ widely in their personality and habits, so some of these behaviors might not indicate pain in every dog. The key for you is to know what is normal for your dog, and then look for differences from the norm, using the listed behaviors as a guide. Have your veterinarian or oncologist help you assess pain in your dog.

There are some circumstances in which you can be sure your dog is in pain. If your dog just had a biopsy or other surgery, he will likely experience temporary pain at the incision site. Good pain management protocols can help a great deal until the pain fades away completely.

The best you can do is to identify possible pain in your dog and bring it to your vet's attention.

Believe it or not, a recent study found that dog owners could be quite skilled at diagnosing chronic pain in their dogs. According to the study, once guardians were educated about the signs and symptoms of their dogs' pain, they could detect it better than any test (heart rate, cortisone levels or other clinical tools). Once you bring the pain to your vet's attention, your vet will try to find the source, which will help her to decide how to manage it.

It's very common to prescribe an anti-inflammatory drug to reduce pain and inflammation. Anti-inflammatories are good for mild to moderate pain and can also be used in combination with the opioid pain medications described below. Current common anti-inflammatories include: Metacam, Deramaxx and Previcox. Rimadyl has been in use for some time and is currently being phased out. As mentioned elsewhere, the ingredients in Apocaps have shown anti-inflammatory effects, also.

Although many opioid drugs can suppress pain, some dogs may experience agitation on these drugs: panting, pacing, whining or weaving and, generally, fighting the effects of the drug. Tramadol usually (although not always) is the exception to this rule. This prescription opioid narcotic not only produces good pain control (especially when used with other medications like NSAIDS), but also is well tolerated. Another useful combination is Tylenol with codeine. All these drugs are to be used under veterinary supervision.

Combining pain control drugs is a very useful strategy (called multimodal therapy). When single drugs are used for pain control, such high doses are sometimes required, that side effects become more likely. By using different drugs together, even though the pain control of each one contributes, since its side effects are often different, they are minimized.

I use this strategy for dogs in pain who have been admitted to the hospital. I often use a constant rate infusion (CRI), where the pain control drugs are used at lower doses, in combination, and given continuously through an IV drip. Low dose ketamine is selected often, along with lidocaine, fentanyl, Dexdomitor or other drugs (the ketamine dose is much lower than that used for anesthesia, see page 120).

For at-home pain control, sometimes a Fentanyl patch is prescribed. This patch looks like an adhesive bandage; it sticks to the skin, so that it can administer Fentanyl steadily, over time. If your dog gets a patch, make sure that she doesn't lick, bite, or eat it, because it's toxic if ingested. To cover the patch you can put a t-shirt on him and use an Elizabethan collar.

These drugs – NSAIDS, Tramadol, Tylenol with codeine, CRIs and Fentanyl patches – are examples of drugs used for controlling what is called adaptive pain. Adaptive pain is a response to specific, direct injury. It can be caused by tumors, trauma, or surgery, and the pain seems to arise from the injured area itself.

There is another type of pain that is not directly related to tissue injury. The nervous system (brain, spinal cord and nerves) can react to the original injury and create neuropathic pain, sometimes called "wind-up." This additional pain adds to the adaptive pain, which worsens both. Anxiety sometimes seems to worsen neuropathic pain and even more with chronic pain. Medications like Elavil (amitriptyline), gabapentin and amantadine can help with neuropathic pain and can be used right along with other pain medications.

Morphine is a popular drug for pain control, especially for advanced, chronic pain. However, I do not generally recommend its use for dogs with cancer, because recent research shows it may support tumor growth, increase metastasis and shorten survival times. These findings in rats are raising red flags for both human and veterinary oncologists. Some severe or chronic pain cannot be controlled in any other way, so you will need to weigh these factors with your veterinary professional.

Another common drug, which I do not generally recommend, is Torbugesic (Torbutrol). Although prescribed as a medication for use at home, it is not strong enough and does not last long enough to offer real relief. It is, therefore, becoming outmoded for a pain medication in dogs.

Other tools that can help with pain are acupuncture, palliative radiation, pamidronate (for osteosarcoma), warm or cool compresses and gentle massage.

It might take a little tweaking to find the right combination of medications for your dog; when you do, it can seem almost miraculous. Dogs can perk up, become more loving, move around more, eat better, and engage more — sometimes so much so that the guardian asks me *What's in that pill?*, as if the drug is a stimulant or a euphoria-inducing hallucinogen. In reality, pain control just makes the dog feel better. If you've ever had a splitting headache and taken an aspirin, you know how good it feels to be restored to your normal state. This is likely how our dogs feel, too.

When pain management protocols work, I always feel a sense of relief and accomplishment. Not only have I have addressed a real problem, but I have also found out more information about the dog's condition. Pain relief — whether it comes from a prescription pain medication such as Tramadol, a nutraceutical such as Apocaps, or from a gentle massage — is very important to dogs with cancer.

Bug for Blueberries

"We use both krill oil and fish oil capsules. We're just too busy to do the home cooked meals, but he gets a mixture of ZiwiPeak Venison (real meat, air-dried, no grains) and Preference foundation mix from The Honest Kitchen to get him vegetables. He often gets raw broccoli florets with his breakfast and if we make a salad, asparagus or cauliflower for dinner he always gets some of the leftovers. He's also a bug for blueberries and blackberries."

- Al Marzetti, Raleigh, North Carolina

Chapter 18: Joys of Life

*I*s my dog happy? How do I know?

These are important questions that deserve careful consideration at any time of life, not only when cancer is present.

It is hard to know for sure whether anyone is happy or not, including our dogs. But there are certainly things that make dogs seem happy. Here is a list of what I call the Joys of Life:

- **The Joy of Eating and Drinking:** Most dogs, like most people, enjoy eating when they are hungry and drinking water when they are thirsty. Hunger and dehydration are unpleasant and uncomfortable conditions for humans, and I think they're uncomfortable for dogs, too.

- **The Joy of Motion:** Most dogs enjoy walking, running, frolicking, frisking and generally moving around. Even if your dog is normally less athletic than others, when he is unable to move freely, he will likely experience a lower quality of life.

- **The Joy of Social Interactions:** Your dog is a social creature, biologically designed to thrive in groups. When something interferes with her ability to interact normally with you or with other dogs, her potential for taking pleasure in social interactions diminishes.

- **The Joy of Having a Fully-functioning Body:** Dogs seem to feel good when their bodily functions operate normally. It may seem simplistic, but if you've ever had problems urinating, defecating, breathing, smelling, seeing, hearing, tasting or sensing the world with your hands, you know how disorienting and unpleasant it can be. Normal bodily functions are important for feeling good.

- **The Joy of a Healthy Mental State:** Depression, stress, senility, chronic pain and other unpleasant altered states, likely decrease life quality for dogs, just like they do for people.

- **The Joy of Play:** Dogs are by nature playful creatures. While they tend to slow down as they get older, they never completely lose their desire for fun, whether it's chasing balls, tug of war or wrestling. If your dog is incapable of playing to the same degree as before, I believe that his quality of life suffers.

- **The Joy of Expression:** Dogs have unique personalities, and they express themselves in many ways. Some dogs are naturally affectionate and helpful. Others are natural watchdogs or protectors. Some are clowns or goofballs. When your dog's normal natural self-expression becomes muted or disappears, there is probably a slipping of life quality associated with the change.

Paying attention to your dog's joys – and what increases or decreases them – can help you to determine his overall quality of life. Go down this list and see which are affected right now, and how many are left. Then ask yourself whether most of the ones that matter to your dog are still there. This assessment is one of your primary responsibilities as his guardian. For some guardians, this will reveal unwelcome and hard truths; for others it will offer reassurance that their dogs still have good life quality.

I understand that sometimes guardians feel that any loss of life quality is bad. While I understand how distressing it can feel to see your dog's quality of life slipping, I have a more nuanced perspective. When only one of your dog's joys is gone, life quality can stay quite good. For example, blind people can have a good overall quality of life, and so can blind dogs. They can still enjoy many other things, including the pleasure of food, physical activity and close relationships.

I will never forget a case, early in my career, when I was forced to amputate a dog's front leg. I was really bothered by it, because I imagined he would be suffering terribly from the loss. Imagine my relief and surprise when he ran through the surf to greet me, just a few weeks later, tail wagging and completely delighted to be alive. It was clear that the loss of one leg did not lessen his quality of life. His guardian told me he was eating, drinking, engaged, playing, and free of pain, depression and stress. (There is a wonderful online community called www.tripawds.com just for guardians of three-legged dogs.)

When two joys of life are significantly affected, it's my opinion that we need to start assessing life quality. And when three joys are gone for good, I believe the scale is tipping and life quality may be dropping significantly.

Your dog is an individual and you are the best person to assess her happiness. I suggest going over the list above and noting any joys of life that are negatively affected at this time. Any joys that can be corrected with supplements, surgeries, medications, lifestyle changes or simple attention, will be considered for inclusion in your treatment plan.

Chapter 19: Average Life Expectancy

*E*very dog is different, of course, and no one can ever predict how long any particular dog will live. I've seen dogs live well past their expected lifespan, including some dogs with cancer. Even so, as you work through the decision-making process, it will be important to have a hard piece of data on hand: your dog's life expectancy, based on the average for her breed and/or weight. Without this comparison, it is difficult to have a truly wide-angle view of your dog's situation.

The following list contains most of the common breeds in the United States and the average life expectancy of each, based on published data and my own clinical experience.

Average Life Expectancy Based on Breed	
Afghan Hound	12 years
Airedale Terrier	11 years
Basset Hound	13 years
Beagle	13 years
Bearded Collie	12 years
Bernese Mountain Dog	7 years
Border Collie	13 years
Border Terrier	14 years
Boston Terrier	12 years
Boxer	10 years, 4 months
Bull Terrier	13 years
Bulldog	9 years
Bullmastiff	8 years, 7 months

Average Life Expectancy Based on Breed	
Cairn Terrier	13 years
Cavalier King Charles Spaniel	10 years, 7 months
Chihuahua	13 years
Chow Chow	13 years, 6 months
Cocker Spaniel	12 years, 6 months
Corgi	11 years, 4 months
Dachshund	12 years
Dalmatian	13 years
Doberman Pinscher	10 years
English Cocker Spaniel	12 years
English Setter	11 years
English Springer Spaniel	13 years

Average Life Expectancy Based on Breed	
English Toy Spaniel	10 years
Flat-Coated Retriever	9 years, 6 months
German Shepherd	10 years, 4 months
German Shorthaired Pointer	12 years, 4 months
Golden Retriever	12 years
Gordon Setter	11 years, 4 months
Great Dane	8 years, 5 months
Greyhound	13 years
Irish Red and White Setter	13 years
Irish Setter	12 years
Irish Wolfhound	7 years
Jack Russell Terrier	13 years, 6 months
Labrador Retriever	12 years
Lurcher	12 years, 6 months
Maltese	13 years
Miniature Dachshund	14 years
Miniature Schnauzer	13 years
Miniature Pinscher	14 years
Miniature Poodle	14 years
Norfolk Terrier	10 years
Old English Sheepdog	12 years
Pekingese	13 years
Pomeranian	14 years

Average Life Expectancy Based on Breed	
Pug	13 years
Rhodesian Ridgeback	9 years
Rottweiler	10 years
Rough Collie	12 years
Samoyed	11 years
Scottish Deerhound	9 years, 6 months
Scottish Terrier	12 years
Shetland Sheepdog	13 years
Shih Tzu	13 years, 4 months
Staffordshire Bull Terrier	10 years
Standard Poodle	12 years
Tibetan Terrier (Lhasa Apso)	14 years, 4 months
Toy Poodle	14 years, 4 months
Vizsla	12 years, 6 months
Weimaraner	10 years
Welsh Springer Spaniel	11 years, 6 months
West Highland White Terrier	13 years
Whippet	14 years
Wire Fox Terrier	13 years
Yorkshire Terrier	13 years, 6 months

It's useful to keep in mind that just as one year in human years is different from one year in dog years, one year in the life of one dog is not the same as one year in the life of another. If your dog is of a breed that usually lives ten years, and he stands to gain one year from a course of treatment, that extra year represents ten percent of his natural lifespan. On the other hand, if your dog is of a breed that usually lives fourteen years, one year gained is equal to only seven percent of his lifespan.

While this breed chart can provide a useful guideline for purebred dogs, it is not helpful for mixed breeds. Generally, dogs of the same weight live about the same length of time, and the smaller the dog, the longer the life span.

| Average Life Expectancy Based on Weight ||
Body Weight	Approximate Life Expectancy
Miniature (up to about 12 lbs.)	14 years
Small (12–30 lbs.)	13 years
Medium (31–50 lbs.)	12 years
Large (51–80 lbs.)	11 years
Giant (over 80 lbs.)	9 years

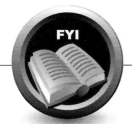

Old Age Is Not a Disease

Age is not a disease, nor is it a pre-existing health condition, like kidney or heart disease. To make a prognosis, or prediction, about the ultimate outcome of a particular dog's cancer, we look for the presence or absence of certain factors (which vary depending upon the cancer type). Old age is not automatically one of those factors. Advanced age does not necessarily worsen a prognosis. The reason to look at your dog's age, compared to her expected lifespan, is because it shows you what you're fighting for.

Chapter 20:
Treatment Plan Analysis

*I*f there were one absolute "cure for cancer," there would be no need for you to analyze your cancer treatment options; you would simply do what we recommend. Unfortunately, we don't yet have the silver bullet that kills cancer, so you have some decisions to make, and those decisions require some thought. This chapter will help you to analyze yourself and your dog's cancer.

I suggest taking notes as you work through this chapter, because you will want to record your thoughts and as much of the data as you can. In Chapter 23, I recommend keeping a journal; your work in this chapter may be the start of it. You may also want to use the companion book *The Dog Cancer Survival Guide Companion Journal.*

Keeping track of your planning, your decisions, your actions and your questions will really help you when you take your plan to your vet or oncologist for input and refining.

By answering the following questions, you will be facing your dog's cancer head on and recording your thoughts in black and white. The truth of what you are up against may become clearer and more "real" to you than it has up to this point. We can't predict what emotions this might trigger; the breathing exercises from Chapter 2 might come in handy.

Although this analysis is straightforward, sometimes guardians feel stumped. If you get stuck or

---

We Are Clearly Type B

"We used your book as a support and guide to determining how we would address the horrible reality that our dog had cancer. Your book gave me the following: 1. Education 2. Channeling energy into action not remorse, regret or second guessing 3. Providing a decision-making platform. My husband and I discussed her condition, her age, her prognosis and what makes her happy. We adopted her at two. She is a very emotionally needy dog, she is "fretful", does not like vet offices (our vet come to our house) and does not readily embrace strangers. We decided that any protocol requiring a lot of time in vet offices would reduce the quality of her life. Your book helped us determine what we are – clearly – Type B."

- Valerie Sachs, Pepper Pike, OH

---

you can't answer a question, it may be because you're feeling overwhelmed. It will help to focus exclusively on your dog for a moment. Be with him and "tune in" to whatever he's experiencing at that time. Once you are tuned in, look at the question again and listen carefully for the answer. Listening from this space of connectedness may help you to relax enough to hear your answer come welling up from deep inside. If you still feel stumped, go to the next question and return to the tough one later. You can always use the exercises in chapter 2, if needed.

Once you have finished answering these questions, you will have a wide-angle view of your dog's cancer and will be ready to consider possible treatments.

Diagnosis and Prognosis

First, let's get an overview of your dog's cancer. Write down your dog's diagnosis, based on what you know from tests that have been run so far. What type of cancer does your dog have and how advanced is it? Has it metastasized? Where?

Now write about your dog's possible prognosis. Does this cancer tend to be aggressive? Is it eligible for curative surgery? Palliative surgery? Chemotherapy or radiation? How long does your vet or oncologist expect your dog to live, with the treatments they recommend? How long without the treatments?

Take some time to review your vet's and/or oncologist's reports (if you don't have copies, you can get them, see page 256). What does Dr. Ettinger say about your dog's cancer in her section of the book? Make notes about what you learn. You may not have the answers to all of these questions; write down what you know so far, and make a list of questions you need to get answered.

My Best Advice: It is worth repeating that the prognosis is neither a promise nor a guarantee. Instead, it's a best guess at how long your dog has, based on what conventional veterinary medicine knows at this time. Some guardians make the mistake of thinking it predicts the day of their dog's demise, as if it's an execution day. Many vets think of it this way, too. Cancer is not an automatic death sentence, and thinking of it that way is not only unscientific, but also distressing and unhelpful.

———— • ————

Cancer is not an automatic death sentence, and thinking of it that way is not only unscientific, but also distressing and unhelpful.

———— • ————

No one really knows when your dog will pass from this world, or what the cause of death will be. I suggest thinking of the time given for a prognosis as a mile marker on a highway – it tells you where you are, in relation to the expectations of the conventional medical establishment. It is a useful way to orient you, but it is not definitive.

Life Expectancy

Another piece of data that can help establish a wide-angle view of your dog's situation is the average life expectancy for her breed or weight. Based on the charts in Chapter 19, how long is your dog expected to live on average? How old is she now? How much more time does she have, based on these conventional expectations – or has she already lived longer than expected?

This calculation can feel coldhearted, but it is important to know where your dog is, in relation to the average length of life for her breed and/or weight. Like the prognosis date, this can help you to orient yourself when considering your options.

My Best Advice: Many guardians get very upset after they try a recommended treatment and their dogs do not live "long enough," as a result. This question is designed to help you set your own expectations for what constitutes "a long time" for your own dog. Particularly for dogs with cancer, "a long time" for a dog may not feel like a long time for us guardians.

For example, if a dog is expected to live for ten years and a cancer that is left untreated will probably shorten her life, that is a tragedy. On the other hand, if a particular treatment could extend her life by a full year, that is **ten percent of her lifespan**. From a veterinary perspective, this increase in longevity is a big success, because we are calculating time in the dog (not human) years *for that dog.*

To put this in a more human context, consider a hypothetical human case. Let's say that Dan is a gentleman who is expected to live to 80 years based on his family history and his overall state of good health. Unfortunately, Dan is diagnosed with cancer at age 70. The prognosis for survival time is one year without treatment and eight years with treatment. In this hypothetical case, the treatment would extend life to nearly the expected lifespan – and provide a gained life expectancy of nearly ten per cent. Is that a long time?

It depends upon your perspective, of course. If Dan spends those years in relative comfort and with few side effects or other health conditions, it could feel short. On the other hand, if those years are spent weak, sick and bed-ridden, they might feel long. We cannot possibly generalize about how long is too long for other humans.

The Best Dog Caregiver

"I did not do radiation or chemo. I did not want to put Jazzie through that. If his cancer were a different kind, maybe I would have. [My best advice is] don't give up on your dog. Read about what kind of dog care giver you are before you make decisions. I wanted to cure Jazzie, but I was unwilling to do things that may have made him feel bad. I was "the best dog caregiver" I could be within my finances and time. [Taking care of you first] is important, because one must be strong and know how to proceed emotionally."

- Jo Anne Kikel, Denver, Colorado

We can't generalize for dogs, either. This is an exquisitely individual matter, and it's important to know where you stand. For some guardians an extra three months is a precious miracle. For others it is the blink of an eye.

Make a few notes for yourself: write down the expected lifespan for your dog, your dog's current age, and the difference between the two. Also write down how many months your dog has left, according to the prognosis (with and without treatment). Two different guardians, looking at this same set of numbers, may have radically different opinions. What's important, of course, is *your* feeling about *your* dog.

Life Quality

Longevity is not our only concern; life quality is also important. List your dog's specific joys of life. Have they decreased in number because of the cancer? Will certain treatment side effects, other illnesses or conditions affect them? If there is life quality loss, is it permanent or temporary? Can life quality be boosted?

These are important questions, because the answers can have a big impact on the type of treatments you choose. For example, managing side effects is imperative when overall life quality is already suffering. Sometimes other health issues or health conditions negatively impact life quality. For example, some dogs get cancer at an advanced age, after they have lost some vision or hearing. In these cases, when quality of life may already be lowered, you could be unable to do much about it.

If you read the earlier "joys of life" discussion with a lump in your throat because you fear that your dog's quality of life is low, I recommend you make a list of the joys you would like to work on and include them in your treatment plan. Also, make a list of any side effects your dog is currently experiencing which will need to be managed.

Pain Management

Life quality certainly goes down when there is unmanaged pain, so take a moment to assess your dog's current pain level. Pain management is an important but sometimes overlooked part of cancer treatment. Managing it effectively can increase overall life quality, which, as we've discussed, can help your dog get an edge on cancer. Based on what you learned in Chapter 17, make a point of discussing any signs of pain with your vet or oncologist, as soon as possible.

Guardian Type

While every guardian loves her dog, not everyone approaches cancer and cancer treatments in the same way. There is no one right way except the way that is best for you. Therefore, one of your most important tasks is to establish your overarching priorities for your dog's cancer. To help you, I've created a device that can allow you to see yourself from a wide-angle perspective: "guardian typing."

Most guardians seem to fit into one of three types. As you read through the three descriptions, see which one is closest to your own personality and point of view. This insight will help you to establish your own priorities and make decisions much easier.

Are you …

Type A: "I will do everything I can to stop the cancer. Quality of life is important, and my main goal is to keep my dog alive for as long as possible, so he has every chance to beat the cancer. I understand that side effects can occur, as a result of treatment and I'm willing to deal with them when they arise. The risk is worth it, because the ultimate payoff is remission and/or more time with my dog."

Type B: "I want to keep my dog's life quality high, while prolonging her life as much as possible. I understand that there may be some side effects with treatment and I'm willing to deal with them as they arise. However, if they are too extreme, I will not be happy. My main goal is to balance life quality and life expectancy."

Type C: "I want to keep my dog as comfortable as possible. I understand that side effects may arise as a result of treatments, and I want to avoid any but the most minor. My main concern is my dog's quality of life, so, I am not willing to prolong life, if life quality suffers."

Which type are you? There is no right or wrong way to be; no matter what, there is plenty you do to help your dog.

Budget

The amount of money spent on cancer treatments is an important consideration for most guardians. Some spend tens of thousands of dollars on their dog's cancer treatments, while others spend far less.

It might seem that people with more money spend more on cancer treatments, but that is not necessarily true. Different guardians have different life priorities, and that is certainly reflected in their budgets.

What seems to matter most is what Type of guardian you are. I know a Type A guardian, with nearly unlimited means, who spent tens of thousands of dollars on his dog's cancer treatments. I know another Type A guardian who works two jobs and refinanced his home in order to pay for treatments; another went into credit card debt.

On the other hand, I know a Type C guardian, with two vacation homes, who chose to forgo expensive treatments and instead focus on relatively inexpensive supplements and dietary changes – not to save money, but because her personal values required it.

Some guardians are willing to spend more money on certain types of treatments, or on treatments with a reliable track record. Others will only spend more money if their dog will not suffer side effects.

Take a moment now to consider how much money you are willing to spend on cancer treatments. Are there certain treatments you will spend money on and others you won't? Write down your answers (there is advice about working with your vet and financial issues in Chapters 22 and 24).

Time

No matter which cancer treatments you choose, it takes time to care for your dog. Trips in and out of the hospital (sometimes daily), cooking for your dog, administering pills and consulting with experts all take time. Dogs with cancer may need extra nursing care, which may be as simple as creating a space for him to heal after surgery or as complicated as hand-feeding him and giving sponge baths. Depending upon the cancer you are treating and which treatments and strategies you choose, your free time – such as it is – could be devoted to cancer-related tasks.

How much time do you realistically have to care for your dog? Once you factor in work and other family responsibilities, what's left? Is there any room for flexibility in your schedule or are you locked in? Is there anyone else in your dog's life, who can help you with your dog, or with your other responsibilities? Can you hire someone to help you with your dog, or with your other responsibilities? For how long?

I know guardians willing to cut work hours and take home less pay, so they can personally care for their dog. I know others so pressed for time that it is difficult for them to cook (for themselves, or for their dog). Take some time now to realistically assess your own availability, so you can choose cancer treatments that fit your schedule. Make sure to write down any relevant data, such as specific hours of availability, upcoming vacations, other helpers and their availability.

Other Health Issues

Other non-cancer health issues can complicate your decisions. Does your dog have diabetes? A liver condition? Heart disease? Allergies? Is he deaf, or blind, or have hip problems? Write down all of his health conditions.

For example, if your dog already finds it difficult to walk due to hip dysplasia, losing a limb to amputation could present a much bigger challenge than it does for a dog who is otherwise spry. Meanwhile, medications used to manage heart disease, liver disease, kidney disease or diabetes may preclude using certain cancer drugs or supplements.

Make a list of your dog's other conditions and any current medications. Make sure to double check with your vet about whether they could interfere with the cancer treatments you choose.

Side effects

There are potential side effects for every cancer treatment; the question you need to answer is which ones are tolerable to you and at what severity.

Nausea, vomiting and diarrhea can happen after conventional treatments; they can also happen when you change your dog's diet or give drugs or supplements by mouth. Are you willing to tolerate some stomach upset, if it helps your dog in the long run? If you can manage it, with medications or natural strategies, does that make a difference to you? If these symptoms are mild or short-term, is that more acceptable?

More severe, but less common, effects, like kidney, liver or heart damage, brain injuries and even (very rarely) death, must also be noted. For every treatment you consider in the next chapter, note its possible side effects and your own tolerance for dealing with them. Later, when you share your plan with your vet, be sure to ask how likely these side effects are to occur for your dog.

My Best Advice: I hate feeling stomach upset, so, managing it in my canine patients is a priority for me. Feeling sick on a regular basis is, in my opinion, a lowering of life quality that I (and many of my clients) find unacceptable. Is this true for every dog and every guardian? Not necessarily.

Although it is difficult to predict with accuracy what a dog will experience during or after any given treatment, we do have educated opinions to guide us. Carefully calculating your own tolerance for side effects and sharing that information with your vet is an important responsibility.

Mission Statement

We've covered a lot of ground by looking at these questions. Now, it's time to articulate your own wide-angle view of your dog's cancer. We're going to do that by reviewing your notes and writing a mission statement. Although it may seem odd, this exercise from the business world can help you choose the right treatments in the first place, then stay on course as circumstances change.

Mission statements are used to demonstrate your commitment to a goal. Businesses and organizations use them to state objectives, articulate how those goals will be attained, and guide future decisions. We often don't fully realize our commitment until we write it down in clear, concise language.

Keeping in mind whether you are a Type A, B, or C guardian, take a few minutes to write a short, to-the-point mission statement that includes the following:

- **Tell why you are treating your dog's cancer.** This may seem blindingly obvious to you, but it may not be to others. Some guardians treat because they think they can get a cure. Others treat because they want their dogs to feel better in the time they have left. Others choose to treat because they feel they owe their dogs love, support and help. Take a minute to clarify your reasons, because clearly articulating your "why" can help you and others on your team to understand the basis for your decisions.

- **Write about your desired outcome or outcomes.** Do you want pain relief? Tumor reduction? Life extension? To avoid amputation? To see your dog play again? List as many concrete outcomes as you can.

- **List the key values, to which you are committed, in regard to your dog's treatment.** This is a broad topic; some guardians want only "the best" treatments, others want compassionate team-members, and others want to spend as much time as possible with their dogs. If nothing leaps to mind, you might try imagining yourself ten years from now, looking back on this time. What is so important to you that, if it is not honored, you will regret it later?

- **List any limits that you place on treatments.** Are there treatments you will not use? Are there budget or time limits? Is there a certain quality of life you are not willing to accept?

You may need to tinker with this mission statement before it feels complete. Take the time you need to make it represent your mind and heart, and then you'll be ready to use it like a compass. A strong, clear mission statement can guide you toward the right treatments, strategies and activities for your Full Spectrum cancer plan. Sharing your mission statement (or a version of it) with your vet, oncologist or any other practitioner or helper, may also be a good idea.

Chapter 21: Choosing Treatments

Now that you've analyzed yourself and your dog's cancer case, it's time to make some preliminary treatment choices. In this chapter we'll review each of the five Full Spectrum steps, so you can record the treatments, supplements and activities you would like to include in your cancer care plan. I recommend you use the same journal or note-taking device you used in the last chapter.

Reviewing each Full Spectrum step is critical, and so is including every treatment you think might help your dog, even if you don't think you can financially afford it, or if you worry you don't have the time to do it. You may be able to get financial help (see Chapter 24), and your ideal "wish list" can be prioritized, tweaked or whittled down later, when you review it with your vet or oncologist. Also, keep in mind that cancer is a fluid condition, and treatment plans change when the disease changes or new information comes to light. Carefully thinking about each recommendation now – and your reason for choosing it or not choosing it – will help save valuable time later, if you have to make a shift.

If you don't know the answers to these questions right now, that's all right. Just write down what you do know and make notes about what you still need to research. You may be able to find some answers online or get them from a knowledgeable friend; write down questions for your vet, oncologist, or other practitioner, so you can refer to them later in a consult. In the next chapter, which covers how to work effectively with practitioners, we'll revisit this important topic.

If you find yourself stalled on a particular step or treatment, refer back to your Mission Statement to clarify your thinking. Ask yourself: does this support my Mission Statement?

Step One, Conventional Treatments

In this step (Chapter 11) we target cancer directly by using the conventional tools: surgery, chemotherapy and radiation. Many guardians use these to target cancer cells, and you may

We Lent Our Vet This Book and Came Up With a Plan

"Read Dr. Dressler's book and educate yourself about options available to you. We were offered radiation treatment as a huge cost. After lending our vet Dr. Dressler's book we came up with a plan of attack together."

- Susan Taniguchi, Avondale, Arizona

have already started doing so by the time you read this. If needed, review what you have learned from your vet and consult Dr. Ettinger's section and Chapter 11. Then, record all of the conventional treatments you are currently using or considering. Add as many details as you know at this time, including the following:

- **Specific surgeries, including expected recovery time and any post–operative care that may be needed.** How many office visits will there be? Include what outcomes are expected from the treatment. Is this outcome desirable? How much it will likely cost, and what follow up care is needed? Also, make a note of possible side effects.

- **Specific chemotherapy protocols or drugs.** Which drugs are involved? How many treatments are needed? When? How many office visits will there be? Include what outcomes are expected from the treatment. Is this outcome desirable? How much it will likely cost, and what follow up care is needed?

- **Radiation treatments.** How many treatments are recommended and how often? How many office visits will there be? Include what outcomes are expected from the treatment. Is this outcome desirable? How much it will likely cost, and what follow up care is needed?

- Also record any other conventional medications your dog takes, and any other health issues, which need to be taken into consideration.

If you choose not to use a recommended treatment, it's worth making a note about why. Later, if your vet or oncologist questions your decision, you will be able to explain your choice. This will also give him a chance to address your specific concerns and suggest alternatives, if appropriate.

Step Two, Nutraceuticals

In this step (Chapter 12), we target cancer cells using plant-based nutraceuticals that may help induce apoptosis and (in the case of Apocaps) may increase life quality. Review Chapter 12, if necessary, and record each of the nutraceuticals you are using or considering using, including:

- **Apocaps.** Does your dog have health issues that preclude Apocaps use? Is she on medications, which should be reduced or avoided when using Apocaps? If you are considering chemotherapy and radiation treatments, do you want to try using Apocaps as a chemo- or radiosensitizer? Include the outcomes you expect, the likely cost, and possible side effects.

- **Artemisinin.** Does your dog have health issues that preclude artemisinin use? Is she on medications, which should be reduced or avoided when using artemisinin? If you are considering chemotherapy treatments, are the protocols compatible with artemisinin? Remember, if you are contemplating radiation treatments, artemisinin cannot be used during treatments or the two months following. What outcomes do you expect? What is the likely cost? What are the possible side effects?

- **Neoplasene.** Does your dog have health issues that preclude Neoplasene use? Is she on medications, which should be reduced or avoided when using Neoplasene? You will need to rely on your vet for application and pain management. How many office visits will this take? Is the tumor in question on the surface, or could it have invaded deeper structures like the bones, which might require emergency medical care to repair after the tumor sloughs off? Include your expected outcomes, how much it will likely cost and the possible side effects.

Step Three, Immune System Boosters and Anti-Metastatics

After targeting cancer cells, your next priority is to strategically boost your dog's immune system, which is likely suppressed, and possibly deranged, by the presence of cancer. Strengthening the immune system can reduce the risk of secondary illnesses and infections and, because the immune system has natural cancer-fighting mechanisms, re-establishing its vitality could enable it to start helping to fight the cancer.

Review Chapter 13 and make a list of the strategies you are considering. There are two free strategies that I recommend for nearly every dog:

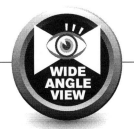

Priority One: Killing Cancer Cells or Boosting Immunity?

Some guardians believe that killing cancer cells directly is a lower priority than boosting the immune system. They hope that if they can stimulate the immune system enough, it will be sufficient to naturally kill the cancer, eventually.

While I agree that boosting the immune system is very important, and that the immune system can kill cancers when it is working effectively, dogs with cancer have likely already suffered severe immune repression. If their immune systems were able to kill the cancer, they would have already done so.

Boosting immune system activity without also killing cancer cells is a dodgy and unreliable strategy, especially with aggressive cancers. No matter what stage your dog's cancer is in, you can take steps to kill it, and I suggest you do.

- High quality sleep: nine hours in total darkness.

- Some sunlight every day, if you can, unless your dog has squamous cell carcinoma or hemangiosarcoma of the skin.

Many guardians have asked me to prioritize the supplements in Chapter 13 in order of their importance, which is done below. You can also see a full listing in Appendix A.

1. **Beta-Glucans:** This is the most important immune-boosting supplement. If you give the supplement called Transfer Factor at the same time, it may enhance the activity of the beta-glucans (Apocaps has some beta-glucans in it, but not as much as what's in K-9 Immunity or many other medicinal mushroom supplements).

2. **Modified citrus pectin**

3. **Doxycycline**

4. **Multivitamins:** Dietary, supplemental doses of multivitamins (not mega-doses). The one possible exception to this is Vitamin C; check with your vet for his preference. Also, if you are feeding a home-cooked diet, I do recommend including a general multivitamin.

Remember to review all of these strategies and supplements for negative interactions with other treatments you are considering, and include those concerns in your journal. Also include how much each will cost, and any possible side effects.

Step Four, Diet

Improving your dog's diet is a very important step in Full Spectrum cancer care. The foods included in the diet (outlined in Chapter 14) may help fight cancer, boost the immune system, or both. Cutting out or reducing processed commercial foods that may contain carcinogens is a relatively easy way to reduce your dog's exposure, and it also may reduce omega-6 fatty acid levels in your dog's diet. Review Chapter 14 and make notes about dietary changes you are considering, including:

- Home-cooking your dog's food, or at least part of it, using high-quality protein, brightly colored low-carbohydrate vegetables, dark green low-carbohydrate vegetables, whole grains, berries, garlic and other potent foods.

- Adding omega-3 fatty acids, including DHA and EPA. The best oils to use are krill and fish oil.

- Adding dietary enzymes to break down your dog's food before he eats it.

Refer back to Chapter 14 to refresh your memory about these supplements and the dog cancer diet. If your dog has a condition that precludes using this diet or any part of it, be sure to note that in your journal. Don't forget to figure out the likely cost of the ingredients, and the time it will take to cook meals every two to four days.

Step Five, Brain Chemistry Modification

Take a moment to review Chapters 15, 17 and 18 and make a list of the treatments and activities you want to include in your cancer treatment plan:

- Exercise
- Play Dates
- Light Training
- Manageable Challenges
- Joys of Life
- Meditation
- Visualization Exercises
- Intercessory Prayer
- Massage or Touch Therapies
- Pain Management (if necessary, see Chapter 17)

Many of these are free; all take some time to implement. Make sure you note what these strategies are likely to cost, and how much time is needed for each.

Other Treatments

If you are considering any treatments not covered in this book, remember to note them in your journal. Include their cost, any possible side effects or conflicts with other treatments. Treatments from Ayurvedic medicine, Traditional Chinese Medicine and homeopathic treatments are better handled by practitioners, skilled in those modalities.

There are many unconventional treatments and supplements purported to help cancer – shark cartilage, Essiac tea, astralagus, and many more – that are specifically not included in this book. This is not an accident. The reasons I excluded them can vary; they may be ineffective, not safe, or impractical to give to dogs, or, in a few cases, they are promising but not yet proven to my satisfaction. If you are curious about which supplements have been excluded and why, check Appendix B (which starts on page 415), where I list the most common ones.

Make Confident Decisions

If you have worked through my system, by this point you will have a fairly solid understanding of the seriousness of your dog's cancer, your own Mission Statement, your financial resources and time commitment and which treatments you would like to try. Review your treatment list and your Mission Statement. Does each treatment support your mission? Put a mark next to the ones which are most important to you or which seem to hold the most promise for helping your dog.

Plan on sharing your ideas with your vet or oncologist. You probably already have some questions for her, and I have more listed in Chapter 22. She may be able to help you identify potential problems with your plan, complications you haven't considered and new treatment options.

Additionally, keep in mind that you will likely tweak this plan as you continue treating your dog's cancer. If your dog doesn't react well to a medication, treatment or supplement, a flexible mindset will help you to adjust smoothly.

Keep your notes from this exercise, because they form the basis of a very important document: your dog cancer journal. Journaling about your dog's progress will help you to make decisions tomorrow, next week, next month and next year. We'll talk more about journaling in Chapter 23.

Take a moment now to look back over the work you just did. Be proud of yourself for taking the time to help your dog. If you feel clear and confident about your plan, that's terrific. If you feel even the slightest hint of doubt or indecision, read the sidebar about how to end "analysis paralysis." The simple exercise outlined there will help you to get clarity and modify your plan, if needed.

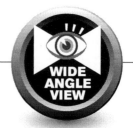

How to End Analysis Paralysis

If you are feeling overwhelmed or anxious and want some extra reassurance about the merits of your Full Spectrum plan, you can do a relatively simple exercise to get clarity.

When you embark on any treatment program, you are doing so because it offers you a possible gain. The hope is that everything will go well and the treatment(s) will have the desired outcome.

Of course, you are also taking a risk. The treatment might not help your dog, or there might be side effects that you cannot manage. In rare cases, the treatment might even harm your dog.

Some people see the possible risks and get scared off. They don't do anything, in case it doesn't work out. Of course, doing nothing has risks, and possibly gains, associated with it, as well. The risks might include your dog's dying sooner than she has to, or living with chronic pain. The possible gains might include avoiding painful

continued on next page

How to End Analysis Paralysis, *continued*

treatments or enjoying a better quality of life. There are risks and possible gains in any life situation – so how do you know, ahead of time, what to do?

You can't know for sure that your plan will work. You can calculate the relative possible gains against the relative possible risks and see which one comes out on top. Please use this calculation anytime you need it.

The basic steps of risk calculation are simple. The first step is to answer the following questions with as much candor and precision as you can (it helps to write the answers down):

What your dog may gain: If you take action on this treatment plan, and it works – when you accomplish the goals in your mission statement – what is the gain? Be specific in your answer. Does your dog feel better? Stop vomiting? Reduce his tumor burden? Live longer? Boost his immune system? Enjoy life more? List every gain you can think of, tangible and intangible. Be thorough, realistic and honest. What is the best-case scenario? Now, answer this: given what you know now, how likely is it that scenario will come true?

What your dog may risk: If you take action on this plan and it doesn't work – if it falls short of the goals you laid out in your mission statement – what do you stand to lose? Be specific in your answer. Does your dog get worse? Feel worse? Suffer? Do you lose time? Money? List everything you can. Put down things that are likely to happen if it doesn't work out. Be thorough, realistic and honest. What is the worst-case scenario? Now, answer this: given what you know now, how likely is it the worst-case scenario will happen?

If you stand to gain more than you risk, follow through with this treatment plan.

If you risk more than you stand to gain, do not follow through with this treatment plan (as it stands).

If you calculate your risk and decide not to follow through on your current plan, I advise you to tweak it to make it less risky. This is a rare situation; the majority of guardians who are reading this book stand to gain more than they would risk, as long as they honestly answered all of the questions above and thoughtfully selected treatments that have real potential to help their dogs.

However, in some cases, this analysis reveals that, even after tweaking and maybe even tweaking again, all plans feel too risky. If this describes you, it may be time to read about dog hospice and euthanasia in Chapter 25.

Chapter 22: Working with Professionals and Loved Ones

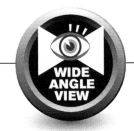

The White Coat Response

Did you know that some people develop temporary hypertension – high blood pressure – just because they are in a medical environment? This is called the White Coat Response.

Some guardians might experience the White Coat Response while going to the vet, too, especially if they are dealing with dog cancer.

If you notice your heart rate go up, you might want to do a breathing exercise from Chapter 2 (perhaps Three Deep Breaths or Fire Bellows Breathing) before you enter the office environment. Bringing a friend along might also help.

Managing your dog's cancer is a big job, for which you are the best-qualified person. Although you are not a vet, you do know your dog best. You have the most to gain when treatments go well, and the most to lose if they don't.

For this reason, I invite you to think of yourself as the leader of a team of individuals involved in your dog's cancer care. Other members of your team include: your vet, your oncologist, any other specialists, and any family members or friends who are available to support you. This chapter was written to help you organize and work effectively with your whole team.

Primary Health Advocate

Human psychological research has shown that we tend to believe what someone in authority tells us. Given this, it's easy to understand why some guardians believe a vet when he says, "your dog can't beat this" or "there is no treatment." Hearing this makes it easier to give up on doing anything to help your dog. However, as you know by now, there are many things that can improve the quality of your dog's life and extend longevity.

Medicine is not an exact science. We learn more every day, which can lead to changes in the way we practice. Even the phrase "to practice medicine" telegraphs this; we don't *perform* medicine, we *practice* medicine. Some vets devour every journal as soon as it's published; others haven't looked at research in years. Some are experts at reading X-rays or ultrasounds, but don't feel confident in surgery. Different levels of experience, different approaches and different philosophies can vastly impact our practices. You might easily get three different opinions from three different oncologists about how to treat your dog's cancer.

When vets and oncologists don't agree – especially about something as serious as cancer, the average guardian becomes confused and frustrated. That's why I advise you to decide, right now, that you are in charge of your dog's health. I call this empowered leadership role Primary Health Advocate. As your dog's Primary Health Advocate, you assemble a team to work with your dog. Your vet, with his specialized training, is an invaluable member – and you are still the one in charge.

(I don't mean to imply that your vet doesn't know what he's doing, or in any way is wrong. Trust his training and experience and take his advice and insights very seriously. This is important for your security and well-being. No matter how wonderful he is, however, you are your dog's guardian.)

Depending upon your vet, you may need to communicate about this role. Researchers conducted an interesting study in which oncologists and their (human) patients were surveyed about decision-making roles. The

> *When vets and oncologists don't agree – especially about something as serious as cancer, the average guardian becomes confused and frustrated. That's why I advise you to decide, right now, that you are in charge of your dog's health.*

results showed that a significant majority of the oncologists thought patients wanted them (the doctors) to make all of the decisions regarding treatment plans. Meanwhile, a majority of the patients wanted the exact opposite: to be in charge or to share decision-making power. As you can imagine, this difference causes needless friction and upset. The study authors recommended oncologists get on the same page with their clients by asking, "Do you want me to make all the decisions, do you want to make all the decisions or do you want to share decision-making?"

Your vet might assume you want him to be in charge of deciding how to treat your dog's cancer, which is why I recommend initiating this conversation, if the topic doesn't come up naturally.

Empowered to Find the Right Vet

"Don't listen to the on-cologist when they say, "He only has __ to live." I had to go on anti-anxiety medication, because I was so afraid of my dog dying! Then I got Dr. Dressler's book. It totally empowered me. I felt like I actually could make a difference in the outcome. Traditional vets only know radiation, chemo, and surgery. If you talk about supplements, etc., they just stare at you like you have two heads. Thank goodness, I found a terrific on-cologist who is open to everything, and actually carries on a conversation about all the alternative things that I am doing for my dog. I know Dr. Dressler strongly recommends talking to your vet before administering any of the supplements. So now, I bring in a whole list of things my dog is eating and taking, and he gives me the thumbs up. I also, because of the book, knew about what to do before surgery, and what questions to ask the vet. Don't ever give up hope."

– Vicki Hagopian,
Hudson, Massachusetts

Medical Files

If you don't have one already, get a copy of your dog's complete medical records, or, at least, whatever your vet has on file. I recommend doing so as soon as possible, so you can read through it in preparation for your next consult. Having your own copy of the file will also help if you consult with another vet, oncologist or other specialist. The information in the files is yours by law, so your vet will have no objection to copying them for you (there may be a small fee to cover costs). The records will include a copy of the biopsy and any other tests that verified your dog's diagnosis. If recent X-rays were taken, your vet will let you borrow the original X-rays to bring to a specialist for review. If the X-rays are digital, they can be emailed or burned to a CD for you.

Keep the file up to date, in future, by getting notes and reports from every vet, oncologist or any other health care professional involved in helping your dog. Ask them to fax their notes and reports to your general practice vet, so that his medical file remains complete.

Set Aside Time to Talk to Your Vet

In order to lead your team, you should have a full understanding of your dog's illness. Hopefully, reading this book has helped you, and discussing the specifics of your dog's cancer with your vet and/or oncologist is still very important. Your treatment plan analysis has probably generated several questions already, and there are many more (listed below), which may also be helpful.

Vets typically have very busy schedules and a great deal on their minds, so the best way to get your questions answered is to make a scheduled appointment, to have her undivided attention. Most vets are happy to schedule courtesy phone consults, and some also give short courtesy in-person appointments.

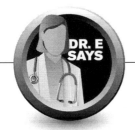

Ask for a Second Opinion

If you have a good relationship with your vet, you might be worried that you are hurting her by asking for a second opinion. Even so, if your vet or oncologist does not have much experience treating your dog's specific cancer, ask for a second opinion. It may help you (and your vet) to think of this second opinion as an appointment to gather more information.

As in any field, different vets are good at different things, and it is very hard to find a vet who does everything well. Most vets know this is true, and they will not be insulted when you want to consult with someone else to round out your team.

Because I'm an oncologist, clients are usually coming to me for a second opinion. However, if they want a third opinion from another specialist or another practitioner, I'm not offended, I'm not insulted and I'm not hurt. I fully support their decision.

During Your Appointment

To make the best use of your time, be prepared with written questions. This may be an emotional meeting, and having a list will help you stay organized. Give yourself permission to ask whatever you need answered. Even if you have dealt with cancer before, there may be gaps in your knowledge. There really is no such thing as a stupid question (and if your vet seems to think there is, or if you get the feeling that you are being treated unfairly or unkindly, it may be time to find a new vet for your team).

If you don't understand something, make sure you ask for clarification. We vets can get preoccupied with the medical details of a "case," and may even forget that you do not understand medical jargon.

It's also a good idea to use a recording device or take notes on paper to make sure you don't have to rely on your own memory later. Bringing a friend or family member with you, preferably someone who is less emotionally involved than you are can help you to stay focused and provide emotional support.

Second Opinions

Ideally, guardians would get a second opinion for most cancer diagnoses, mainly because it's always good to get another perspective. If you can do this, I recommend it.

If your vet is a conventional practitioner, I recommend seeing a holistic or alternative vet for your second opinion, even if you are sure that you want to follow what your current vet recommends. You may get something out of that visit that you would never have learned any other way. You can find holistic vets in your area by visiting the American Holistic Veterinarians Medical Association's website www.AHVMA.org and using the "Find a Holistic Veterinarian" feature. You can also look at the Veterinary Institute of Integrative Medicine's website www.VIIM.org.

I have the same advice for guardians who use holistic or alternative vets. Getting the perspective of a conventional vet or oncologist may offer you new insights, or serve as confirmation for your plan.

If you are even considering using chemotherapy or radiation (and some of the more complicated cancer surgeries), I recommend bringing an oncologist onto your team. Oncologists spend all day, every day, treating cancer with conventional tools. There is no doubt that they have more experience than any general practice vet, and there is no substitute for their expertise in conventional cancer care.

Unfortunately, there are only about two hundred small animal veterinary oncologists practicing in the United States as of this writing, and most of them practice near large cities, so finding an oncologist in your area may be difficult. Some offer phone consults to guardians, and others can consult with your general practice vet. You can find an oncologist by going to the American College of Veterinary Internal Medicine's website www.ACVIM.org and using the Search for a Specialist feature. There is also a company called Oncura Partners which can be contracted to review your dog's case and help your veterinarian manage his cancer. You can find out more at www.OncuraPartners.com.

Of course, getting a second opinion will not always yield a consensus about how to care for your dog – because there is no clear consensus on how to treat some tumor types. As frustrating as this can be when you want "the one answer," that just may not be possible. If you find yourself torn between opinions, you'll need to remember that you are your dog's Primary Health Advocate. Center yourself and use your discernment to proceed.

Other Practitioners

Other opinions that may be valuable could come from veterinarians who practice something other than traditional western medicine, such as Ayurvedic (a system of medicine from India), homeopathy or Traditional Chinese Medicine. Although I can hear some of my veterinary colleagues gnashing their teeth as I write this, I keep an open mind to other disciplines, as you now know. Western medicine does not have the "cure" for cancer – so who are we to exclude treatments that might help?

Acupuncture is a branch of Traditional Chinese Medicine (TCM). Acupuncturists use extremely fine

Western medicine does not have the "cure" for cancer – so who are we to exclude treatments that might help?

Extremely Supportive and Open-Minded Vet a Blessing

"I was really blessed to have an extremely supportive and open-minded vet during my Ellie's battle with cancer. I was able to show him parts of Dr. Dressler's book and discuss which natural products I wanted to use (K-9 Immunity, for example), and he was totally open to writing prescriptions for whatever else I needed to get from him (doxycycline). I know some people might not be as lucky to have such a flexible vet. My vet was a very important part of my having access to the full range of cancer-fighting agents."

— Sarah N. Bertsch, Hudson, Wisconsin

needles to stimulate certain points on the body and increase the flow of life energy (*qi*, pronounced *chee*) to body parts, associated with the needled points. Although to the western mind, acupuncture and Chinese herbal formulas can seem mysterious, dangerous or downright wacky, TCM has been in use for thousands of years in Asia and has a strong historical record for dealing with many illnesses, including cancer. Even the most diehard western skeptics are usually impressed by studies showing acupuncture is helpful for non-pharmaceutical pain management and nausea suppression. When we western types look for a physical mechanism to explain the way acupuncture works, we note that there are important clusters of nerves (nerve bundles) along some of the meridians, or channels, that hold *qi*.

The needles are fine – slimmer than sewing needles – and the sensations they generate range from a slight tingling to heat to a heavy feeling. Pain is rarely felt when working with a skilled acupuncturist, which is why I recommend that you consult with a veterinarian who is certified in acupuncture. You can find one in your area by using the search features on the American Holistic Veterinary Medicine Association website www.holisticvetlist.com and the American Academy of Veterinary Acupuncture website www.AAVA.org.

Homeopathy is a European system of medicine, based on the Principle of Similars or "like cures like." According to this theory, symptoms (cough, fever, headache, pain, swelling, etc.) are the body's way of releasing an illness, and are, therefore, supported, rather than suppressed. Giving a remedy, which, if given to a healthy individual, would cause the same symptoms, deliberately increases symptoms. While this seems counter-intuitive to many Americans (especially when they find out that homeopathic remedies are extremely high *dilutions* of substances), there is strong evidence that homeopathy, used in conjunction with traditional treatments, helps (human) brain tumors shrink. It may also be useful for other cancer cases.

Homeopathy is a complicated system, and I would look for a highly trained and experienced vet for your team. You can find a homeopath in your area by going online www.HolisticVetList.com.

Questions to Ask Practitioners

If you have already completed your treatment plan analysis and made your preliminary treatment choices, you probably have a list of questions you need answered. In addition, consider asking your vet, oncologist or any other practitioner, any of the following questions for which you need clarity.

Diagnosis

Are you absolutely sure that this is cancer? How did you make the diagnosis?

What tests have you run? What other tests are available?

Is this cancer rare or common? How many cases have you seen?

Has the cancer spread? To where? How do you know?

Treatments

What do you expect to happen as a result of the treatment(s) you recommend? What is the best possible outcome? What is the worst? How likely is either of those to happen?

If this treatment works, how much time do you think it will gain us?

If this treatment works, how much quality of life do you think it will gain us?

What are the odds this treatment will not work?

Why are you recommending this treatment? Are there any negatives in using this?

What is the probable outcome if we decline this treatment?

Are there other treatment options, and what are the positives and negatives about each one?

Do you have any written material I can take home to read?

How long will this treatment last? How often do I have to come in?

Do I stay with my dog during the treatment, or do I have to leave him with you?

Does my dog need sedation or any other medications during treatment?

Is this treatment uncomfortable in any way for my dog?

Is there any special care I need to give after this treatment? Do I need to be home the rest of the day? The next?

Are there any supplies or over-the-counter medications I will need at home for after-treatment care?

What are the side effects of this treatment? How often do they occur? What do they look like?

How do I know if a side effect is severe enough to warrant calling you for emergency care?

How likely is that?

What do I need to do to prepare my dog for this treatment?

How do dogs normally feel after this treatment? Immediately afterward? In the days that follow? When do they feel normal again?

Are there any foods, supplements or anything else to avoid before or after the treatment?

Are there any new treatments or clinical trials to consider?

How much does this treatment cost? Is the cost mostly up front or spread out over time?

Does my dog have any other (non-cancer) health issues that limit our treatment choices or may affect her outcome?

Does my dog have any other (non-cancer) health issues that may affect her life quality?

If I have a limited budget, which treatment or treatments are my first priority?

Pain Management

Do you think my dog is in pain? How would you treat that?

Do you think this pain is chronic or short-term?

Is there anything else I can do to minimize her pain?

Vet-Client Dynamics

What's the best way for me to contact you when I have more questions?

Do you provide a written cost estimate and may I have one?

What types of payment do you accept? May I spread my payments out over time?

May I have a copy of my dog's medical files and images?

Are you comfortable with my getting a second opinion, if I need one?

Are you comfortable with my making the final decisions about my dog's care? Even if I don't follow your recommendations?

Do you consider yourself conventional? Alternative? Holistic? Will you share your professional guiding principles with me?

Even though that last question may feel awkward, asking it is important, because the answer will reveal a lot. My philosophy is that dogma of any kind does not belong in medicine. If a treatment may help and is safe, I am all for it, no matter where it comes from. If you agree with

Dogma of any kind does not belong in medicine.
If a treatment may help and is safe, I am all for it, no matter where it comes from.

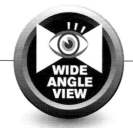

Always Ask Why

When speaking with vets, oncologists, specialists, herbalists, energy healers, or any other practitioners you bring onto your team, make sure you ask these important questions:

Why do you recommend doing this? What is the ultimate outcome you expect?

It can be easy to get caught up in the details of a particular treatment, or in the emotional anguish of the situation, and completely forget the goal that you have set as your dog's guardian.

Asking the "Why?" question will help you to assess whether the treatment will get you what you really want (whether you want tumor reduction, pain relief, increased energy, or some other specific outcome).

I recently noticed that the word "compass" is contained within the word "compassion." Asking "why do this?" on a regular basis can be a compass for us, as we treat our dogs with the compassion they deserve.

me, you might pay close attention to both the words and body language the practitioner uses when sharing her philosophy. Her bias might be revealed in subtle ways. If she is privately thinking "those holistic guys are all quacks" or "Western medicine does more harm than good," it's important that you know it so you can proceed appropriately.

Be sure to share your own philosophy with your vet, too. This helps him to know how to serve you best. If you feel comfortable, you can share your mission statement. Some guardians would rather keep that private. At least, make sure you share:

• Which benefits you find most important.

• Which side effects you can tolerate and which you cannot.

• Any options you are considering in addition to what has already been discussed.

Getting on the same page with your vet is critical to having a good working relationship and helping your dog. Dealing with dog cancer is hard enough without feeling uncomfortable with your veterinary professional.

Working with Loved Ones

Health care practitioners are not the only members of your Full Spectrum team. Reaching out to friends and family members can be a great way to get emotional support while you deal with your dog's cancer. Your spouse, child or close friend can be an active member of your team. However, even if you have a truly exceptional group of people in your life, you may run into a few who just don't "get it".

Lack of Understanding

Many people don't have the psychological skills to help us at a time like this – and maybe we should not expect them to. A guardian told me that one of his best friends refused to speak with him during his dog's cancer ordeal. "I lost my mother, my father and my uncle to cancer," she said. "And my son died last year. I just can't stomach how upset you are over a *dog*."

That may seem heartless and it certainly hurt my client's feelings. I suspect, however, that this otherwise loving friend was still grieving her own losses. For whatever reason, she just couldn't be there for my client at that time.

Often friends and family members who behave with insensitivity may actually be very worried about you. Their comments could be designed to help you by "shaking you out of it." What they most likely really want is for everything to be all right, for you.

Of course, that's what you want, too. But if you love your dog the way that Dr. Ettinger and I love our dogs, it may not be possible for you to act like everything is all right. If your friends and family are not dog lovers, they may never understand what you are going through. For some people, dogs are animals, not loved ones. The sooner that you accept this, the sooner you will find peace of mind and maybe even forgive them for hurting your feelings. Releasing those hurt feelings is important.

If someone is really hurting your feelings on a regular basis, intentionally or not, it's absolutely all right for you to say something like "I appreciate your advice, but I'm going through a really tough time right now. Can we talk about this later?"

Dismissive Comments

Sometimes friends or family try to be supportive by saying something like "Everything is fine, you're fine." This can actually feel a little dismissive. I know that if my dog Björn had cancer, I would not feel "fine."

It's all right to be honest about how you feel. You can say "Thanks, but right now I feel [angry, sad, afraid, guilty, frustrated, etc.]." Agreeing that you're "fine," when you don't feel "fine" can actually set you up for trouble.

According to experts, sadness that is repeatedly avoided turns into a more intense form of grief, which, if it continues to be avoided, turns into depression. Sadness is an emotion that ends after a while. Depression, on the other hand, is a recurring, life disrupting disorder. Also, because of the emotional feedback loop between you and your dog, your depression might even put your dog at risk for depression.

The bottom line is this: be a guardian at all times. Do not assume that your best friend, your mother, your sister, or your favorite uncle can be as supportive as you may wish. Remember that they love you and want what is best for you, and try to see their good intentions behind any insensitivity. If you can, drop your expectation that they be perfect, and if you need to, protect yourself. Right now, your priority is your dog – right?

Children

What if you need to protect someone else? Children and teenagers often blame themselves for a dog's cancer. And sometimes they blame the adults – in other words, you. This can be really hard on guardians.

Remember, there is an emotional feedback loop between you and your children; your mood influences them. Be as kind and supportive as you can be, and include them in important decisions to demonstrate to them that you are taking charge and helping your dog. In my experience, some of the best cancer caretakers are teenagers. They will often do more for their dogs than they would for themselves. Depending upon their personalities, maturity, sensitivity and skills, young people can make valuable members of your team.

Although it may be difficult, it's also important to have a conversation about the possibility that your dog could die as a result of this cancer. The purpose is not to plan for or to focus on it. The purpose is to have a complete and intimate conversation. For example, it can be very helpful for children to find out that you believe your dog has an indestructible soul (if this is what you believe). As a child, I found this idea very comforting when a beloved pet was sick and facing death.

Professional Support

No matter how strong you are, if your dog has cancer, you are scared. I've never met a guardian who wasn't, even those of us who tend to tough it out. Who wouldn't be afraid of losing her dog?

If you have been in therapy before, or if you regularly talk to your spiritual leader, you probably don't need to be reminded to call him and let him know what is going on. Do not underestimate the impact your dog's cancer can have on your emotional and spiritual life. At the very least, it's draining. You can use the support.

If you are a stiff-upper-lip-type, listen up. You must admit that this is hard, even if you only admit it to yourself. If you are fighting to stay tough, you are using valuable energy that is better spent helping your dog fight cancer.

Talking to someone, like a priest, pastor, rabbi or other religious figure, can help you a great deal. Professional counselors and therapists can be very helpful, also. It can be a relief to speak with someone trained to listen.

Some veterinary schools (Cornell, University of Minnesota, University of Tennessee and others) offer support hotlines, supervised by professionals and staffed by vet students with good "bedside manners." Speaking with one of these compassionate students can be very helpful. The best way to find these support lines is to go online and search for the keywords "veterinary school support line."

Other Sources of Support

There are several good online support groups for guardians whose dogs have cancer. One that readers have found very helpful is the yahoo.com group named "Canine Cancer" http://pets.groups.yahoo.com/group/caninecancer.

Speaking with a good friend can also be very restorative, and remember the emotional management exercises in Chapter 2.

The bottom line is this: there are a lot of people going through the same thing. Reach out for help and get the emotional support you need; you are worth it. You're also helping your dog when you help yourself.

Chapter 23: Keep a Journal

O nce your plan is in place and you're in motion, you'll need to stay organized. You'll need a place to record your schedule, treatments, side effects, diet changes and many other factors. Doing this in an organized fashion helps you to chart your progress over time.

By using a journal, you'll be able to accurately discuss your dog's cancer case without having to rely on your memory. The act of keeping a journal also sharpens your observational skills; small changes that happen gradually won't be missed this way.

Many guardians start a new diet, new drugs, new supplements and new therapies immediately after a cancer diagnosis; that's when it is especially important to keep notes. Because any change in a dog's diet or routine can cause stomach distress, for example, knowing what changes you made and when will help you to figure out what may be causing problems, if they arise.

Keep your journal in a way that makes sense to you. Some guardians already have a daily journal; they just add this information to it. Others get a special notebook or binder or a bound journal. There are computer tools available, too, and even Smartphone applications. You can also use the companion book to this one: *The Dog Cancer Survival Guide Companion Journal.*

The best time to write in the journal is usually at the end of the day, when you have a full day's worth of information to enter. You may not be able to journal every day; every two to three days is still helpful.

Starting Your Journal

You may have already started your journal as you worked through your treatment plan

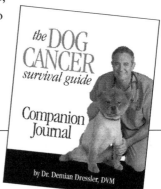

Dog Cancer Survival Guide Companion Journal

This handy journal is a great place to record your insights. It helps you to analyse and plan your dog's cancer treatments. It also features journal pages formatted with Full Spectrum cancer care in mind, so you can track your dog's health.

analysis. In addition to those notes, it is also helpful to record a general description of your dog when she is healthy. How much does she eat and when? How often does she drink? Take a walk? Sleep? Add as many details as you can about her normal play habits, attitude, personality, likes and dislikes. You will find this very helpful later, when you want to chart her progress. Reading through this description, and comparing it to her current condition, can really help you to understand her world.

What to Track in Your Journal

Here is a list of things for you to track in your journal, on an ongoing basis. Not all of these items are necessary to note all the time, of course, and some may be totally unnecessary for your dog's case.

- Mealtimes: including what she ate, new foods or changes to her diet, any positive effects (for example, did she like it? Did she perk up afterward?) and any problems, like digestive upset. Was anything turned away? Was her appetite good?

- What medications were given, how much and when. Make a note of any good effects (for example, increased energy, pain relief) and bad effects (vomiting, diarrhea, etc.).

- How did you manage side effects? Did you have to call your veterinarian or oncologist? What did he do?

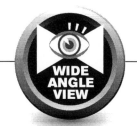

How to Take Your Dog's Temperature

Dogs with cancer have a suppressed immune system, which leaves them at risk for infections. Infections tend to raise the body temperature, so knowing how to take your dog's temperature can alert you to the presence of a problem in time to address it quickly.

It is not necessary to take your dog's temperature unless she seems depressed or lethargic, and especially if she has recently had chemotherapy. A normal resting temperature is 100.5°-102.5°. If your dog is panting, excited or has just come in from a run, her temperature can go up to 103.5°. If your dog's resting temperature is over 102.5°, or over 103.5° when excited, contact your veterinarian or oncologist.

You have to take your dog's temperature in the rectum. It sounds worse than it is, I promise, but you may want to use disposable gloves.

The best thermometers to use are the flexible, digital thermometers that get readings in seconds, rather than old-fashioned

continued on next page

How to Take Your Dog's Temperature, *continued*

glass thermometers, which tend to break and are very slow. Smear the thermometer generously with lubricating jelly, which you can get at the drugstore.

Just as most people would, your dog will almost always react when you insert the thermometer. Most will automatically sit, look back at you, or turn their butt away from you, but more aggressive dogs may even snap at you.

To avoid this, you have to hold her in place. If you are right-handed and your dog is small enough to sit on your lap, the easiest way to take her temperature is by putting her rear end to your right and tucking her head under your armpit, with your left hand palm up, underneath her belly. From there you can access the rectum and insert the lubricated thermometer. Lefties with small dogs can do the same thing in the opposite direction, facing her to the right, rear end to the left.

If your dog is larger, it's a little more difficult to do this by yourself. I do it in the corner of a room. I put my dog's head into the corner with his right side against the wall. I crouch down and slide my left knee under his abdomen, holding him to the wall with the left side of my body, his head behind me. Then I lift up his tail with my left hand, lubricate the rectum, and insert the thermometer with my right hand.

As soon as it's in, I cradle his body with my left hand, like I'm hugging him, until the reading is over. Lefties can put the dog's left side against the wall and reverse all the other directions. It can be really helpful for someone else to hold the front end, especially while you practice.

Of course, if you think your dog may react badly and bite you, seek help with a vet or a vet tech.

- Thirst: was more water gone from the bowl? Less?

- Temperature (you do not need to take your dog's temperature unless she is feeling poorly, especially in the days following a chemotherapy treatment): any change?

- Energy Level: Alert? Tired? Spunky? Really low?

- Weight (weighing your dog every five to ten days is recommended): Gain? Loss?

- Vomiting: When? Color? How often? How did you manage it? Did you need to call your vet or oncologist for help?

- Stools: Diarrhea? Mucus? Blood? Amount of stool? Straining? Color?

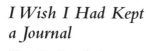

I Wish I Had Kept a Journal

"Per Dr. Dressler's suggestion, keep a journal with every little bit of information and observation. I did not and have wished many times that I had. Don't give in or give up. Be hopeful and determined. Put in the time and effort and try the things Dr. Dressler recommends. Do this. Do it with 100% commitment because you have absolutely nothing to lose and everything to gain. Even if you can't implement everything, implement all that you can."

– Kim Gau, Stow, Ohio

- Coughing: When? Moist? Dry?

- Sneezing: Nasal discharge? Clear or yellow/green? Any blood?

- Panting: When? For how long?

- Labored breathing: When? For how long?

- Vocalizations: Was she barking? Whining? Moaning?

- Coat quality: hair loss? Sores or ulcers?

- Mobility: Any limping or reluctance to move around?

- Color of gums: Salmon pink (normal)? Pale? White? Yellowish?

- Changes in cancer (if visible): Measure the size of any visible tumors, or compare to another object, like a pea or a golf ball. Any surface changes?

- Surgical site: is the incision healing well?

- Mind-body: What is your read on your dog's overall feeling? What is the look in

I Have Referenced My Journal Countless Times

"I have a lot of advice for the reader. Become your dog's personal advocate. Research, research, research. Combine what you've found and learned into a program that you believe intuitively is best for your dog. Think positively. Consult experts, but make your own decisions. Never let a vet/other animal professional push you into treatment or a lifestyle change or otherwise, that you are not comfortable with or don't believe in yourself. Read this book cover-to-cover. Find an integrative veterinarian, and/or a veterinarian that is open to options above and beyond surgery, harsh drugs and radiation. Feed your dog the best possible diet you can afford. Stay up-to-date with research and information. KEEP A MEDICAL JOURNAL SPECIFIC TO YOUR DOG - I can't tell you how many times I've referenced mine for my dog. Love your dog. Be grateful for the time you have together. Ask the universe, friends and family for positive thoughts and prayers - every little bit helps. Most of all, enjoy every minute you have with your dog and try really, really hard not to dwell on the illness or diagnosis. Positive thinking works miracles!"

- Tammy McCarley, Sacramento, California

your dog's eyes? What do you think she's going through today? What steps have you taken to improve her life quality?

- Self-Care: Did you take care of your dog's guardian today? Did you meditate with your dog, or exercise? Talk to a counselor, get a massage?

Chapter 24: Financial Help

Conventional cancer care costs an average of $5,000 to $8,000, and if all three treatments (surgery, chemotherapy and radiation) are used, the bill can easily exceed $10,000. For many guardians this is a real financial burden, and for many others, the price tag makes any treatment prohibitive. Whether that number makes you gulp or yawn, spending your dollars wisely is important. Every dog deserves the best care her guardian can provide and, luckily for all of us, every kiss, hug and caress you give your dog makes a difference.

Unfortunately, kisses and hugs don't pay the vet bills; if you need help, there are several organizations that may be worth contacting.

Organizations That May Help With Medical Bills:

- **Magic Bullet Fund:** For dogs with cancer, whose treatment may extend life a year or more www.themagicbulletfund.org

- **Angels for Animals:** General financial help www.angels4animals.org

- **United Animal Nations Lifeline:** General financial help www.uan.org

- **Canine Cancer Awareness:** Help for dogs in need of cancer treatment www.caninecancer-awareness.org

- **Cody's Club:** Financial help for dogs in need of radiation treatment codysclub.brave-host.com

- **Riedel & Cody Fund:** Provides an online community site where you can raise funds, apply for a grant and network with others www.cancerpets.org

- **Help-a-Pet:** General financial help www. help-a-pet.org

- **In Memory of Magic:** General financial help www.imom.org

- **Pet Fund:** Non-emergency financial

> ### *An Individual Decision*
>
> "Treating our boy was expensive, emotionally and financially. There are a few things that we said we would never do this again with another dog, but other times that we feel that it was completely worth it. It is a very individual decision based on your dog, your circumstances and your available resources."
>
> *- Candice Lapa, Fresno, California*

help www.thepetfund.com

- **Pigger's Pals:** Financial help for owners seeking oncologists or surgical specialist services www.piggerspals.org
- **AAHA Helping Pets Fund:** General help for sick pets, if your veterinarian is a member of AAHA (American Animal Hospital Association) www.aahahelpingpets.org
- **Helping Harley Working Dog Cancer Treatment Grants:** For working dogs with cancer (service dogs, assistance dogs, etc.) www.grants.landofpuregold.com
- **OSLF Fund for Orthopedic Cases:** Financial help for pets needing amputations or treatment for help in movement www.oslf.org
- **Labrador Lifeline:** Financial help for labs www.labradorlifeline.org
- **Save Us Pets:** Financial help for pets in New Jersey www.saveuspets.org
- **Animal Cancer Therapy Subsidization Society:** For pets with cancer in Alberta, Canada www.actss.ca
- **Greedy or Needy:** A make-a-wish site www.greedyorneedy.com

These links were all operational at the time of this writing, but, as you know, things can always change on the internet. I cannot guarantee any of these sites will help you, but they give you a place to start your search. There may be other resources available, too; common search terms include your breed's name, "cancer bills," "vet bills," and "help."

Clinical Trials

Veterinary schools and research facilities are often actively conducting clinical trials for new techniques or medications. Participating in these can be a good way to get new treatments, at reduced cost. Calling organizations or schools in your area directly is the best way to find out about local trials, and you can also check the Veterinary Cancer Society's website for an index www.VetCancerSociety.org

Barter

An old-fashioned practice has regained popularity: barter. Although not everyone is a fan, I have heard from some readers that this solution worked for their vet and other caregivers. Perhaps you can work off your bill by trading your professional services, such as accounting, building contracting or consulting. The owner of a corporate chair massage business traded a day's worth of chair massage, for the veterinarian and his employees, in exchange for an equivalent reduction in her medical bill. Another reader bartered a reduction in the bill for cleaning and repainting the vet's parking lot, shampooing the carpets and waxing the office floors. An owner of a popular restaurant gladly fed her vet and his family, without charge, until her bill was paid down.

If you suggest barter to your vet, I strongly recommend a dollar-for-dollar trade to avoid quibbles over how much is owed or paid. You should also consult with your accountant, because bartered services may be taxable.

CareCredit

Some veterinarians and oncologists accept CareCredit, which is a healthcare credit card that can be used to pay off your veterinary bills in monthly payments, over time. As long as you pay your bill according to the terms of your agreement with CareCredit, there are no additional costs, upfront fees or pre-payment penalties. CareCredit can do this because practices pay fees to participate, plus, the bank's penalties for late or missed payments on your part are hefty. Depending upon your needs and which promotional packages your veterinarian offers,

Don't Worry If You Can't Afford Expensive Treatments – Your Dog Is Stronger Than You Are

"If you are facing the challenge of cancer with your beloved canine, please know that you are not alone. Your emotional pain is singular, yet it is shared by so many. Love your dog as much as possible each and every day. Do whatever you need to do in order to spend as much time together as possible, even if it's just riding around in the car or lying on the floor together. Take photos. Lots and lots of photos. No matter what the outcome, this is a precious time. Speak in terms of positive things and tell your dog how great s/he is. There will be moments when you may feel overwhelmed with conflicting information, various treatment options, and differing opinions. Gather as much knowledge as you can at any given moment, and then make a decision based on what you know (at that moment) and how your heart feels (at that moment). If you have honestly done this, then do not second guess yourself as that can be excruciating. If a treatment plan isn't working, be open to trying something else. And always be open to trying less rather than more. Never forget that your dog will tell you what you need to know, but you may have to be very patient and pay very close attention. Don't worry if you cannot afford very expensive treatment options. Embrace what you are able to do and do not focus on the "what ifs". Be thankful. Be thankful every time you hear the paws patting across the floor or feel the warm tongue on your hand, every time you see the glistening eyes and feel the soft ears. Give extra-long tummy rubs or neck scratches. Rejoice if you are given a good prognosis. And if you are not, remember that your dog is stronger than you are. Together you will be able to get through whatever comes next. Keep track of how enjoyable life is from your dog's perspective. If the time comes when you must make a decision to help your dog through the end of this struggle, be there to love him/her throughout the process. It is a privilege to love a creature that much. Never forget that cancer cannot rob you of all the happy times. Keep the memories alive. Always remember that love is stronger than cancer. Always. No matter what."

- Sarah N. Bertsch, Hudson, Wisconsin

this could be a good option for some guardians. Although there is an application process, and your credit history will be reviewed before you get approval, even guardians with less-than-great credit may still be qualified. You can have a co-applicant with better credit scores apply with you or for you, also. If you have ever purchased furniture or electronics on a line of credit, this is a very similar process. You can find out more online www.CareCredit.com.

Chapter 25: End of Life Choices and Care

There may come a time when you need to let your dog go; this chapter is designed to help you through this unfortunate time. It covers how to provide hospice care for your dog, what to expect if you choose euthanasia, and offers a few thoughts on grieving. If you are not ready for this chapter right now, you can skip it. Otherwise, please accept my heartfelt sympathy, and also my congratulations for having the strength of mind and heart to contemplate this final act of kindness.

For many guardians, this time is filled with crushing pain and deep sadness. I've also noticed that guardians who feel prepared for the end find more than just pain. Some also feel a deep sense of relief that their dogs' struggles are over. A few feel a strangely vibrant, fierce sense of connection with their dogs.

First, the most common question I get. How do you know when it is time to let go?

How to Know When "It Is Time"

In my experience, guardians know when the end of their beloved dogs' lives are near. Some guardians see a pleading look in their dogs' eyes, as if they are literally begging them to stop the pain. Others take an honest look at their quality of life and just cannot imagine their having to live this way for much longer.

Many guardians feel a *click* inside – a sudden realization that it is time to let their dogs

"I Did My Absolute Best Today"

"... every night, say to yourself " I did my absolute best for my dog today." When things start to get bad, and there isn't much you can do for your dog, still say" I did the best I could for my dog today." How you, your family, your vet help your dog leave this life is what you will remember about the whole experience of his disease. Have a plan ready. I was so grateful that my vet came to my home, my grown children could be there, a service came to take him for cremation and returned his ashes. Everyone was so caring and respectful. I know it is very hard to think about this ahead of time. Believe me, it is worth it. On that day, you can again say "I did the best that I could for my dog, and myself." "

- Mignon Owens, Jessup, Maryland

pass. Sometimes others – your spouse, your vet, your children, your friend – feel the *click*, too.

How you handle that click is going to depend upon your own personality, beliefs and desires.

You feel the *click*, but think your dog still has some time left. If this is you, you may look at your dog's quality of life and feel that it still has more positives than negatives, or that certain positives outweigh the negatives. In this case, you may choose to continue with cancer treatments, while also acknowledging the click and emotionally preparing for the end.

For example, one guardian named Nancy despaired when Fergus lost his ability to walk, although he still ate with relish, and thumped his tail and smiled when she walked in the room. For her, that was evidence that he still wanted to "hang on." She discontinued expensive chemotherapy treatments and continued all treatments that were minimally invasive and provided palliative support. A few weeks later, when his tail no longer thumped, and his smile didn't last as long, she was emotionally ready to contemplate hospice and euthanasia.

You feel the *click* and know it is time to start hospice. If this is you, you may look at your dog's quality of life and feel that it has more negatives than positives. Although you feel that your time with your dog is limited, you do not want to shorten it – you simply want to make his last days with you as comfortable and pain-free as possible. The best choice for you may be to start providing hospice care for your dog.

For example, when Poppi stopped wanting to go for walks, had lost his appetite, and his other joys of life were slipping away, Jesse chose to start hospice care. He eliminated all cancer treatments and just focused on palliation, making Poppi comfortable and pain-free. He was surprised at how the hospice care seemed to give Poppi more time than he was told to expect – two whole weeks (more about this in the hospice section).

You feel the *click* and know it is time to put your beloved friend to sleep. Guardians who feel that their dog's quality of life has suddenly and sharply dropped often contemplate euthanasia. The quick release can seem very attractive when there is intense pain or a life-threatening, seemingly irreversible condition.

When Sue's Chopper came to the end of his life, his health took a very sharp decline. He spent much of his time sleeping, breathing heavily and fitfully. Once it became clear that he would no longer get any more joy out of life, and that living had become, instead, a burden, Sue decided to euthanize her dear Chopper.

You feel the *click* and ignore it. A few guardians resist the idea of their dog's lives ending. If this is you, I recommend dealing with your resistance before trying to decide how to handle the *click*. It may be time to revisit Chapter 18 and look at your dog's Joys of Life.

Although we cannot control our dogs' state of health, exercising what choices we do have can help us look back on this time with no regrets. As your dog's guardian, it is important to identify the next step. Everyone has a voice inside that, if listened to, gives the best direction. The irony is that in a time of great emotion, it might be difficult to hear that voice.

When You're Still Not Sure

You may need to take some time to clear your mind and listen to yourself. This is a time to consult your compass(ion).

This short exercise can help you if you do not hear your still, small voice.

1. Go to a place that feels safe and protected. If you have a friend or family member who is supportive and helpful, you might want her or him with you.

2. Let yourself feel your emotions, as honestly and deeply as you can. You might find yourself crying, yelling or lecturing out loud. Whatever comes up is normal and fine and you can handle it. Don't stop until you are truly finished.

3. When you are finished, you might feel your emotions burn out, like a candle that has run out of wick, or you might just suddenly feel "done." When you are truly finished, a sense of calm will likely well up in you; here will be a sense of clarity, fullness, and stillness. Your own emotions may still be present, and they will feel less intense and more manageable. You will be able to place them to the side for the next step.

4. Think of your dog and focus all of your attention on him. Ask yourself whether or not he wants to be here any longer. Feel yourself inside his experience, as much as you possibly can. Mentally review his life in the past, and compare it with his current experience. From this calm, connected state, allow the answer to your question to bubble up. It will come.

5. If you have any other questions, such as whether your dog wants hospice care or euthanasia, ask them while you are still in this state.

6. Take action on what you've learned.

In the end, the decision about how to finish your dog's days cannot be made by anyone but you. The calmer you feel as you make the decision, the more confidence you will have in it.

Dog Hospice

If you are ready to stop focusing on treating the cancer and start focusing only on your dog's quality of life, dog hospice might be a good choice for you. There are several practical things you can do for your dog to make him comfortable in his last days. First, I want to tell you about a fascinating phenomenon described in the *New England Journal of Medicine:* human cancer patients may both live longer and live better with palliative hospice care.

In a study that looked at human patients with non–small–cell lung cancer, those who received early palliative care with reduced chemotherapy treatments lived an average of almost two months longer than those who received standard chemotherapy treatments alone. Other studies, which looked at breast, prostate, colon, pancreas and other cancers, revealed that patients who received palliative care along with standard treatments lived longer than patients who received just standard treatments – with gains ranging from averages of twenty to sixty-nine days.

Palliative care attempts to shore up quality of life. Longevity is not the main goal; the emphasis is whether the patient feels good physically, psychologically and emotionally. While I recognize that this research has all been done in humans so far, I think that we can safely make the case that palliative hospice care may be very helpful to our dogs.

From a conventional mindset, stating that palliative care can extend life doesn't make much sense. However, when we look at this from a Full Spectrum mindset, it does. Chronic pain creates a lot of unhealthy circumstances in a dog's body. If you've ever had a headache that just wouldn't quit, you are familiar with the emotional, physical and psychological stress that accompanies this kind of chronic pain. As you'll remember, stress may suppress cancer-fighting white blood cells, like the natural killer and cytotoxic T-cells. Aggressively relieving pain, as is done in palliative care, may relieve that stress and allow more of these helpful cells to flourish and do their jobs.

Sometimes guardians worry that starting palliative care is giving in to cancer, or giving up on their dogs. Maybe, in light of this research, it is the opposite. It might be helpful, at a certain point, to stop trying to "fix the problem" of cancer and allow the body to just feel good.

To start palliative hospice care for your dog, shift your focus away from life extension and move it toward providing comfort and pain reduction. There are several areas to address:

> *It might be helpful, at a certain point, to stop trying to "fix the problem" of cancer and allow the body to just feel good.*

Cleanliness

If your dog isn't both clean and dry, she is probably uncomfortable and at risk for developing skin irritation and even sores. If your dog soils herself, make sure to give her a gentle sponge bath with slightly warm water and a soft cloth, to remove urine and feces. If incontinence is a routine problem, she might need sponge baths two to three times a day.

Bedsores

Most dogs in hospice care cannot move easily and spend most of their time lying down. Unfortunately, staying in one position for a long time reduces circulation to the part of the body in contact with the ground. This can cause ulcers, or bedsores, which are painful and hard to heal (this happens most often in larger breeds). To prevent bedsores, make sure your dog is lying on a thickly padded surface and rotate him from side to side so that he doesn't lie on one side for too long. At least every six hours, gently gather his legs to his belly and roll him over onto his front, and then onto the other side. (Do not roll your dog onto his back, particularly if he is a deep-chested breed, because this can cause a condition called gastric dilatation and volvulus (GDV), also known as "twisted stomach" or "bloat." GDV is a veterinary emergency.)

Pads in the shape of donuts can also be helpful: secure them to sensitive, high pressure areas like the elbows and knees with light tape.

Appetite

Some dogs in hospice care have completely lost their appetites and refuse most food. Appetite stimulants, like B-complex vitamins, prednisolone, mirtazapine, MegAce (megestrol acetate), Winstrol (stanozolol) and cyproheptadine are sometimes used, although they may not help that much. Many dogs, however, will still be tempted by food that seems interesting. Throw away all of the rules you learned about what to feed

She Gave Me One Last Gift, a Gift of Love

"Your book gave me hope and the knowledge of what and how I could help Kristi in her final days. Every morning we would pray together then we would go back into time and remember our life together. From the first day I met her, carrying her in my arms, training her every day, playing ball and catching Frisbee, we were inseparable. She would listen and lick my face, wiping my tears away. Remembering and talking about it with her, made the sad moment turn into happy times. It would even perk her up and we'd play for a while. (Her memory will never die.) She was a puppy at heart and would wonder what was wrong with her. I explained why she would get tired so easily and couldn't run and play like she used to. I told her about the place called heaven and there would be endless fields to run in. When the time came for her to go, I told her she would get all her strength back and could play again, but I wouldn't be there. Papa would be waiting for her, and one day, we would all see each other again. As much as I tried, I couldn't hold back my sadness and turned to wipe away the tears. When the time came to put her down, she knew it would break my heart, so she gave me one last gift, a gift of love. We played tug of war with one of her favorite shredded, busted up toy one last time, and then Kristi passed away quietly in her sleep the next morning. I am so glad that we had that and many other moments to share and the time to remember our lives together. Thank you!"

- Lois Boesing, Ewa Beach, Hawaii

your dog with cancer and give him whatever his heart desires. Whether it is meat, broth, angel food cake, junk food or cat food, go ahead and tempt your dog with anything that moves him to take a bite (the only exceptions are the foods that we know to be poisonous for dogs: chocolate, onions, grapes and raisins). Indulging your dog's remaining appetite is an important life quality treatment.

Dehydration

Dehydration is both painful and dangerous, so prevent thirst and entice your dog to drink about one ounce per pound of body weight over a twenty-four hour period (for example, a ten pound dog would drink ten ounces over twenty-four hours). If plain water does not tempt him, try using chicken or beef broth, soup, or any other liquid. If you can't get your dog to drink, you can try using a turkey baster to squirt fluids into the back of his mouth. If even this isn't working, injecting subcutaneous fluids may be your best bet. You can get fluids from your veterinarian, who will show you how to administer them at home by injecting them under the skin.

Pain Control

Pain management is a priority in palliative hospice care. In addition to the pain measures outlined in Chapter 17, you might consider sustained-release oral morphine. Some dogs don't like it and get whiney. If your dog tolerates it, it may be his new favorite pill.

Fentanyl patches can be used for a few days of pain relief. It is important to ensure that the patch is not chewed off and consumed, or a dangerous dose of Fentanyl may be absorbed. Usually these are placed in an area that is hard to reach, or covered with a bandage, and an Elizabethan collar may be needed. Your vet or oncologist will help with the application of the patch.

We veterinarians have just started to explore the idea of using medical marijuana in dogs. We don't yet have studies about its use in dogs, but we do know that about 25% of the dogs who take the prescription gel-cap form, Marinol, become quite agitated and vocal. It's very expensive, and using it in dogs is very "outside the box;" if this is something you want to explore, your vet may be able to prescribe it, depending upon where you live.

Apocaps has also helped several dogs in my practice feel better in their final days.

Your vet or oncologist will be helpful in coming up with a pain management strategy that works for your dog. Keep in mind that combined medications might be more effective than single agents.

Life Quality

Even dogs with limited mobility can enjoy fresh air and sunshine, massages, petting, going for a drive, or gentle play sessions with favorite toys. Acupuncture has a good record for providing some pain relief and nausea management, and a session or series of sessions might really help. Do anything you can to fill your dog's life with connection, warm feelings and closeness.

Dealing with Difficult Emotions

To help yourself prepare for your dog's passing, it might be helpful to do one or two of the exercises from Chapter 2. Pledge of Thanks and Life Story can be especially meaningful at this time.

Some guardians struggle with guilty feelings. One way to help cope is to take some time to apologize to your dog for everything you feel you could have done better in his life. Although it may sound sentimental, expressing your regrets to your dog directly, out loud, can help you feel you've really apologized from the heart. Dogs have a way of letting us know they forgive us for even our deepest faults, and that can be healing.

Even if you don't feel guilty, this exercise can be helpful during this time of transition to say your last words.

Spending quality time with your dog in her last days can be moving. It can also be exhausting and sad and just plain hard. It is normal to feel lots of different emotions and have many stressful thoughts during this time. Be kind and compassionate toward yourself, so that you can stay focused and help your dog.

Euthanasia

Sometimes dogs die naturally, in their sleep, at home. Most guardians, however, come to realize that what is best for their dog is to put her to sleep. If you are contemplating euthanasia, this section is for you.

Making the Appointment

Sometimes euthanasia is suggested during a vet appointment, or after an overnight stay, but very often you can schedule the appointment in advance. Schedule the appointment for a time when the vet is not likely to be terribly busy or rushed. The receptionist will probably ask you how you would like your dog's remains to be handled, after death. You will have the choice of taking them home with you or leaving them with your vet for burial or cremation.

Preparing for the Appointment

To prepare yourself, it is helpful to remember that you may see healthy pets in the waiting room. I also recommend asking a family member or friend to come with you. Even if you don't want them present during the procedure, you may need their help getting home. Having a loving presence with you at a time like this can ease the suffering a little.

Some guardians do not want to be present for the euthanasia. There is nothing wrong with this, however, the majority of people do not regret being with their dogs in their last moments. If you are worried that you will be too emotional, remember that the vet and her staff have probably seen many people react to the death of their beloved dogs, and it's unlikely they will judge you. If you are having trouble deciding, it may help to imagine yourself a year from now, looking

> ### Your Dog Will Let You Know
>
> "If and when it comes time to help them cross the bridge, they will let you know and they will, in their own way, convey their appreciation to you for a life well lived."
>
> *- Jill Stout, Medford, Oregon*

back at this time, and ask yourself from that vantage point, whether you will regret being present or regret being absent.

Some guardians feed a "last supper" immediately before the euthanasia appointment. Although I understand this impulse, a very full stomach can sometimes cause nausea or vomiting, particularly if a sedative is given prior to the euthanasia solution. For this reason, try to schedule that delicious meal at least two hours before the appointment.

At the Appointment

Euthanasia is a very simple procedure, with a profound impact on everyone involved. There are several things for you to know.

The euthanasia drugs must be administered directly into a vein, so it is important that your dog doesn't move around during this final procedure. To ensure that your dog is both extremely comfortable and calm, many vets use a sedative before actually injecting the euthanasia solution. Depending upon the circumstances, it may be possible for you to hold your dog or cradle him while this happens. Once the dog is sedated, the vet finds a vein, usually in the foreleg, and slips a very fine needle into it. He slowly injects the euthanasia solution into the blood. This solution is, most commonly, an overdose of a rapid-acting barbiturate. According to what we know of humans who received drugs like this, there is no pain.

Six to twelve seconds after the injection is complete, the dog usually takes a deep breath, relaxes, and then quietly passes away. Your dog may release his bowels and bladder during this time. There may still be some involuntary movements or a few more breaths taken before death occurs. However, most guardians are surprised by how quick and painless euthanasia is. Vocalization is very rare.

Most vets will give you a few moments alone with your dog after she has passed, which many guardians appreciate. At my practice we also take an impression of the dog's paw in clay and give it to the guardian as a memento. Some guardians collect a little fur as a keepsake.

After the Appointment

If you have opted to bring your dog home, you can bring a casket or box with you or your vet will have a box or a blanket ready.

If you are leaving your dog's body, the staff will probably wait until after you leave to handle the remains. If you choose cremation, it can take a few days or longer to get the body to the crematorium. Make sure to ask your vet how long it will take to get your dog's ashes, and any other questions you have about this process. One question I get a lot is "how do I know whether those are my dog's ashes?" Most crematoriums are very sensitive and careful about making sure that the ashes delivered belong to the right guardian. If you have any questions about the process, be sure to ask them.

The journey home may be a tough one for you, so if someone else can drive, that might be best. Everyone handles euthanasia differently, and we often can't predict our own responses ahead of time. It can be normal to cry, laugh, scream, feel numb or have any other emotional response.

Home Euthanasia

Sometimes guardians want to have the euthanasia performed at home, and some vets do perform this service. While home euthanasia can be less stressful than going to the clinic, there are things to consider. Some house call veterinarians do not have support staff, which means that you may have to take on the task of restraining your dog, cleaning up soiled blankets and linens, and handling your dog's body after the vet leaves. Depending upon your emotional state, this may be difficult, especially if your dog is less compliant on his home turf. Make sure you ask if your vet will bring an assistant, and whether they can bring the remains to the crematorium for you. Keep in mind there may be extra fees for after-hours or in-home visits, transportation, or assistants.

Grieving

I am not a psychiatrist or a therapist; however, as a veterinarian and a dog lover, I am all too familiar with loss. I would like to offer a few words about the grieving process, which may help you as you face the death of your own beloved dog. Loss of any kind results in grieving of some kind, and no one is exempt. We all experience our grief in our own ways, and it is hard to predict exactly how.

Most of us feel sad. This is completely natural and expected, and you need to accept it. Give yourself permission to feel your own sadness — it's a way of honoring your love for your dog, and it's not a sign of weakness or mental instability. If you are like me and many other guardians, you consider your dog to be a family member, and you have experienced a genuine loss. Let yourself feel it.

Grief can manifest in many ways. For example, some people feel physical pain like a stomach-ache or a headache, while others feel terrible emotional sadness. Some people cry continuously, while others grow quiet and reserved. Some sleep all day, while others stay up all night.

Some guardians may hear a sound that reminds them of their dogs' running through the house or even catch a glimpse of something out of the corner of their eye that registers as their dogs. Sometimes a scent or a visual reminder will trigger a memory so vivid that it feels unbearably intense. This is a lot more typical than you might think, and it's not a sign that you are crazy.

Sometimes the sadness is terrible at night, when the house is quiet. Other times it is worse during work hours, or when you're doing an everyday chore. Sadness, anger and upset feelings are normal and natural. Feeling them as they come up is important for the grieving process. Trust yourself.

It is not uncommon to struggle with the loss and have a really hard time. You may even need the help of a professional to get through the grief, and if you do, there is no shame in getting it. For many guardians, our dogs are true family members, and we take our grieving seriously. Counselors, psychologists and psychiatrists help people dealing with emotional hardships of all kinds, and this certainly qualifies. Friends, family members, online support groups and spiritual leaders can provide help, too.

As time passes, those intense grieving sessions usually shorten, become fewer and farther apart. Things will start to feel normal again, and you will stop thinking about your dog as much as you did at first. This is normal, too. It's not a betrayal of your dog – it's just what happens as we heal from grief.

If you successfully grieve (as awkward as that sounds) and really feel your feelings as they arise, without holding on or wallowing in them, your feelings of grief will diminish. Most people never stop missing their dogs, and yet, you may find that if you think about her, a few months down the road, you feel mostly all right.

At some point, many guardians are able to remember the time they shared with their dogs with joy rather than pain at the memory of their death.

Some people grieve in stages, and begin long before actual death occurs. Although it's a little unusual to think about it this way, some guardians receive the news of the diagnosis and can't help but immediately imagine what life will be like when their dogs are gone. What they imagine can be upsetting enough to actually trigger feelings of pain, loss and separation, even months or years before the actual death occurs.

This isn't true for everyone, of course. Some shove the sadness down deep while treating the cancer, only to be surprised later by the intensity of their grief after their dogs' death. Other guardians never fully realized how much their dogs meant to them until they are bowled over by the loss.

Hopefully you have taken time to get in touch with some of your feelings by using the exercises in Chapter 2. Guardians who have done this seem to have an easier time grieving and letting go of their dogs at the end of their lives.

As you move through this exquisitely tender period of time, remember this: There is no one way to experience grief. There is no standard process for the loss of anyone – let alone man's (and woman's) best friend.

One of the greatest gifts our dogs have for us is their unconditional love. Some of us feel that unconditional love strongly at the end of life, and it opens our hearts wide. I know some guardians who feel that the death of their dogs, more than any other life experience, made them truly human, open and loving.

For me, there seems to be some divine design to all of this, some arrangement of machinery where the earth spins and the heart beats, and everything makes sense in the long run. In this grand design, there is a point for each of us to enter the world, and a point at which we leave it. In between, we connect and love. If your dog could speak to you right now, I imagine I know what he would say. The next chapter features the loving message I feel I have heard many times from dogs in my care.

Chapter 26: If Your Dog Could Speak

*I*f your dog could speak, this is what I think you would hear:

"Thank you, thank you. Thank you, thank you, thank you, thank you!"

As a lifelong dog-lover and a veterinarian, I have heard this message and felt waves of gratitude from many dogs.

Their natural enthusiasm can be a gentle reminder to us to treasure our time together, no matter how short or long it may be.

Throughout their lives, dogs pack their To Do Lists with the very best experiences life has to offer:

Cuddling with loved ones…

Plenty of time outside in the fresh air…

Long and peaceful naps…

Running at top speed…

Playing with the most entertaining toys…

Exploring new places…

Eating delicious food…

Standing next to your side.

We can learn a lot about living the good life, if we pay attention to our dogs. They keep offering us teachings right up until their deaths, and even beyond.

My childhood dog, Bogart, runs through my memories when a certain breeze blows through the fields near my house. The same breeze used to lift his red hair as he caught a delicious scent and took off, tail wagging. This memory reminds me to stop, right now, and enjoy myself. I can hear Bogart, telling me:

"It is good to be alive. It is good to be here. **It is good to be with you.***"*

I think every dog on this planet feels this way. We humans tend to forget what dogs are eager to remind us:

> We live.
>
> We breathe.
>
> We smell the breeze and it feels good.
>
> We hold each other and we like each other.
>
> We play and walk and run.
>
> This life is good.
>
> I am good.
>
> You are good.

Becoming your dog's guardian is a great gift. His trust in you is justified by your loving him as deeply as he loves you.

> He thanks you for that.
>
> She thanks you for that.

If your dog is with you right now, take a moment to look at him. Gaze at her with soft eyes and a melting heart.

> This is why she was born – for this moment, right now.
>
> This is why he is with you – for this moment, right now.

If your dog could speak, she would tell you that her love for you is bigger than you can imagine.

> He would remind you to always remember:

"You are loved. You are loved by me, your dog, and you always will be. Our love lasts forever."

Chapter 27: The Rest of the Book

Thank you for reading and learning about Full Spectrum cancer care. Dealing with dog cancer can be challenging (to say the least) and I congratulate you for your strength of mind and heart. My best wishes are with you.

The next part of the book, From the Oncologist, is written by my co-author, Dr. Susan Ettinger. She'll give you nitty-gritty details about twelve common dog cancers, including how they start in the body, how they are diagnosed, prognostic factors and the current "best of breed" conventional protocols. There is also a section about the most common chemotherapy drugs. Make sure you look up your dog's cancer in her section, as well as chemotherapy drugs she recommends, if any. Read her introductory remarks, which start on the next page.

Following Dr. Ettinger's section, you will find several helpful appendices. Appendix A contains all of the supplements I recommend, in the general order of their importance. It answers the question "If I can't give my dog every supplement, which ones are the most important?"

Appendix B describes supplements which are not included in Full Spectrum care, and why. This is not a complete list of the supplements I have considered and rejected, but it does contain the most common.

Appendix C contains the resources I recommend for purchasing supplements, finding out more information, or doing further research.

Many guardians who read this book want to know not just how to treat their dogs with cancer, but also how to prevent their other or future dogs from getting cancer, in the first place. My advice for how to prevent cancer would be very different from the advice given in this book; that advice requires a book of its own. There are, however, some common sense steps you can take today to make sure you are caring for your healthy dog or dogs in the best way possible. That advice is in Appendix D.

Every concept and recommendation in this book is backed by thorough, extensive, scientific and medical research. Those references are contained in Appendix E, organized by topic. We are including these references so that veterinarians and other scientifically minded individuals can read the primary sources upon which Full Spectrum cancer care is based.

Finally, at the end of the book, you will find a comprehensive Index.

Part V:

From the Oncologist

In this section, Dr. Ettinger writes about her experience as an oncologist, treating dogs with cancer. Each of the major canine cancers is covered: lymphoma, mast cell tumors, mammary tumors, osteosarcoma, hemangiosarcoma, transitional cell carcinoma, oral tumors, nasal tumors, soft tissue sarcomas, brain tumors, anal sac tumors and melanoma. She also discusses each of the major chemotherapy drugs, including side effects.

Chapter 28: Message from the Oncologist

by Dr. Susan Ettinger, Diplomate AVCIM, Oncology

f I'd known back in veterinary school that I'd someday be co-authoring a book on a Full Spectrum approach to canine cancer care, I would have been very surprised. When I was a student, and later a resident, we learned little about these Full Spectrum treatments. There was little emphasis on the role of diet in cancer care, for example. Chemotherapy, radiation and surgery were the primary solutions we valued.

Luckily, medicine evolves, and I have evolved, too. In addition to what I learned at Cornell University's College of Veterinary Medicine and my subsequent oncology training, it turns out that fatty acids, a high-protein low-carbohydrate diet, and other strategies covered in this book, have been shown to be valuable for canine cancer patients. While they haven't supplanted the main tools we use, they have caught our attention.

At this point, my bottom line is this: Consider everything. If it's not going to hurt, and it might help, let's try it …

… Including surgery, chemotherapy and radiation.

As a board-certified oncologist, practicing in an urban medical center with several oncology colleagues, I am proud of how conventional treatments help dogs with cancer. I am well aware that many dog owners do not opt for these treatments, and many may not even consider them viable options. The purpose of this section is to give you my most up-to-date recommendations for conventional cancer treatments for each of the major canine cancers.

I hope to dispel some of the myths that have built up around conventional treatments, and quiet some of the trepidation you may be feeling as you consider chemotherapy, surgery and radiation.

You may find out that conventional therapies are something to consider for your dog and, if you decide they aren't, at least you will be making an informed decision.

There is one important thing to know about me, before I continue: like you, I am a dog lover through and through, and I will do just about anything for my dog. If it could have helped my beloved Black Labrador, Paige, I would have given her my own kidney.

How an Oncologist Can Help You

If you are even *thinking* about using conventional cancer treatments, I strongly urge you to consult with a board-certified cancer specialist.

Oncologists have more expertise in both diagnosing and treating cancer than general practice vets do. We have completed extra years of extensive training in general medicine and surgery, then even more time in our oncology specialty. We must pass rigorous examinations to achieve board certification from our college. In addition to this in-depth, focused education and training, oncologists see cancer patients exclusively. Because we spend all day, every day, using conventional tools to treat cancer in animals, general practice vets or specialists in other fields can't match the breadth and depth of our clinical experience, using these tools.

There may be different cancer specialists involved in managing your dog's cancer. For example, I am a medical oncologist, which means I am a specialist in the treatment of cancer via chemotherapy drugs. There are also surgical oncologists, who are board-certified surgeons, specializing in cancer surgery. Also, there are radiation oncologists, who specialize in the treatment of cancer with radiation. Each of these subspecialties is distinct, and the amount of knowledge each subspecialty requires is vast.

Your veterinarian is likely a well-educated, skilled and experienced practitioner, but, in my opinion, when it comes to cancer, dogs, just like humans, need to see an oncologist.

Although most cancers cannot, at this time, be cured, they can usually be managed with proper care. An oncologist can help you understand your dog's prognosis and offer a more nuanced and comprehensive conventional treatment plan than one you might get from a general practice vet.

Diagnosing cancer, and using chemotherapy, radiation and surgery to treat it, is not something that can be learned over the phone or from a book. There are no "recipes" that I can give you or your general practice vet that will ensure a positive outcome for your dog.

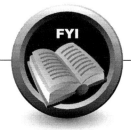

FYI

How I Think About Cancer

It's difficult for clients to feel positive about treating cancer when they think of it as "incurable." That's why I often tell dog owners how I view cancer: as a chronic condition, like diabetes. Even though your dog may need chronic medical care and medications, the cancer can be managed, and the dog often lives both longer and well in spite of it.

Your best bet, if you are considering chemotherapy, surgery or radiation, is to consult with an oncologist directly. Receiving the right care from the start can have a dramatic effect on your dog's outcome.

I realize your access to an oncologist may be limited by distance and/or budget. Oncologists usually practice in urban centers, where there is a larger population of patients and better access to state-of-the-art facilities, and they are more expensive than general practitioners. To find an oncologist in your area, visit www.ACVIM.org and use the "find a specialist" search feature.

If physically visiting an oncologist is not possible, keep in mind that your vet can consult one by phone. Many labs have oncologists on staff and private practices often offer phone consults to veterinarians, and occasionally to owners.

Some clients worry that using a specialist will cut their regular vet out of the loop. Some also wonder, "who should I follow up with?" as they start to consult with specialists. I am not in any way urging you to replace your family veterinarian with an oncologist. Your own vet, who is the expert on your dog's overall health, best manages all general care. When I see a new client, I always call the veterinarian that day to discuss the case, and I keep her in the loop with constant communication. I fax updates for her files after every single visit, and I send all the lab results and paperwork over, so she remains in the loop. If she calls with questions or new information, I take those calls promptly. I consider myself a specialist, called in just for the cancer treatments and follow-up appointments, strictly related to that illness.

Cancer's Cost

One thing that stops many dog owners from consulting with an oncologist is a very common assumption: oncologists cost too much, and the treatments they use cost too much.

That may be true for owners who are on a very tight budget, but in my experience, if you're choosing to treat the cancer, bringing an oncologist onto your team can actually save money in the long run.

When I run diagnostic tests on cancer patients, I often order blood work, urine tests, lymph node or mass aspirates, chest X-rays, abdominal ultrasounds and sometimes, a bone marrow test. I may ask a colleague for an informal consult or get a formal second opinion on a biopsy. These tests can total over $1,000, just to stage the cancer.

The tests are important. Knowing the stage of the cancer helps me to predict outcomes and decide which treatments to use. Most general practice vets would order the same tests I do, with a similar price tag. So what's the difference? Expertise.

If an owner tells me her budget is limited, I can weed out tests that may be less necessary, saving money for actual treatments. If the family veterinarian can perform those treatments – for example, a surgery that does not require a board-certified surgeon – I send the case back the regular vet. I can do this because I have expertise: I have seen so many dogs and so many cancer cases and analyzed so many pathology reports and created so many cancer treatment plans. Without all of that experience, I would not be confident in my decision to limit some testing and start treating.

Extra tests, especially when a dog owner chooses not to treat the cancer with conventional treatments, are a waste of money. I am too often in the uncomfortable position of having to tell a new client that the battery of tests that have already been run was unnecessary. This is especially frustrating when the client decides not to treat the cancer. In those cases, the money spent on those tests could have been spent on some form of treatment or saved altogether. It's better to understand what your dog is actually battling before running too many expensive tests.

An oncologist's experience and knowledge allows him to evaluate the necessity of each test to create a plan that fits into the owner's budget. This is why I recommend that, after the initial diagnosis, you consult an oncologist, if possible. The perception may be that calling in a specialist costs more money, but in my experience there is less waste and more value for each dollar spent.

An oncologist can evaluate your dog's case and weigh the specifics against what is known about the cancer's remission rates and median survival times. He can compare protocols and make a recommendation for what will give the best outcome.

Oncologists are not just cold, scientific specialists. They tend to be compassionate about budgets and personal circumstances. A good oncologist will be willing and able to create a plan that takes your budget and time into account and to talk about the possible side effects and potential risks involved in the treatments she recommends. A good oncologist will be able to go over the options and work with you to find a protocol that takes all of these things into consideration.

> *An oncologist's experience and knowledge allows him to evaluate the necessity of each test to create a plan that fits into the owner's budget.*

Chemotherapy and Radiation Side Effects

Many dog owners get an emotional charge when they hear the words "chemotherapy" and "radiation." This is understandable, because many people have had to endure those treatments themselves, or watched a loved one go through them.

It's a mistake to think that our dogs experience the same things humans do. Chemotherapy in particular is *very* different for dogs from how it is for people. Most protocols do not make dogs seriously ill, because we use doses that are lower than those used in people. In my practice, many owners express their surprise at how well their dogs feel during and after chemotherapy treatments. Most side effects are mild and manageable, and the majority of my clients have told me they're happy they took the leap and chose chemotherapy.

If you're particularly worried about side effects, make sure to tell your oncologist about your concern. He may be able to prescribe supportive medications, or there may be new treatment options available for you to try, instead.

Review Chapters 11 and 41 for more general information on surgery, radiation and chemotherapy, and for specific strategies on how to manage common side effects such as nausea, vomiting and diarrhea. Your dog's comfort and quality of life is a high priority for me, both as an oncologist and as a dog lover. I want your dog to live as long as possible and I want your dog to *live well*.

Median Survival Times

Some dog owners feel the amount of time likely to be gained by using chemotherapy, surgery and radiation is too little. I empathize, because I have felt the same way. Every dog dies too early – even those who outlive the normal life expectancy for their breed.

I include the most recent statistics about each canine cancer in the chapters to follow. It's important that you understand what these statistics really mean.

In canine cancer, we often use a statistic called the median survival time. Median survival times tell you the length of time past initial diagnosis at which half of the dogs were still alive. For example, if a study looks at sixty dogs, and the median survival time is twelve months, that means twelve months after diagnosis, thirty dogs were still alive and thirty were not.

Using this statistic is advantageous because it is less likely to be skewed by very unusual cancer cases. For example, some clients wonder why we don't use average numbers: add up the total survival times for all sixty dogs in the study, and then divide the result by sixty. While this average – also called the mean survival time – might seem like a useful statistic, it may not always be so.

Averages can be skewed by even one or two unusual cases. For example, if one dog in the study was an extremely long-term survivor, adding that in the average survival time might give the impression that most of the dogs in the study lived much longer than they actually had. The opposite could also be true: if one dog, sadly, died very early, averaging in his short survival time might give the impression that most of the dogs lived a much shorter time.

It's important to remember as you read statistics that the numbers do not necessarily apply to your dog. Each case is different, and statistics only tell us part of the story. We can't know what any statistic means for your dog at this time; they're included to help you form a general expectation.

Keep in mind the undeniable fact that dogs do not live as long as humans. For example, an extra year of time, for a dog whose breed has a ten-year life expectancy, is 10% of her normal lifespan. When we're looking at survival times, we must remember: time is relative.

Specific Cancers

The twelve most common cancers (in my experience) are covered in the next twelve chapters. I share what we know about each cancer's cause, effect on the body, diagnosis and prognosis, including statistics on survival times with and without treatment.

I present information about how to treat each of these major cancers, using surgery, chemotherapy and radiation. This advice, of course, is general and not intended as a recipe or a treatment plan. I recommend you take what you learn here, and then consult with your vet or oncologist to make a plan that takes your dog's cancer and other health conditions into account.

Some cancers have common protocols that, when followed, yield fairly consistent outcomes. Unfortunately, for most cancers, there are no standard protocols. In these cases, I offer the best of what we know at this time. This can be disheartening and frustrating for dog owners, of course. It's also frustrating for oncologists. Cancer is a complex and intricate disease; giving you honest facts and helping you to form realistic – or cautiously optimistic – expectations is part of my job.

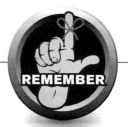

Read Everything

Empowered and educated clients make the best decisions, so, the more you know and understand about your dog's cancer, the better off you'll be.

When Dr. Dressler first invited me to co-author this book, I did not say yes immediately. I'm very busy with my practice, and my husband is also a very busy veterinarian. Add two children under the age of five, and you get an idea of my life. I even had to think carefully about whether contributing to this book was worth the time and effort necessary.

After reading the first edition and reviewing Dr. Dressler's blog, my loyalty to dogs and to my profession inspired me to say yes. I'm not a veterinarian by accident, and I didn't become an oncologist because it's easy. I work with animals because I love them, and I practice oncology because I believe in it. I'm also a dog lover, just like you are.

I have participated in this entire book, from cover to cover, including Chapter 11 (which is also about conventional cancer

continued on next page

While the most common canine cancers I see are covered in this section, there are many more types of cancer in existence, and some of those can develop in dogs. If your dog has one of these very rare cancers, I strongly recommend you bring an oncologist onto your team, because he or she will be best able to advise you with the latest strategies.

From My Heart to Yours

I see dogs with cancer day in and day out, and I see the toll the diagnosis and treatment takes on owners who worry over their dogs. My heart goes out to each and every one, and to you, the reader, as well. Here's what I tell my own clients about worry:

"Worry doesn't help your dog get better. It's wasted energy. Try not to worry about outcomes, or whether he will live up to or exceed the statistics. Let me worry about those things – that's my job! Meanwhile, you should be focusing on caring for your dog in ways I can't: enjoying your time together. Reporting back to me how he's doing is enough work for you – leave the rest to me." I hope the information in this book allows you to worry less, and enjoy your time with your dog more.

Read Everything, *continued*

treatments). As you can tell from reading the sidebars, I don't always agree with Dr. Dressler. Even so, I respect his work and know him to be a well-trained Cornellian (Cornell University grad). He doesn't recommend voodoo, and he's exhaustive in his literature research. He uses science to back up his work, and only recommends what has been shown to have value.

Important: if you haven't yet read the rest of this book, make it a priority to do so. There is important information there that isn't covered in this section.

Chapter 29: Lymphoma

Lymphoma is an aggressive cancer; it occurs in the lymphatic cells and quickly spreads throughout the body. Also called lymphosarcoma and malignant lymphoma, it is called non-Hodgkin's lymphoma when it occurs in humans.

Despite its aggressive nature, oncologists consider lymphoma one of the most treatable of canine cancers because it is highly responsive to chemotherapy. Dogs receiving chemotherapy have a median survival time of thirteen to fourteen months. During that time, most dogs live well, even during the chemotherapy treatments.

Early detection and treatment are vital to this happy outcome.

Without treatment, symptoms worsen and interfere with normal life functions, such as eating and drinking. Lymphoma negatively affects vital organ function. Most affected dogs will succumb to the disease in one month, on the average, while for some it can be a matter of days.

What is Lymphoma?

Lymphoma occurs in tiny cells called lymphocytes, specifically in the T-cells and the B-cells, which are part of the immune system. These specialized white blood cells circulate in the clear body fluid called lymph, which flows through the lymphatic system. T- and B-cells, along with other lymphocytes, are responsible for fighting and destroying bacteria, viruses and other foreign substances in the body. When these normally helpful immune system cells

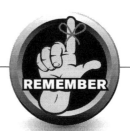

When you need to look up the definition of a word or phrase, find it listed in Chapter 5, which begins on page 46.

undergo a malignant transformation and become cancerous, they lose their ability to function normally and are called lymphoma. Lymphoma can develop in T-cells, in just the B-cells, or in both.

To understand this cancer, you must first grasp the complexity and vastness of the lymphatic system. It is a vast network of tubes and tissues, similar to the circulatory system in structure: large vessels lead to smaller and smaller ones, as they branch into most body tissues. Inside the network is the lymph, which carries the lymphocytes, as well as nutrients, to the cells, and wastes away from them.

If a map of the lymphatic system looks a little like a subway map, then the lymph nodes are the subway stations. Lymph nodes (or lymph glands) are "filters," located throughout the body. As the lymph flows through, the nodes trap bacteria, viruses and other foreign substances, so they can be contained and destroyed by lymphocytes. Organs that contain a lot of lymphatic tissue are sometimes called lymphoid organs: examples include the spleen, thymus and bone marrow. Lymphocytes also originate in these tissues.

Lymph nodes can become swollen when there is an infection (viral, bacterial, etc.) in the body, because they are filled with white blood cells, including B-cells and T-cells, fighting and destroying the infection. You are probably already familiar with this phenomenon from your own life experience, especially if you have ever had strep throat. As you may remember, this infection creates "swollen glands" in the neck, which can be felt through the skin and may cause pressure or discomfort in the throat. These glands are actually lymph nodes.

Lymphoma is thought to start (and is often first detected) in the lymph nodes. However, in some cases, it is not detectable in the nodes, but in other places, such as the kidneys or central nervous system. Regardless of where it begins, lymphoma is, by definition, a systemic cancer, one that is everywhere in the body, because lymphocytes circulate everywhere the lymph goes. This spreading nature also means lymphoma tends to progress rapidly.

About 80% of dogs with lymphoma have the "multicentric" form, in which multiple lymph nodes are cancerous. Often, the first involved lymph nodes are on the outside of the body, just under the skin. As lymphoma progresses, it can also involve the internal lymph nodes in the chest and abdomen, and also the liver, spleen and bone marrow. Less commonly, lymphoma will spread to the digestive tract, skin or nervous system.

Advanced lymphoma can infiltrate the bone marrow, where blood cells are produced. When this happens, blood cell production can be affected. As the cancer fills the space inside the bone, normal blood cells become crowded, resulting in low red blood cell count (also called anemia), which leads to low energy; low white blood cell count, which can lead to infections; and low platelet count, which leads to blood clotting difficulties. Sometimes only one cell line is affected, sometimes all three.

Which Dogs Are at Risk for Lymphoma?

A few specific breed lines, or families, of Rottweilers, Otter Hounds and Bullmastiffs have been reported to be genetically predisposed for lymphoma, which means the genes that cause lymphoma can be passed down through their breed lines.

Studies also show that some breeds are generally at an increased risk for developing lymphoma. These include the Boxer, Basset Hound, St. Bernard, Scottish Terrier, Airedale, Labrador Retriever and the Golden Retriever.

Those same studies show the following breeds at decreased risk: Dachshund, Pomeranian, Pekingese, Toy Poodle, Chihuahua and Brittany Spaniel.

Intact (non-spayed) females also appear to be at decreased risk for lymphoma.

In 1994, a study linked herbicides (particularly 2,4–D) and canine lymphoma. However, a subsequent study re-analyzed the results and failed to confirm them. For this reason, the jury is still out on whether herbicide exposure creates a proven risk for developing lymphoma.

Other environmental factors are reportedly associated with canine lymphoma, including electromagnetic radiation exposure (like the exposure from high voltage power lines), proximity to industrial areas and exposure to paints or solvents.

What are the Signs of Lymphoma?

The major sign of lymphoma is one or more enlarged lymph nodes. These are often discovered by the owner while petting the dog. There are several common sites for these masses, including under the jaw, in front of the shoulder and behind the knee. Because many dogs are otherwise healthy in the early stages, swellings under the skin may be the first sign that something is wrong.

Swollen lymph nodes typically feel firm and can be moved back and forth under the skin. They are generally not painful to the touch, and your dog will usually not seem to mind if you touch them. If lymphoma is present, lymph nodes will typically increase in size rapidly over the span of weeks, or even days. As the nodes grow, larger masses may feel more fixed, or anchored, in place.

Sometimes, cancerous lymph nodes can hide deep in the body, where they cannot be felt through the skin. When organs with a lot of lymphoid tissue, such as the spleen, liver or thymus are involved, there may be additional symptoms specific to those organs. For example, if the skin is involved, dogs may have ulcerated, oozing skin lesions, usually in multiple locations. If lymph nodes within the chest or lungs are involved, the dog may cough or have difficulty breathing.

Sometimes, a palpably swollen lymph gland is not the first sign there's something wrong. An owner may bring his dog in because he is experiencing general symptoms, such as weight loss, decreased appetite, lethargy, vomiting, diarrhea or fever. In these cases, a vet will typically do a physical exam and run routine blood work to discover the cause of the symptoms. The vet may find a lump during the physical exam.

Even if she doesn't, elevated blood calcium levels may show up in the blood work, warning her of the possible presence of lymphoma. Blood work can also be quite normal, even in advanced lymphoma.

Elevated blood calcium levels are associated with both B-cell and T-cell lymphoma, particularly with T-cell lymphoma. This is, in part, because cells in a special lymph node in front of the heart, called the mediastinal lymph node, can produce a hormone, which raises blood calcium levels. This special node cannot be seen or felt on the surface of the body, so, the owner would not have known it was enlarged.

How Is Lymphoma Diagnosed?

The nature of the lymphatic system is movement, which is why lymphoma spreads so quickly, and so widely. This is why I strongly recommend that new lumps in a dog's body be tested, measured and recorded in the dog's records for later comparison.

Lymphoma is highly treatable if caught early, so I recommend getting suspicious lumps checked out with a fine needle aspirate to determine if cancer is present. This is especially true when the dog is already not feeling well, or more than one lymph node is enlarged. No one – not even experienced oncologists – can be sure that a suspicious lump is benign, just by feeling it.

Lymphoma can usually be confirmed with this fine needle aspirate. A lymph node close to the surface of the skin is selected, as it is safer to access and does not require sedation or surgery. Typically, organs are not aspirated, especially if their appearances on ultrasound images are normal. On the other hand, if peripheral lymph nodes are normal on exam and these organs are abnormal on ultrasound, they will need to be aspirated to make the diagnosis. Because there are so many places lymphoma can occur, the aspiration site is decided on a case-by-case basis.

If the aspirate comes back "inconclusive," a biopsy will be done. If either the aspirate or the biopsy comes back positive for lymphoma, I recommend starting treatment immediately; that day, if possible. With many other cancers, owners may have a few days to deliberate treatment options. In the case of fast-moving lymphoma, any delay can cause problems. Once positive results on the aspirate or biopsy are received, I recommend you see an oncologist as soon as possible, and that you be prepared for her to recommend treating the cancer on that day or the next.

I strongly recommend consulting with an oncologist when your dog has lymphoma, because most have successfully treated many, many dogs with this disease. By "successfully," I mean dogs have an excellent quality of life and significant life extension.

The next step an oncologist will take is to run tests to determine how far the lymphoma has advanced, or what stage it is in. These tests are critical to developing the best treatment plan, custom-tailored to your dog. Tests may include blood work, urine tests, chest X-rays, abdominal ultrasound, immunophenotyping (testing for whether B-cells and/or T-cells are malignant) and, sometimes, a bone marrow test.

These tests are useful because knowing the stage of the cancer can help in gauging survival times. In addition, these tests provide a baseline, so that as treatment progresses, we can observe how the lymphoma is responding. Careful examination and thorough staging can help your oncologist decide how to treat the lymphoma, and you to decide whether to treat it.

One thing I look for in particular is a large

"tumor burden" – in other words, a lot of lymphoma showing up in nodes, organs, and/or the bloodstream. If the patient has a large tumor burden, he is at risk for developing "acute tumor lysis syndrome" within forty-eight hours after the first chemotherapy treatment.

Ironically, this syndrome arises because the chemotherapy is very effective for lymphoma. As massive numbers of cancer cells die, the substances that were once inside them (intracellular electrolytes and metabolic by-products such as phosphorous and potassium) are released quickly into the bloodstream; so quickly that the body is overwhelmed. This syndrome is characterized by vomiting, diarrhea, lethargy, collapse, increased or decreased heart rate, heart arrhythmias, renal failure, muscle twitches and breathing problems. This is especially serious when the dog is dehydrated because of not eating and drinking well, or because she has been vomiting from the lymphoma.

When I see large tumor burden in the staging tests, I tailor the dog's treatment plan to include hospitalization for a day or two, after treatment. This allows us to administer IV fluids prior to and after treatment. The fluids flush out the system and remove the metabolic wastes from circulation. Typically, dogs do not need to be hospitalized for subsequent treatments.

If a dog does not have a large tumor burden, this kind of reaction to chemotherapy during and immediately after treatment is rare, as is the need for hospitalization. Staging tests and examinations help determine which dogs are at risk.

As useful as these tests are, they can cost over $1,000 – and they do not treat the cancer, only tell us more about it. If you ultimately decide not to use chemotherapy to treat the lymphoma, these extra tests could seem like a waste of money. If you have received a positive biopsy or aspirate, and are not sure that you want to treat the lymphoma with chemotherapy, tell your oncologist about that possibility. If owners tell me this, or if they tell me that funds are limited, I may advise them to skip some tests or even staging altogether and, instead, put that money toward treatment.

Canine Lymphoma Test

There is a test available from PetScreen called the Canine Lymphoma Test (CLT). It uses advanced technology to detect certain lymphoma biomarkers, present in a dog's blood serum, which indicate a high likelihood of lymphoma. Despite the manufacturer's claim that this test provides a minimally invasive alternative to a fine needle aspirate, in my opinion, it is not necessary for the average dog with lymphoma.

One reason is: using a fine needle to aspirate a lymph node just under the skin is no more invasive than collecting the blood needed for this test.

Also, lymphoma is not technically difficult to diagnose in most dogs, as their lymph nodes are close enough to the skin to allow an easy aspiration. (Lymph node aspiration is no more invasive than the blood draw required for CLT.) CLT may have more use in cases where lymphoma is suspected, but not detectable, after the routine staging I describe above.

This test may have more promise as a monitoring tool used during the monthly rechecks that are necessary after chemotherapy treatments end. It may help to detect lymphoma relapse, although the expense might be burdensome. It is unclear whether using this test to find relapsed lymphoma will lead to longer survival times; if you consider using it, keep these limitations in mind.

What Is the Prognosis for Lymphoma? B-cell or T-cell?

There are many factors that we consider in order to arrive at a prognosis. The most consistently predictive factor is the lymphoma's immunophenotype: does it occur in the B-cells, the T-cells, or both? B-cells typically respond better to chemotherapy than T-cells do, and a dog with B-cell lymphoma survives longer, statistically. Therefore, a dog with B-cell lymphoma has a better prognosis than a dog with T-cell lymphoma.

The second most consistent prognostic factor is the substage: whether the dog is feeling sick at the time of diagnosis. In general, if the dog feels sick at the time of diagnosis, the prognosis is negatively affected.

Substage (a): no clinical signs related to lymphoma – in other words, the dog does not feel sick, at time of diagnosis.

Substage (b): there are clinical signs related to lymphoma – in other words, the dog feels sick at time of diagnosis (lethargy, vomiting, diarrhea, weight loss, anemia, fever, etc.).

Lymphoma, like most cancers, has a staging system associated with it. As a general rule, the higher the stage is, the worse the prognosis, although stage is less consistently helpful for prognosis than it may be in other cancers; studies vary. Even so, I include the staging system for your information:

Stage I: one lymph node is involved.

Stage II: multiple lymph nodes are involved, on the same side of the diaphragm

(The diaphragm is located between the chest cavity and the abdomen, so lymph nodes above the diaphragm are in the "head end" and those below the diaphragm are in the "tail end" of the body.)

Stage III: multiple lymph nodes are involved, on both sides of the diaphragm.

Stage IV: the liver and/or the spleen are involved, with or without stage(s) I, II or III present.

Stage V: the bone marrow and/or blood are involved, or there is extranodal (outside of the lymphatic system) involvement (for example in the eye or the gastrointestinal tract), with or without stage(s) I, II or III present.

There are several other independent predictive factors we look for to arrive at a prognosis. These are also reliable, statistically proven predictors:

How does the lymphoma respond to treatment? If the lymphoma responds well to treatment, the prognosis improves. If the lymphoma does not respond well the prognosis worsens. Obviously, your dog's response cannot be known until treatment is started, so this indicator won't help you until after treatment begins.

Is the dog on prednisone? If a dog is already on prednisone before chemotherapy begins, the prognosis worsens. Prednisone tends to activate a protein in the walls of cancer cells, called a multidrug resistance (MDR) pump (see page 130). This protein pump kicks toxins out of cells on contact. For cancer cells, chemotherapy drugs are the toxins. If the dog is already on prednisone, this pump may be active, which means that it could interfere with the effectiveness of chemotherapy protocols. This is not an absolute rule, as some of my patients on prednisone, even those with other negative predictors, have outlived others. Ironically, prednisone is often used in chemotherapy protocols, and also has an anti-cancer protocol of its own. The problem is *use prior to starting chemotherapy,* so inform your oncologist if your dog is

on prednisone and, if you have to start using prednisone for some other disease, do so in consultation with your oncologist. Despite this negative predictor, I recommend starting treatment, even if your dog is on prednisone already, as any delay in treatment worsens the overall prognosis.

I'd like to pause for a moment to remind you that every dog is different from every other dog, and that every cancer case is different from every other cancer case. Being acquainted with the stages and the predictors can help you nurture more accurate expectations about your dog's possible outcome. Lymphoma moves quickly and can end a dog's life in a matter of weeks, if left untreated. However, it is highly responsive to chemotherapy, especially in its early stages.

What Are the Available Protocols for Lymphoma?

Much is known about lymphoma in dogs, and there are several published protocols on how to treat it. Because lymphoma is so sensitive to chemotherapy, it is the treatment of choice. The goal of treatment is to achieve a complete remission of the lymphoma while maintaining an excellent quality of life for your dog. I will outline the most important – in my experience, the most successful – protocols below.

Keep in mind as you read my recommendations that there is no "one right way" to treat lymphoma. Every patient is unique, so, the best treatment for one dog and his owner may not be the best treatment for another dog and her owner. As always, consider your preferences, budget, and other factors, as you review your options (hopefully, with your oncologist).

As tempting as it may be to think of these recommendations as "lymphoma recipe" chemotherapy treatments, it is impossible for me to give that to you. Cancer is not predictable. In any given case, in my own practice, I may tweak the starting protocol at each successive visit, in response to the dog's progress.

The highest remission rates and the longest survival times are achieved with combination protocols, so I will begin with the one with which I have had the most success.

University of Wisconsin CHOP Protocol

The University of Wisconsin (UW) CHOP protocol is my treatment of choice for just about every dog with lymphoma (except, perhaps, T-cell lymphoma), especially if money is not a concern.

Any multi-drug protocol that combines cyclophosphamide (C), doxorubicin (hydroxy-daunorubicin or H), vincristine (Oncovin or O) and prednisone (P) is known as a "CHOP" protocol.[9] These combination protocols have had the best success rates, so the nineteen- or twenty-five-week protocol, published by the University of Wisconsin, is what I currently recommend.

Over 90% of afflicted dogs go into complete remission on the UW CHOP protocol, usually within the first few weeks. The typical protocol lasts five to six months, and once it is completed and treatments end, the remission typically lasts another four to six months. If a relapse occurs during this treatment-free time, approximately 90% of dogs achieve a second remission when the same protocol is repeated. The median survival time for treated dogs is thirteen to fourteen months from the time of diagnosis.

The rate of complications relatively low. Most dogs will ex of digestive upset (vomiting, diarrhea or nausea) at least once or twice during the course of the protocol. These side effects are usually managed with the home care (described in chapter 11) and don't require an office visit. The few (less than 5%) dogs who have more severe symptoms may need hospitalization for IV fluids, antibiotics and injectable anti-nausea medications. Most of these can still continue the protocol, although doses may need to be adjusted or preventive medications used.

Some dogs experience low white blood counts on these protocols. When this happens, doses may need to be reduced, or treatments delayed, to get those white blood cell counts back up (see page 131). Interestingly, a recent study found a silver lining in this scenario: dogs with moderate to severe low white blood cell counts during chemotherapy treatment actually experienced longer first remissions. This suggests that the dosage reductions and treatment delays did not affect the length of the first remission (longer first remissions indicate longer survival times). On the flip side, dogs that did not develop low white blood counts had shorter first remissions (which are associated with shorter survival times). Would these dogs have done better in the long run with higher doses of chemotherapy, and lower resulting white blood cell counts? This is an intriguing area that needs more study. I cannot say for sure that using higher doses with the goal of inducing low white blood counts will definitely translate to longer remissions and survival times; however, based on this study I do consider that strategy on a case-by-case basis with my own patients. If this approach is inter-

Handwritten note in left margin: DRUG COMBO

---

[9] The original University of Wisconsin CHOP protocol also included L-asparaginase (Elspar) in the induction (beginning) phase of the protocol. However, a follow-up study found that including this agent did not affect response or survival rates. For this reason, some oncologists do not use Elspar. Personally, I think Elspar can be a good choice because, in my experience, it works well for most dogs with few side effects. I do not use it for every dog, and always decide whether to include Elspar (and any other drug) on a case-by-case basis. Even if I do not include Elspar at induction, I consider using it at relapse.

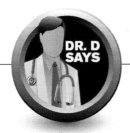

The conventional treatments that Dr. Ettinger recommends for lymphoma may be considered part of step one of Full Spectrum cancer care (Chapter 11). Please review that chapter for more general information about surgery, radiation and chemotherapy and handling their common side effects.

For more information on all other Full Spectrum steps, including nutraceuticals, immune boosters, dietary changes and brain chemistry modification strategies, review Full Spectrum cancer care, which begins on page 103.

You will also find information about specific chemotherapy agents in Chapter 41.

esting to you, I would discuss it with your oncologist.

During most CHOP protocols (including the UW), dogs get weekly treatments. Depending upon the specific version of the protocol chosen, treatments may decrease in frequency to every other week. Lymphoma typically responds quickly to treatment, so most dogs who are sick at the time of diagnosis are feeling better, or even back to normal, within two to fourteen days of the first session.

Given the number of treatments and how

many agents are involved, CHOP protocols are some of the costliest lymphoma treatments available.

Alternative Chemotherapy Protocols

Your oncologist may outline alternative lymphoma protocols, some of which may be less expensive and require fewer visits than CHOP. As usual, there are trade-offs to consider when looking at other options.

One protocol I offer is the single-agent doxorubicin protocol. This protocol has a 60-80% response rate (compared to 90% with the UW CHOP) and median survival times of seven to nine months (compared with thirteen to fourteen). As there is also a potential for cardiotoxicity (heart problems) after six to eight doses of the doxorubicin, oncologists typically stop treating with this agent after five or six doses.

Some of my clients choose the COP protocol (cyclophosphamide, vincristine or Oncovin, and prednisone). The complete remission rate is about 70%, with a seven-month median survival time. In the first six months, this protocol is certainly less expensive than the twenty-five-week UW CHOP protocol. Treatments continue during remission. If the dog stays in remission for a year (which of course makes us happy), the cost, over time, may actually exceed that of the UW CHOP protocol. Some clients prefer that the cost and the visits are spread out, while others wish they had gone with the UW CHOP to begin with, so that their dog could have had more intense treatments up front, yet enjoyed more treatment-free time in remission.

Other Treatments for Lymphoma

While chemotherapy is the treatment of choice, there are a few other treatment options.

Prednisone is a steroid often prescribed for its anti-inflammatory effects. However, it also has anti-cancer properties, and can help kill some of the lymphoma cells. The complete remission response rate is only 50%, much lower than those of the chemotherapy protocols mentioned above, and the median survival time is two to three months. Nevertheless, prednisone helps the dog feel better, and steroids are very inexpensive. Because prednisone can interfere with chemotherapy if started prior to treatments, using it is not recommended unless chemotherapy has been totally eliminated as an option.

If radiation is available in your area, palliative radiation can be useful in treating lymphoma, especially when it is directed at a single area, to relieve symptoms associated with an obstruction. For example, if a lymph node under the jaw is very swollen and large, it can obstruct the upper airway and impede breathing and/or swallowing. Radiation can reduce the size of the lymph node and ease these symptoms, markedly improving the quality of life. Palliative radiation can also ease breathing, by shrinking a swollen mediastinal lymph node in the chest cavity. In another example, if spinal lesions are pressing on the spinal cord, there can be symptoms like pain or paralysis. In these cases, palliative radiation can shrink those lesions and help improve symptoms. Palliative radiation protocols for lymphoma typically require four to six weekly treatments and should be used in combination with traditional chemotherapy protocols.

Another type of radiation treatment is called "half-body" radiation. During this protocol, the dog's body is irradiated one-half at a time, first from the mid-section up, and then from the mid-section down, without overlapping the treatments. Dogs who receive both this half-body radiation and the stan-dard twenty-five-week UW CHOP chemotherapy survive five extra months (in addition to the thirteen or fourteen from the UW CHOP). However, some oncologists question whether the increased cost and toxicity from the radiation are worth the extra time. Every dog, every cancer and every owner is different, so this is a topic for you to consider and discuss with your oncologist.

You may have heard about a human treatment for lymphoma: a bone marrow transplant with total body radiation treatments to put the cancer into full remission. The goal of this treatment is to cure the lymphoma, and the cure rates in people with Non-Hodgkin's lymphoma are 50-66%.

This treatment is also offered for dogs, with the same intent to cure. In order to qualify for this procedure, the dog must already be in remission, so most dogs have to get chemotherapy for two to twelve months prior to the treatment. It's offered at very few places, including North Carolina State University (NCSU).

The first step in the procedure is to give dogs very high doses of chemotherapy to clear lymphoma from the blood. This usually takes two weeks. Next, a medication called Neupogen is given for eight days, which drives healthy stem cells out of the bone marrow and into the bloodstream. After that, a complex series of procedures harvests those healthy stem cells from the blood (this is called leukaphoresis). Once the stem cells are safely out of the body, the dog is given total body radiation to kill all the lymphoma cells. This is a very intense procedure, lethal to more than 95% of dogs if they do not receive a bone marrow transplant immediately afterward. During the transplant, the healthy stem cells are re-planted into the bone marrow by transfusion (the stem cells do not have to be implanted directly back into the marrow, they enter the body through a vein). This is done soon as the radiation is complete, in the hope that the marrow will replenish the blood with healthy red blood cells, healthy white blood cells and healthy platelets.

This intense treatment is not for every patient. For one thing, it is very expensive (about $15,000-$17,000, plus the costs of all of the prior chemotherapy treatments) and requires two to three weeks of hospitalization. During this time, dogs must often be in total isolation, because they will temporarily have no white blood cells or platelets, leaving them at risk for infections and bleeding disorders. Also, the toxicity of this protocol varies from manageable to lethal, depending upon the patient. As it is still fairly new, it is too early to know what the cure rate is in dogs, but it could be a good option for the right dog and the right owner. If you are interested, consult with Dr. Steven Suter at NCSU, who has done the most research and treated the most dogs to date.

What If Lymphoma Relapses?

A good outcome for lymphoma protocols is a four- to six-month complete remission after completing the CHOP chemotherapy. However, relapses can occur. One possible reason for this is that lymphoma cells have become increasingly resistant to chemotherapy agents during the course of treatment (survival of the fittest).

At the beginning of chemotherapy, the cells most sensitive to the agents are the first ones killed. As treatment wears on, however, the remaining cells tend to be stronger and more resistant. These "survivor" cells are more likely to express the gene encoding for P-glycoprotein, which is associated with multi-drug resistance (MDR). You may remember this protein from our discussion about prednisone,

North Carolina State University Is a Very Special Place

"We heard about the stem cell bone marrow transplant program at North Carolina State University and – after doing a lot of soul searching – decided to make the commitment so LP could have a chance for a longer life. While LP was there for three weeks, we also used so many things we had learned in your book and found the staff at NC State so accommodating. They were so open minded about LP's diet and even have a nutritionist who worked with us. They have one person who spent time just sitting with LP during the extended time when we couldn't see him. I stayed in Raleigh for a couple of weeks and kept doing my visualization exercises and I am sure it helped LP and me. My husband is an equine vet and we deal with vet schools all the time. North Carolina State University is a very special place that we both highly recommend."

- Susie, Millwood, Virginia

above, or from the sidebar on page 130. This special protein acts as a pump in the membrane or outer layer of the cell. When chemotherapy agents come in, this protein literally pumps them back out, rendering them ineffective.

Another possible reason for lymphoma relapse is infrequent and inadequate doses of chemotherapy. If drugs do not achieve high enough concentrations, they cannot be effective. This can happen, particularly in sites deep in the body, such as the central nervous system (the brain and spinal cord).

If a dog has relapsed, the owner usually wonders whether to start chemotherapy again (called a rescue protocol). It is helpful to know that, in general, the likelihood of a second remission (or re-induction) is 50% and the second remission usually lasts 50% as long as the first.

A small number of dogs, especially if off chemotherapy at the time of relapse, after experiencing a complete remission, enjoy a longer second remission. For example, I have treated dogs who experienced an eleven-month remission, relapsed, and then enjoyed a nineteen-month remission. One patient, Lola, was put on prednisone by an emergency clinic to treat her lymphoma, and then came to me for a twenty-five week UW-CHOP rescue protocol. It has now been over two years since her last chemotherapy, and she has even developed a low-grade soft tissue sarcoma, which was successfully surgically removed during that time. I have another client who just celebrated her dog's eleventh birthday; I treated Jabba the Mutt six years ago with two UW CHOP protocols. Cases like Lola's and Jabba the Mutt's, while not the statistical norm, give us real reason to be cautiously optimistic about lymphoma rescue protocols.

Another relevant decision is whether to repeat the same protocol, or to try new drugs. This depends upon how long the dog's remission lasted. For example, if your dog completed a protocol like the UW CHOP protocol and experienced a long remission, I typically recommend using the same protocol again, because it worked the first time. This way you can save new drugs for a possible future relapse. However, if the dog does not achieve what is called a "durable remission" – a remission that lasts fourteen to twenty-one days – I recommend switching drugs. If your

> ### Fight If You Have To
> "Do everything you can, read the book, cook the food and pray. We enjoyed nearly three times as much time with Tyler as originally diagnosed. Fight with your own vet over treatment, they are not aware of this research and will tell you there is nothing that can be done. THEY ARE WRONG."
>
> *- John Arquette, Fayetteville, New York*

dog responds for only a few days or a week, this is not considered a good response, and I would look for another rescue protocol. Similarly, if your dog comes out of remission one month after completing the CHOP protocol, I typically recommend moving on to a new protocol. Common rescue protocols include: MOPP, MVPP, oral lomustine, doxorubicin, mitoxantrone and actinomycin-D.

The Bottom Line

From my perspective as a veterinary oncologist, lymphoma is highly treatable. Owners in my practice are typically extremely pleased with their decision to treat this cancer.

I rarely answer the question "would you treat this cancer, if this were your dog," because I cannot compare my resources to those of clients: I'm an oncologist, my husband is a veterinary internist, one of my closest friends is a veterinary surgeon, and I have the support of many specialists at my disposal. Yet, I make an exception in the case of lymphoma and readily answer "yes, I would treat this cancer, if this were my dog."

When aggressive chemotherapy treatment is balanced to maximize tumor kill and minimize serious side effects, dogs generally tolerate treatment well and live much, much longer than they would if they did not receive treatment.

During the weeks of chemotherapy treatments, most dogs' experiences parallel their normal lives. Interestingly, owners often report that dogs have more energy during treatment than during the previous months, even year, when lymphoma was not clinically present.

Dogs may get sick from treatment, but, in order for them to live longer (and well), they require chemotherapy. I truly believe the benefit of treating dogs with lymphoma easily outweighs the risk of side effects. Even if the dog gets sick, he typically recovers and can continue therapy. Treated dogs live significantly longer, are happy, run, play, sleep and eat, much as they did before they got sick.

Chapter 30: Mast Cell Tumors

Mast cell tumors (MCT) are cancers of mast cells, special immune system cells, heavily involved with inflammation and allergic reactions. Tumors most commonly develop in the skin, especially on the trunk, and can occur anywhere in the body. Mast cell tumors are also known as mastocytoma, mast cell sarcoma and systemic mastocytosis (or metastatic MCT).

While long-term survival is more common with MCT than with other dog cancers, MCT is a tricky cancer to predict. For example, some dogs with low or intermediate grade MCT have tumors that can be cured with surgery. They never recur or metastasize, or, if they do, it can be two to five years after the initial treatment.

Other dogs – about 10-15% – develop multiple skin tumors all at once, or over the months or years, never experiencing internal metastasis. Others develop multiple skin tumors over time, then internal metastasis eventually occurs. Still other dogs experience a higher grade of MCT with aggressive, malignant tumors that cause a rapid deterioration in health within months, and occasionally, within weeks. Because of this wide variance in outcomes, proper staging of MCT is important to determine your dog's prognosis.

Traditionally, MCT is first treated with surgery to remove the primary tumor. The use of radiation therapy after surgery is very effective to prevent recurrence, especially if the tumor is on a limb; chemotherapy can also be helpful for some dogs. Especially for lower grades, I consider MCT a highly treatable cancer. Exciting new treatment options have recently come on the market, including Palladia, a new tyrosine kinase inhibitor, designed especially for dogs with MCT.

What are Mast Cell Tumors?

Mast cells play an important role in inflammation. While other immune system cells tend to circulate throughout the body, mast cells don't – once they mature, they take up residence in specific tissues. Many live in tissues that mark the boundary between the outside environment and the internal environment, for example: the skin, the mouth, the digestive tract, the nasal passages and the lungs.

Mast cells contain structures inside their cell walls, called granules, which are like little sacks. These granules are filled with substances, or cytokines, including heparin and histamine, which help the im-

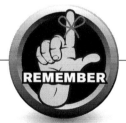

When you need to look up the definition of a word or phrase, find it listed in Chapter 5, which begins on page 46.

mune system respond to problems. Heparin is a blood thinner which helps defend the body against foreign invaders, and histamine is a chemical that triggers inflammation. Normal mast cells release these substances when prompted by the immune system. In addition to their role in inflammation, mast cells are involved in allergies, anaphylaxis (systemic inflammation), the healing of wounds and defense against outside pathogens.

Mast cell tumors are cancerous accumulations of mast cells with a malignant potential. While MCT is very rarely found in humans, it is the most common malignant skin tumor in dogs, accounting for 15-20% of all skin tumors. Mast cell tumors first occur in the skin and the subcutaneous tissues beneath the skin. It's very rare to find MCT in internal organs without a primary skin tumor, and skin tumors do spread to the regional lymph nodes, the spleen, the liver, other places deep in the abdomen and to the bone marrow.

Which Dogs Are at Risk for Mast Cell Tumors?

The cause of MCT is not known, although we do know a few things about what can predispose a dog to developing it. Dogs of any age, and either gender, can develop MCT; we see it more commonly in the following breeds: Boxers, Boston Terriers, Labradors, Golden Retrievers, Pugs and Staffordshire Bull Terriers. Boxers tend to develop low and intermediate grade tumors.

Chronic inflammation of the skin may predispose dogs to develop MCT, as can repeated application of skin irritants. Also, about one-third of dogs with MCT have a genetic mutation in a protein called the c-kit oncogene.

Although we tend to associate skin cancer in

humans with sun exposure, studies have found no link between sun exposure and MCT in dogs.

What are the Signs of Mast Cell Tumors?

Most dogs do not seem sick when they are diagnosed with MCT. They usually have a lump, or mass, on or just under the skin. These lumps are often found by the owner, and sometimes by the vet, during a routine exam.

MCT tumors usually look like raised, hairless, pink bumps – and their appearance can vary widely. Because of this, MCT is called "the great impersonator." Tumors can look like benign skin tags or harmless lipomas. Some are mistaken for insect bites because they get bigger and smaller on their own (this is due to the cyclical building up of and subsequent releasing of histamine, which causes inflammation and swelling and then a reduction). The tumor can be ulcerated (an open sore), swollen and inflamed or relatively benign looking. Tumors can be found anywhere, the trunk and the limbs being the most common locations.

Some tumors are present for months or even years, with little change in growth or appearance; others appear suddenly and grow very rapidly.

Some MCT masses itch and dogs may scratch or lick them to relieve the sensation. If your dog chews, scratches, or bangs the tumor against the ground, it can open up and release inflammatory chemicals from the granules. This is called degranulation, and the release of histamine can cause a localized swelling that looks like a hive. Massive degranulation can also provoke system-wide symptoms, like full-body swelling or, in very severe cases, anaphylaxis (shock).

Because of the wide variation in the appearance of MCT, I strongly advocate that every skin mass be aspirated for microscopic evaluation as soon as it is found (see below). With this evaluation, MCT might be caught early.

If MCT has spread to the internal organs, symptoms other than skin masses can occur. For example, internal tumors can release histamine into the bloodstream and cause the stomach to produce excess acid. The resulting stomach irritation and ulceration can lead to a decrease in appetite, vomiting with a small amount of blood, dark tarry stools and weight loss. Massive degranulation of internal tumors can also produce low blood pressure. Dogs with MCT of every grade tend to experience delayed wound healing because of the excess histamines and other chemical substances in the MCT granules.

How Are Mast Cell Tumors Diagnosed?

MCT are typically diagnosed with a fine needle aspirate, which has proven very reliable in confirming their presence. No one – not even experienced oncologists – can be sure that a suspicious lump is benign just by feeling it, which is why every skin mass (and those just below the skin) must be aspirated. The results allow your vet to then formulate an accurate treatment plan.

The most important factor in treating MCT is the grade of the tumor, which cannot be discovered via aspirate. Once the malignancy of your dog's MCT is found, your vet will likely want to do a surgical biopsy before planning curative surgery or other treatments. Let's look at how to grade MCT.

Grading MCT

If possible, the entire visible tumor is removed, along with a wide margin of surrounding normal tissue, because it may be possible to "get it all out" with the biopsy. (Wide margins in these tumors are two to three centimeters on all sides and a layer of tissue underneath.) These margins are not always achieved, of course, and must be confirmed with the pathologist's report.

If there is more than one tumor, it is recommended to biopsy each one, because each separate tumor could be of a different grade and need a different course of treatment. If there are many tumors – more than four or five – I will often biopsy the two largest or the ones which have grown most quickly, depending upon the specific case, the location and size of the tumors, and my own discernment.

The pathologist will look at several criteria to grade MCT (see below) and assign one of three grades to each biopsied tumor: grade I, II or III, according to what is called the Patnaik grading system.

Grade I tumors are the easiest MCT to deal with, and account for 33-50% of all MCT cases. These tumors are also referred to as low grade. They do not invade surrounding tissues, are well differentiated and they rarely metastasize. If your dog has a single Grade I tumor, further staging before surgery is probably not necessary.

Further Staging for MCT

In all other cases – two or more tumors of any grade, a Grade II or III tumor, a recurrent MCT tumor, or lymph node metastasis – further staging is necessary before deciding upon a course of treatment. For these tumors, staging will include, at minimum, an aspirate of lymph nodes in the region of the tumor or tumors (even if they are of normal size) and an abdominal ultrasound to check for internal metastasis. A bone marrow aspirate may also be needed.

Vets often perform lymph node aspirates first, because they are minimally invasive, do not require sedation and are relatively inexpensive. If cancer cells are found in the aspirate, even when they are not numerous enough to confirm actual metastasis, a lymph node biopsy will be done (usually the entire lymph node will be removed). If either the aspirate or the lymph node biopsy is positive, local metastasis has already occurred and the lymph node(s) will be scheduled for removal or radiation. Meanwhile, the internal organs will be checked before the first surgery is scheduled.

If no cancer cells are found in regional lymph nodes, it is probably safe to go ahead with surgery to remove the primary tumor, and wait to do the ultrasound (and maybe a bone marrow aspirate) later. This holds true only if there is enough room around the tumor for a wide excision (two to three centimeters) of normal-seeming flesh and if the tumor is not in a location with a higher risk of metastasis (see the prognosis section below). The advantage of going ahead with a surgery at this point and leaving further staging for later is that the tumor is excised sooner and its biopsy can provide useful information about the cancer's grade.

In addition to spreading to the draining lymph nodes, MCT tends to spread to the liver, spleen and, sometimes, internal lymph nodes; an abdominal ultrasound will reveal suspicious lesions or enlarged, infiltrated organs. If these are found, it does not necessarily mean that

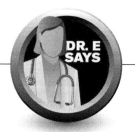

New Grading System for MCT

Currently, we are still using the Patnaik grading system, but that may change soon because of studies conducted by Michigan State University. According to those studies, twenty-eight different pathologists who separately examined the same ninety-five MCT tumors didn't classify their grades consistently.

For example, 75% of the pathologists agreed on which tumors were grade III, but only 63% agreed about which tumors were grade I and II, which means that pathologists may not be classifying tumors in real life in a consistent fashion. If this is true, their assessments based on grade may be less reliable in determining prognosis.

The study also revealed a tendency to grade tumors on the borderline between I and II as grade II. This makes a grade II tumor assessment less valuable as a prognostic factor.

This inconsistency matches my clinical experience, and is why I generally recommend getting a second opinion on MCT biopsies. The study has also prompted the creation of a new system for grading MCT.

In the new system, there would be two, rather than three, grades, and it would be based on the mitotic index (how much replication is going on),

continued on next page

New Grading System for MCT, *continued*

the presence of bizarre or multiple nuclei cells, or karyomegaly (which is increased nuclear size). Tumors would be classified as either low-grade (longer time until metastasis, and more than two years median survival time) or high-grade (shorter time until metastasis, higher death rates due to the MCT, and median survival times of less than four months).

This streamlined system is still quite new and being validated, but it would not surprise me if it is adopted in the future.

there is metastasis; the organs must be aspirated to confirm the situation. In most dogs, these aspirates can be done without sedation, using ultrasound as for guidance.

Before aspirating internal organs, a blood-clotting test will be performed, and if the blood is not clotting properly, steps will be taken to boost clotting for the aspirate. I have heard vets express concern that aspirating internal organs suspected for MCT can cause bleeding problems; this very rarely happens in my experience. Because mast cells contain granules filled with heparin, which is a blood thinner, their concern is that a sudden release of this chemical into the body could keep the blood from clotting properly. While this is true, there typically is not enough heparin to cause an issue, so the actual risk is low. Information is power when it comes to this unpredictable cancer – and with each case being so very different, the information gained by aspirat-

ing these organs is valuable, necessary, and worth the slight risk involved.

In addition to lymph node aspirates/biopsies and abdominal ultrasounds, I often recommend a bone marrow aspirate. I always recommend this test for Grade III MCT, and sometimes for Grade II tumors, or recurrent tumors. This procedure requires sedation, so I usually perform it while the dog is already under anesthesia for a biopsy or curative surgery. It is also an additional expense, so I usually discuss its inclusion with owners before scheduling it for Grade II tumors.

Every removed tumor should be submitted for a post-surgical biopsy. In addition to looking for clean margins (clean margins usually indicate that future recurrence is less likely), the pathologist can find more definitive information to make a prognosis.

For example, the pathologist will look at the mitotic index, or how many MCT cells are dividing. In a recent study, it was shown that the higher the mitotic index, the poorer the prognosis: if the score is over five on the mitotic index, the median survival time was only two months, regardless of grade. If the score was under five, however, the median survival time was seventy months (over five years), regardless of grade. Other studies put the bar higher, even up to a score of ten, and the new grading system discussed in the sidebar on page 312 uses a score of seven as the bar. As we continue to use this score to evaluate MCT tumors, I expect we will come to a firmer consensus. For now, knowing the mitotic index can really assist your oncologist to plan treatments, and formulate a prognosis.

The pathologist can also discover other information that may be helpful. There are certain markers, which help to evaluate cancer proliferation and

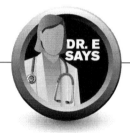

Do you really have to run all of these tests?

MCT is a complicated cancer and there are many ways it can spread in the body. Some owners choose to stage the cancer without knowing the grade of the primary tumor, because if spread is found, they might not attempt to treat the primary tumor with surgery.

There is no one right way to handle MCT, and I recommend that you carefully and closely consult with your veterinarian or oncologist to decide what is right for you and your dog.

cell division: AgNOR, PCNA, Ki-67, c-Kit and c-Kit mutation status. Only a handful of laboratories have the special stains and expertise needed to analyze these markers, so I recommend consulting with your oncologist to see if this information is necessary before adding these expensive tests to the biopsy. I find this panel especially informative for Grade II and grade III tumors, so if budget is a concern, this may be more helpful than a bone marrow aspirate when dealing with Grade II.

There are a couple of screening tests that were historically used for MCT diagnosis which have proven unreliable. A buffy coat evaluation (a blood sample is spun in a centrifuge so that the white and red blood cells are separated) can reveal mast cells circulating in the blood. This is not evidence of MCT, however; other conditions that can cause the same result include inflammatory skin disease, parvo, regenerative anemias, traumas and even other cancers. Because of all these possibilities of false positives with buffy coat evaluations, I do not use them to screen for MCT (rarely, I use them to monitor MCT patients over time).

Another test sometimes used to screen for MCT involves an examination of the eosinophils in the blood. Eosinophils are a type of white blood cells often associated with mast cells, and sometimes MCT can cause an elevation of their concentration, as can allergies, parasites, and other cancers, including lymphoma. Therefore, I do not consider eosinophil levels to be a useful test for MCT in general, but if, in your dog's case, eosinophil levels rise and fall along with their MCT, I may use that information to monitor him, over time.

What Is the Prognosis for Mast Cell Tumors?

It is very difficult to definitively offer a prognosis for MCT, because there are so many variables to consider. Each dog's case should be considered individually, and several factors should be weighed.

Grade is the most consistent predictor of outcome. Here is the current grading system:

- **Grade I** tumors are usually confined to one tumor in the skin and do not recur once they are surgically removed, with clean margins. These account for approximately 33–50% of all MCT.

- **Grade II** tumors account for approximately 25-45% of all MCT, are locally invasive (have gone into the deeper layers below the skin) and are more likely to disseminate to other parts of the body. They are also more likely to recur, especially if they have incomplete or narrow margins.

- **Grade III** tumors are usually very malignant, have invaded deep into the body, and are highly aggressive, with a 55% to 95% rate of metastasis. Grade III tumors are also extremely likely to recur and account for approximately 20-40% of all MCT cases.

When I say that MCT is unpredictable, I am particularly thinking of Grade II tumors. Some act like Grade I tumors and are highly treatable. Others, however, act more like Grade III tumors and have a greater likelihood of spreading. Plus, some dogs present multiple, new tumors over time. This unpredictability requires us to look at as many prognostic factors as possible, beyond grade. When the lymph nodes are involved, if there has already been metastasis, if the proliferation scores are high, or if the mitotic index is five or higher, the prognosis worsens.

Another factor that affects the prognosis includes stage – the location(s) where MCT actually appears in the body. Here is the World Health Organization's (WHO's) Clinical Staging System for MCT:

Stage 0: One tumor, which has been removed for a biopsy, but still has microscopic cells left at the surgical scar (this is also called an incomplete removal), *without* regional lymph node spread.

Stage I: One tumor, completely confined to the skin (no spreading into deeper subcutaneous layers) *without* regional lymph node spread.

Stage II: One tumor, completely confined to the skin (no spreading into deeper subcutaneous layers) *with* regional lymph node spread.

Stage III: Multiple skin tumors, or large tumors which infiltrate deeper layers, *with* or *without* regional lymph node spread.

Stage IV: Any tumor with distant spread, including blood and bone marrow involvement.

In general, the higher the Stage number, the worse the prognosis.

Please note that, although multiple tumors do indicate a higher stage, according to this official staging system, many oncologists – including myself – believe the Stage III classification is outdated. In our experience, multiple MCT tumors do not indicate a more advanced disease. Although counterintuitive, it is our experience that MCT presenting with multiple tumors are not skin metastases, but new skin MCT. Therefore, it is not necessarily more aggressive and does not have a worse prognosis than a Stage II single tumor. WHO's official staging has not yet been modified to reflect this new understanding.

Another factor we consider, when offering a prognosis, is whether your dog is feeling sick.

Substage (a) means that there are no systemic clinical signs related to MCT – in other words, your dog does not feel sick at time of diagnosis. In that case, the prognosis is better.

Substage (b) means there are systemic clinical signs related to MCT – such as decreased appetite, vomiting, bloody stools, and swelling or edema associated with MCT degranulation. If your dog feels sick at the time of diagnosis, the prognosis worsens.

There are several other predictive factors that can help form a prognosis. The most reliable are:

- **Proliferation Rate:** If mast cell tumors are

rapidly multiplying, the prognosis worsens.

- **Recent Rapid Growth:** If there has been recent, rapid growth of a tumor, the prognosis worsens.

- **Tumor Size:** The larger the tumor, the worse the prognosis.

- **Recurrence:** If tumors have been removed and recur, the prognosis worsens.

- **C-Kit Mutation:** If a c-Kit genetic mutation is detected, the prognosis worsens.

- **Location in the Body:** Certain locations have been associated with a higher rate of metastasis. Mast cell tumors located in the internal organs, on the genitals, scrotum, muzzle, ear and gums all have a greater tendency to metastasize. While this makes these MCT tumors more aggressive, it does not necessarily mean that they are untreatable. For example, a recent study of muzzle MCT showed that while metastasis was more likely, it occurred later in dogs with lower grades of cancer. The overall mean survival time was still two and a half years with aggressive (not palliative) treatment.

Let me remind you, here, that every dog is different from every other dog, and that every cancer case is different from every other cancer case – especially if your dog has MCT. As you can tell, it's a tremendous task to pull all of this information together and formulate a prognosis and treatment plan. There is a lot to consider, and if you can't absorb all of this right now, that's OK. Your vet or oncologist can help you understand your own dog's case.

What Are the Available Protocols for Mast Cell Tumors?

Surgery is the treatment of choice for MCT, and often the only treatment needed. The goal is to completely excise (remove) it and prevent its recurrence. The surgeon should aim for a minimum margin of two centimeters all the way around the tumor, including at least one deeper tissue layer. A surgical biopsy is necessary to determine whether the margins are complete. When they aren't – or if they're dirty – the surgeon will consider a second surgery (a scar revision) to remove more tissue. The tissue from the second surgery will also be biopsied to check for clean margins, because a completely removed tumor is less likely to recur or metastasize.

If your dog has more than one MCT, both should be completely removed. Although, in my experience, more tumors do not indicate more aggression or a worse prognosis, I still advocate removing as many as possible. For the uncommon case of many MCT all at the same time, this surgery may not be realistic and, in that case, I recommend a systemic chemotherapy protocol (see below). Even then, I recommend removing at least one tumor for biopsy, to obtain the grade and other prognostics from the lab.

Additionally, if a tumor is really huge, I may try to shrink it before surgery, so that we can remove it more easily. For this, I use chemotherapy or radiation treatments (see below).

For some MCT, especially those located on the lower leg, surgery cannot achieve the necessary clean and wide margins because there isn't sufficient tissue surrounding the tumor. If wide excision is not possible, or if the margins are contaminated with tumor cells, radiation therapy will be considered.

Post-surgical radiation provides excellent long-term MCT tumor control for dogs with microscopic cells remaining after surgery. The vast majority (85% to 95%) of dogs with low- or intermediate-grade MCT remain tumor-free two to five years after treatment. Even grade III MCT cases can benefit: in a recent study, 70% of these dogs were still alive one year after radiation treatment. Radiation treatment protocols usually involve fifteen daily treatments (Monday through Friday for three weeks). These will be scheduled two to three weeks after surgery, before MCT has a chance to recur and after the surgical scar has healed. The radiation should be directed to the area three centimeters around the scar.

While radiation therapy can be helpful for treating microscopic cells post-surgery, it is less successful as a primary treatment. Statistics show that treating measurable tumors (tumors large enough to see and measure, also called macroscopic) with radiation therapy alone leaves only 50% of dogs still alive after one year. If radiation is being considered as a primary treatment, an increase in the amount of radiation and the addition of chemotherapy and steroids may improve the response rate and duration.

Radiation can also be used for non-resectable, or inoperable, tumors. In these cases, a palliative approach of four weekly treatments, combined with steroids, has produced a response in an impressive 88% of all dogs with MCT. In this study, the MCT tumors did not progress (grow) for a median time of thirty-four months – almost three years! This is an extremely positive outcome for an inoperable tumor. It's also worth noting that dogs with non-resectable MCT on the leg did better than those who had non-resectable MCT on the head.

Radiation therapy can also be helpful when it is started prior to surgery, with the goal of shrinking very large tumors. This approach may allow more complete removal of the remaining tumor and also slow tumor progression (growth).

In many MCT cases, I do not recommend chemotherapy at all, because it is not as effective as surgery and radiation for a primary tumor in the skin, especially if the cancer is of a lower grade and/or confined to one local area. Sometimes, I use chemotherapy instead of radiation for large MCT tumors which need to be shrunk prior to surgical removal, and I would also consider palliative chemotherapy for non-resectable tumors, if radiation therapy is not available in your area or if you have decided against radiation.

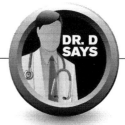

The conventional treatments Dr. Ettinger recommends for mast cell tumors are to be considered part of step one of Full Spectrum cancer care (Chapter 11). Please review that chapter for more general information about surgery, radiation and chemotherapy and how to handle their common side effects.

For more information on all other Full Spectrum steps, including nutraceuticals, immune boosters, dietary changes and brain chemistry modification strategies, review Full Spectrum cancer care, which begins on page 103.

You will also find information about specific chemotherapy agents in Chapter 41.

For more advanced MCT cases, I may recommend chemotherapy in addition to surgery and radiation, and occasionally instead of those therapies. This is common for grade III MCT, for example. However, I sometimes also use it for grade II MCT with high proliferation marker scores or for multiple skin MCTs, which is a less common, and even controversial, practice. I decide this on a case-by-case basis, and have had success with vinblastine, prednisone, Lomustine, and the new tyrosine kinase inhibitors, Palladia and masitinib (Kinavet CA-1).

Two of these are worth special mention, because they can be very beneficial for MCT. Masitinib, trade name Kinavet CA-1, is a new drug in the United States (conditionally approved by the FDA in December of 2010) but already approved in Europe for MCT. Prior to approval, U.S. oncologists were able to get it through the FDA's compassionate use program, so most are familiar with the drug.

Palladia is available in the U.S. and is FDA-approved specifically for dogs with recurrent, Grade II and Grade III MCT, with or without regional lymph node involvement. Palladia works in two ways to fight MCT: it cuts off blood supply to MCT by blocking angiogenesis, and it also inhibits tyrosine kinase, a protein which stimulates tumor growth. One-third of dogs with MCT have a genetic mutation (c-Kit) that leads to tyrosine kinase being stuck in the "on" position, leading to increased survival for mast cell tumors. Palladia's is particularly helpful for these dogs. In fact, Palladia (along with masitinib) is part of a new class of drugs named for this ability: tyrosine kinase inhibitors (TKI).

Overall, 60% of the dogs treated with Palladia alone in clinical studies had their MCT disappear, regress or stabilize (stop growing), and this result was seen even in dogs who did not have the c-Kit muta-tion. In addition to the effect on the tumors, quality of life improved for these dogs, who experienced more energy and better attitude.

Palladia is a relatively new drug and I'm excited about its results, so far. Because drugs often work even better in combination, Palladia's use in combination with other chemotherapy drugs is now starting to be evaluated to see if it helps microscopic cancers and metastatic cancers. Of course, the risk of possible side effects increases when you combine drugs, so if you contemplate this, I recommend doing so with an oncologist's supervision.

Additional Considerations for Mast Cell Tumors

In addition to surgery and radiation, and possibly chemotherapy, you may want to consider supportive medications to counteract the effects of possible degranulation (when the mast cell tumor breaks open). The following are especially helpful for dogs with large tumors, detectable spread, and systemic signs such as vomiting: anti-histamines (such as Benadryl), antacids (such as Pepcid) and proton pump inhibitors (such as Prilosec). These can often be stopped after surgery, if the tumor has been successfully removed and spread has not occurred; some dogs may need these drugs long-term to control their symptoms.

Follow Up

Ten to fifteen percent of canine MCT cases (all grades) develop additional masses after their first mass is removed, and metastasis is also possible. Because of this, I recommend all dogs with MCT receive rigorous check-ups every three to six months for the rest of their lives to check for new masses, recurrence and spread. If a new mass is discovered in between check-ups, definitely get it aspirated and evaluated.

The Bottom Line

From my perspective as a veterinarian oncologist, mast cell tumors are highly treatable. Aggressive surgery is required, with wide margins, and may be the only treatment needed. Radiation treatments and/or chemotherapy might be needed; dogs generally tolerate treatment well and live longer. The addition of tyrosine kinase inhibitors like Palladia to our treatment arsenal makes me even more optimistic about MCT. While there may be recurrence and/or metastasis, long-term control and survival is definitely possible.

I believe the benefit of treating dogs with MCT easily outweighs the risk of side effects. Treated dogs live significantly longer, are happy, run, play, sleep and eat much as they did before they got sick.

She Was Not Receptive ... But She Could Not Dispute It

"I am so sorry that you have to experience this; but don't give up hope. You are your pet's #1 advocate and as such it is your duty to research the current medications available and what research that is being conducted to combat this disease. My oncologist was not receptive to Dr. Dressler's book but had never read it. Every bit of info I brought out in our initial conversation that I took from the book was info she could not dispute and often agreed with. I believe that the more knowledgeable the owner is about their pet's situation, the more willing the doctor will be to pursue other avenues. This is merely my opinion, but it makes sense that doctors are more willing to try different medications with owners who are more interested in their pets' health than with other owners who merely "go with the flow." Also, many owners are capable of asking very intelligent questions that their doctor may not have considered."

- Debbie Granger, Chesterfield, Missouri

Chapter 31: Mammary Tumors

Mammary tumors can develop in several types of cells found in the mammary glands of female dogs. These tumors are also called mammary gland tumors or simply, breast cancer.

Many mammary tumors are responsive to treatment because about half are benign, and about half of those that are malignant, do not metastasize. Surgery is the primary treatment for mammary tumors.

Survival times vary widely, depending upon several prognostic factors. Generally, dogs with benign tumors have significantly longer survival times than those with malignant tumors.

What are Mammary Tumors?

Mammary tumors are among the most common tumors found in female dogs – in fact, dogs are three times more likely to develop mammary tumors than are human women. As you probably know, mammary glands produce breast milk for nursing young. While male dogs do have these glands, they rarely develop mammary tumors; only one percent of all cases occur in males.

Most dogs have ten mammary glands, five on each side (or "chain"). Mammary glands are complicated structures, made up of several types of cells, all working together. Tumors can develop in any of these cells, so, mammary tumors come in many different forms.

About fifty percent of all mammary tumors are benign. The most common are: adenomas, which arise in the epithelial tissue lining the glands; cystoadenomas (also called cystadenomas), which arise in the epithelial tissue in the milk-producing structures, and often form fluid-retaining cysts; and mixed mammary tumors, which develop when tumors arise in both epithelial and connective tissues.

The other fifty percent of mammary tumors are malignant, and of those, fifty percent will metastasize. The most common malignant mammary tumors are: carcinomas, adenocarcinomas (malignant versions of adenomas) and cystadenocarcinomas (malignant versions of cystoadenomas).

Another malignant mammary tumor is the inflammatory mammary carcinoma (IMC). This aggressive tumor is noteworthy (even though it is less common than other malignancies) because of its high rate of growth and rapid metastasis.

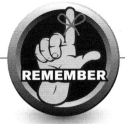

When you need to look up the definition of a word or phrase, find it listed in Chapter 5, which begins on page 46.

All malignant tumors have the potential to spread, especially when left untreated. Breast cancer can metastasize to the lungs, regional lymph nodes, abdominal organs (such as the liver) and bones.

Which Dogs Are at Risk for Mammary Tumors?

Mammary tumors are very rare in male dogs and very common in females. Also, they are quite prevalent in several specific breeds: Cocker Spaniel, Brittany Spaniel, English Springer Spaniel, Pointer breeds, Toy and Miniature Poodles, Dachshunds, Maltese, German Shepherds and Yorkshire Terriers. Both Boxers and Collies have a decreased risk for mammary tumors.

There are several other factors that may determine which dogs become afflicted. The biggest factor seems to be whether she has been spayed or not, and when. Females, spayed before their first heats, decrease their risk to only half a percent for developing mammary gland tumors. The risk increases to eight percent when the spay is performed between the first and second heats, and it jumps to 26% after the second heat cycle. In other words, females spayed after the second heat and intact females are seven times more likely to develop a mammary tumor than those spayed before six months of age!

The protective benefits of early spaying seem to derive from arresting the normal development of mammary glands, as the dog matures from puppy to adult. The early hysterectomy removes the ovaries, resulting in vastly reduced levels of the female sex hormones, estrogen and progesterone. Both of these have been associated with mammary tumor development; research has found both benign and malignant mammary tumors sometimes feature estrogen receptors, which seem to help transform normal mammary cells into cancerous cells (these receptors may be targets in future mammary cancer treatments).

The longer your dog's body is exposed to the female sex hormones, the more likely she is to develop mammary cancer. Even dogs who were not spayed early can still get some benefit from a later surgery; spaying just before the age of two and a half years, while not completely preventative, affords some protection against developing mammary tumors later in life. Studies also show that when an intact female develops mammary tumors, spaying her will typically result in longer survival time.

Early obesity seems to play a role in mammary tumor development; dogs with lean bodies from age nine to twelve months are at decreased risk, while overweight dogs are at increased risk. In this same study, females fed a homemade diet were also at higher risk, and so were those that ate a lot of red meat, especially beef and pork, and little chicken.

Does this mean you are not to feed your dog the dog cancer diet Dr. Dressler recommends? I wouldn't object to feeding the dog cancer diet, based only on this study. It's important that you are aware of this link, and it's important to know that diet plays a vital role in mammary cancer. However, diet is a very complex subject. If you feed the dog cancer diet, I certainly recommend you feed chicken (and other lean meats) and skip beef and pork for these dogs.

I would also modify your dog's intake of dietary fat. Dietary fats are a significant contributing factor in mammary cancer. For example, low-fat, high-protein diets are associated with longer survival times than low-fat, low-protein diets. In the same study, survival times were not affected either way by a high-fat diet, regardless of protein intake. High levels of dietary fat tend to increase blood estrogen levels in women, leading to higher risk for breast cancer; the same thing may occur in female dogs.

Genetic mutations seem to be involved in the development of mammary cancers. Although the specific mutation has not yet been identified, candidates include: p53, c-erb-2 (HER-1/neu) and BCRA1 and BCRA2. In the future, as problematic mutations are identified, we may be able to target treatments to specific genes.

A direct association has recently been found between anaplastic (particularly aggressive) carcinomas and COX-2, an enzyme responsible for inflammation. The anaplastic tumors express a lot more COX-2 than adenocarcinomas, for example. If your dog has an anaplastic tumor, using a COX-2 inhibitor (like NSAIDs) may help control the tumor.

In human women, pregnancy provides some protection from breast cancer; this is not true for dogs. Whether your dog has lactated or not also does not affect her risk of developing mammary cancer.

What are the Signs of Mammary Tumors?

Most mammary tumors are found by owners or by vets, during a routine physical exam. The mammary glands line up along both sides of the chest and abdomen chains. Most dogs have ten glands in total, five on each chain. Each gland is referred to by number, one to five on each side, with number one toward the head and number five toward the tail.

Tumors usually feel like small, discrete, firm balls right at the nipple; in the softer breast tissue, they feel more like diffuse masses. Most dogs do not seem sick when the tumor is found, and blood tests are usually normal.

More than one tumor is found in 60% of cases, although multiple tumors do not exacerbate

her prognosis. Because the tumors can develop from more than one kind of mammary tissue, it's important to examine each one to find out what cancer is present. The most common glands for cancer development are the fourth and fifth of either chain (located towards her tail end).

While benign tumors often feel like they are superficial and unattached to any other tissue, malignancies often seem attached or rooted to underlying tissues. Other hallmarks of malignancies include: ill-defined borders, ulceration (open sore), pain and swelling. Malignancies may also increase rapidly in size.

Although these characteristics have often been found in malignant tumors, their presence does not definitely indicate that the tumor is malignant. Conversely, their absence does not mean the tumor is benign. Every tumor should be biopsied, submitted to a lab, and examined for malignancy under a microscope.

Regional lymph nodes should also be examined. They can become enlarged due to normal inflammation, to metastasis or to a secondary infection from an ulcerated tumor. The most commonly affected nodes are the inguinal (inner thigh) and axillary (armpit). As the mammary tissue includes a complex lymph drainage system, the prescapular nodes in front of the shoulder, the popliteal nodes behind the knee, the sternal nodes in the chest cavity and the abdominal lymph nodes should all be examined, as well.

If breast cancer has spread by the time of diagnosis, your dog can show general signs of weakness, lethargy, and weight loss. The uncommon, aggressive inflammatory mammary carcinoma (IMC) can cause these same symptoms, plus others. As the name suggests, these tumors contain many inflammatory cells, and are associated with swelling, pain and rapid metastasis. They often involve the skin, which can become swollen, warm and red. IMC is frequently confused with mastitis (an inflammation of the breast tissue) because the breast becomes painful to the touch and can even ulcerate.

How Are Mammary Tumors Diagnosed?

Once a tumor or tumors are found, each is measured and possibly aspirated, with a fine needle aspirate, to find out whether the mass is a mammary tumor, an infection or an inflammation. When the presence of a mammary tumor is confirmed, the aspirate can almost never show whether it is benign or malignant. To get that information, a biopsy must be performed.

The biopsy surgery will remove the entire mass, which is then examined under a microscope to check the margins and see whether it is benign or malignant. If the tumor is benign and margins are clean, this biopsy becomes the curative surgery.

If the tumor is malignant, further staging should be done to determine whether there is metastasis. When a tumor has the hallmarks of malignancy (it is very large, inflamed, stuck to underlying tissues, or regional lymph nodes are enlarged), your vet or oncologist may want to stage it, even before removing it with a biopsy.

To stage the malignancy, your vet may order a complete blood count (CBC), a chemistry panel, urinalysis, chest imaging (to check for spread to the lungs), an abdominal ultrasound (to check for spread to the abdominal organs) and aspirates of the draining lymph nodes, deep in the abdomen.

Enlarged lymph nodes can occur because of factors other than metastasis, so their size is not a good predictor of outcome. However, all regional lymph nodes should be checked for metastasis when malignant breast tumors are present.

What Is the Prognosis for Mammary Tumors?

The outcome for mammary tumors is extremely variable, because some are benign, others are malignant and each tumor type is so distinctive. With treatment, the overall median survival time is about fifteen months for all tumors (benign and malignant), and survival times of two years occur for 25–40% of all dogs with mammary tumors.

Dogs with benign tumors have significantly longer survival times than those with malignant tumors. The median survival time for dogs with benign tumors, removed with surgery, is approximately twenty-six months or over two years. (The reason there are median survival times associated with benign tumors is that even these tumors can recur if they are not completely removed.)

Dogs with malignant tumors have a more varied outcome. Low-grade malignant tumors, which are removed with clean margins, may be cured altogether – as if the tumor were benign – while others may recur and spread within the first year. Higher-grade tumors may recur and metastasize even sooner. In general, dogs whose malignancies are removed with surgery experience a sixteen-month median survival time.

Because of the many variables at play, each dog and each case must be considered carefully; however, we do have a few prognostic factors to review.

The stage – location where mammary tumors appear in the body – can be helpful in forecasting your dog's outcome. Here is a modified version of the World Health Organization's (WHO's) Clinical Staging System for Mammary Gland Tumors:

Stage I: Tumor(s)★ are under three centimeter in diameter, with no regional lymph node involvement and no metastasis.

Stage II: Tumor(s) are three to five centimeter in diameter, with no regional lymph node involvement and no metastasis.

Stage III: Tumor(s) are over five centimeter in diameter, with no regional lymph node involvement and no metastasis.

Stage IV: Tumor(s) are any size, with regional lymph node involvement.

Stage V: Tumor(s) are any size, with regional lymph node involvement and metastasis.

★multiple tumors do not worsen the prognosis

In general, the higher the stage, the worse the prognosis becomes. The biopsy results offer you a great deal more information to consider, including the type of tumor (adenocarcinoma, cystadenocarcinoma, etc.) and its grade (aggressive characteristics). Other prognostic factors include: whether there is invasion into the lymphatics or the vascular system, whether estrogen or progesterone receptors are involved, and whether tumors are invasive or ulcerated.

Dogs of advanced age tend to have a less favorable prognosis, as do dogs that are not spayed. Small breeds tend to have more benign tumors than malignancies and live longer than larger breeds.

What Are the Available Protocols for Mammary Tumors?

Surgery is the treatment of choice to remove

mammary tumors, with the exception of IMC (see below). It's important to remember that benign and malignant tumors can both develop at the same time, so every tumor should be addressed.

The number, location and size of tumors will determine the extent of the surgery. For each one, the entire tumor and all affected tissues should be removed with a wide (two-centimeter) margin. All masses will be submitted for biopsy, so that the type of each tumor can be determined, and the margins can be confirmed as clean. Radical mastectomies are usually not necessary for spayed dogs – a lumpectomy or a simple mastectomy (which removes just the mammary gland involved in the tumor) can suffice, as long as the excision is complete. Remember, 100% of benign and 50% of malignant tumors are cured with surgery alone, so approximately 75% of dogs with mammary tumors are treated with simple surgeries and then, potentially, are cured.

If your dog is intact, however, you might consider a radical mastectomy, which removes the entire chain associated with the tumor. A 2008 study reported that almost 60% of intact dogs who had a regional mastectomy later developed a secondary mass on the same side, in the same chain. This study's results directly contradict what veterinary oncologists are traditionally taught about mammary cancer, which is that they should just remove the tumor with an adequate surgery. Since 75% of those secondary masses were malignant, discussing radical mastectomy with your oncologist is a good idea. Further studies are needed to look at whether radical mastectomies actually improve survival times for intact dogs, but they should be considered, based on the results of this study.

Would so many dogs have developed a second tumor if they were also spayed at the time of the first surgery (see below)? Unfortunately, we can't know without another study; if your dog is intact, I recommend discussing spaying and/or a radical mastectomy with your oncologist.

The lymph nodes should also be considered for removal. For example, if your dog has a tumor at the back end of the chain – down near the rear legs – the inguinal lymph node will also be removed, even if it looks normal. The axillary (armpit) node, on the other hand, need only be removed if metastasis is confirmed or suspected. If there is metastasis in any lymph node, or if it is suspected, removing it should be seriously contemplated.

If your dog has IMC, or inflammatory mammary carcinoma, surgery may not be helpful because the surgical incision often does not heal well, due to the inflammatory nature of the cancer. Blood clotting abnormalities and edema can also occur. Treatment for IMC is usually palliative, not curative. NSAIDs can be used, as well as palliative radiation and palliative chemotherapy protocols. Surgery can still be considered, as sometimes just removing the inflamed, ulcerated mass will make your dog feel better.

The role of chemotherapy in treating mammary cancer in general has not been fully established, and there are no standard recommendations from the literature to share with you. One study looked at a small group of dogs, who had surgery along with a course of 5-FU and cyclophosphamide. They experienced significantly improved survival times, when compared to the control group, which had surgery only. Doxorubicin is commonly used in dogs with a high risk of metastasis. If you are contemplating chemotherapy, I strongly recommend consulting with a boarded oncologist who understands mammary cancer, because each case is so distinct.

In my experience, chemotherapy, for dogs with

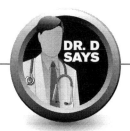

DR. D SAYS

The conventional treatments, which Dr. Ettinger recommends for mammary tumors, should be considered part of step one of Full Spectrum cancer care (Chapter 11). Please review that chapter for more general information about surgery, radiation and chemotherapy and how to handle common side effects.

For more information on all other Full Spectrum steps, including nutraceuticals, immune boosters, dietary changes and brain chemistry modification strategies, review Full Spectrum cancer care, which begins on page 103.

You will also find information about specific chemotherapy agents in Chapter 41.

advanced stages of mammary tumors with a high risk for metastasis, can help maintain a good quality of life and delay or even prevent metastasis. I typically recommend post-operative chemotherapy, based on several prognostic factors, including: tumor size, stage, ulceration and full histopathology (which includes the tumor type, malignancy, vascular and/or lymphatic invasion, invasive nature and margins). Chemotherapy is best used when the disease is still in a microscopic form, because once metastasis has developed, chemotherapy is typically less effective. A careful consideration of your dog's complete pathology is necessary to determine whether chemotherapy can be helpful or not – so make it a point to discuss this with your oncologist.

Radiation therapy is not widely used in dogs with mammary cancer, but it may be useful when a surgery results in incomplete margins and a second surgery is not possible. Also, radiation could be helpful when the mammary tumors are sarcomas, which are more likely to recur after surgery than other tumor types. Inoperable tumors may also benefit from a course of palliative radiation.

Additional Considerations for Mammary Tumors

In addition to surgery and possibly chemotherapy or radiation, consider spaying your dog, if she is intact at the time of diagnosis. I mention this again because this topic is controversial among vets, however, two recent studies have shown that spaying at the time of surgery may increase survival times. Spaying may be particularly helpful for tumors with estrogen hormone receptors, because the spay removes the ovaries, and therefore the main source of estrogen. It's possible that the variable outcomes in studies can be explained by this phenomenon: spaying helps if the tumors are estrogen responsive and doesn't if they are not. Checking the status of estrogen receptors on your dog's tumor would help you make this decision; unfortunately, this test is not commercially available. In general, I recommend spaying at the time of surgery or, when that is declined, a radical mastectomy, for intact dogs.

Hormonal therapy is the use of a drug to help block estrogen's stimulation of the mammary tissue. Anti-estrogen therapies like tamoxifen, which are of-

ten used in human women, may not help your dog because, while your dog may have an estrogen-receptor positive tumor, these tumors tend to be benign and less-aggressive in dogs, and are often well-controlled by adequate surgery. More aggressive tumors in dogs do not usually have estrogen receptors and are less hormone-dependent. The side effects of anti-estrogen therapy can include: vulvar swelling, vaginal discharge, stump pyometra (a severe, possibly life-threatening infection of the "stump" of the uterus left after spaying), signs of heat and urinary tract infections. Because of these potentially severe side effects and the lack of evidence for efficacy, I do not generally recommend anti-estrogen therapy as a treatment.

Follow Up

All malignant mammary tumors have the potential for developing metastasis. For this reason, every dog with a confirmed malignancy should be re-checked periodically for new mammary tumors, even after a complete excision of the original tumor. Also, every dog should be staged periodically, for spread.

The Bottom Line

From my perspective as a veterinarian oncologist, mammary tumors are highly treatable with surgery. With 50% completely benign and only half of the malignancies prone to metastasize, your dog can really benefit from conventional treatments.

Early detection is critical. Stay vigilant about checking your dog for new masses, as the benefit of treating dogs with mammary tumors easily outweighs the risk of side effects. Treated dogs live significantly longer, are happy, run, play, sleep and eat, much as they did before they got sick.

Chapter 32: Osteosarcoma

Osteosarcoma accounts for the majority of bone cancers (85%) in dogs. Although it can develop in any bone in the body, three-quarters of these tumors develop in the limbs, with the front legs twice as likely to develop osteosarcoma as the hind legs.

Osteosarcoma (OSA) tumors grow fast and metastasize quickly. Ten to fifteen percent of dogs with osteosarcoma (OSA) already have detectable lung metastasis when they are first diagnosed and 90% have micrometastasis (spread that is not detected on chest X-rays). This incredibly high rate of micrometastasis makes systemic chemotherapy treatments just as important as tumor removal. Despite its aggressive behavior, OSA is considered a highly treatable tumor.

The standard of care treatment for OSA is surgery, performed quickly, on the affected area, and then, chemotherapy to control the likely metastasis. Because so many OSA tumors are located in the limbs, the surgery is nearly always an amputation. Palliative radiation treatments can help to control pain, if surgery is not an option. Newer, alternative options for local control include limb-spare procedures and stereotactic radiosurgery, such as the CyberKnife.

OSA cases treated with amputation alone have a median survival time of four to five months, with 90-100% dying in one year and only 2% still alive after two years.

Median survival times for OSA cases treated with amputation and chemotherapy increase to ten

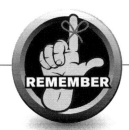

When you need to look up the definition of a word or phrase, find it listed in Chapter 5, which begins on page 46.

to twelve months, with 20-25% of dogs still alive after two years. Several factors useful to help you determine your own dog's prognosis will be reviewed in this chapter.

What Is Osteosarcoma?

Depending upon where they are located in the skeleton, bones are called axial (bones in the head and trunk) or appendicular (bones in the limbs). Osteosarcoma tumors, which can occur in the cells of any bone, typically arise in appendicular bones (the long bones of the limbs).

OSA tumors are usually found at the end of the bone (called the metaphysis) and this location differentiates them from bone tumors that have metastasized from other cancer types, which most often occur in the middle of the bone (called the diaphysis). The most common locations for OSA are "towards the knee and away from the elbow": the top of the shoulder (top of the humerus bone), the wrist (bottom of the radius bone) and the knee (bottom of the femur bone or the top of the tibia bone). Another common site is the bottom of the tibia bone, at the ankle or hock joint. There is usually only one tumor, and it typically does not invade other bones through joints. OSA can sometimes be found in the middle of bones and, less commonly, in torso bones.

OSA tumors can generate excessive new bone growth (production), bone lysis (destruction) or both. Both types of activity can usually be seen on X-rays, although the appearance can vary widely from tumor to tumor, which can make misidentification possible. Fungal and bacterial infections can look like OSA, for example, so, in areas where fungal infections are prevalent, it is wise to get a bone biopsy evaluated both for cancer and for a fungal infection. Veterinarians in areas near rivers or other waterways with sandy, acidic soil are particularly vigilant about the fungus blastomycosis, which can involve the bones of about 30% of dogs who incur the infection. While OSA does not typically make a dog feel sick, blastomycosis infections usually do. If your dog is not eating well, has a fever or suffers from weight loss, coughing, depression, eye problems, lameness or skin problems, make sure you rule out blastomycosis as a cause for any bone changes you see on X-rays. Blastomycosis is a special concern for dogs exposed to water in the late summer and the fall in endemic areas such as Ohio, Mississippi, and the St. Lawrence River Valley.

OSA bone tumors can cause weakness and even severe bone fractures at the primary site. The risk of a pathological fracture – a sudden and painful bone break – is real, which is why amputation is the most prudent immediate course. OSA most commonly metastasizes to the lungs and 10-15% of dogs

have detectable spread at the time of diagnosis. Less often, tumors can metastasize to other bones. The regional lymph nodes can be involved, also, although this occurs in only 5% of dogs.

Micrometastasis is not only possible with OSA, but has probably already happened by the time of diagnosis. Ninety percent of dogs with OSA have microscopic cancerous lesions that cannot be detected by chest X-rays (the most common and widely available test used to look for lung spread). If available and used, advanced imaging tools, such as CT scans, can detect smaller masses otherwise missed on chest X-rays. Even when the primary tumor is successfully removed, these tiny metastases will grow and eventually be the cause of death for dogs with OSA. This makes systemic treatments aimed at controlling micrometastasis a critical part of conventional care.

Which Dogs Are at Risk for Osteosarcoma?

OSA is usually seen in middle-aged and older dogs, age seven to nine, and we also see a smaller peak of incidence in dogs between the age of eighteen months and two years. Axial OSA can be seen in any breed at any time; appendicular OSA is usually seen in the front limbs of large and giant breeds, including Great Danes, Saint Bernards, Irish Setters, Rottweilers, German Shepherds, Golden Retrievers and Doberman Pinschers.

Breed is not as important as height and weight; heavier and taller dogs are more likely to develop OSA. For example, dogs that weigh more than sixty-six pounds are sixty times more likely to develop OSA than dogs weighing less than twenty-two pounds. For dogs weighing more than eighty-eight pounds, 95% of primary bone cancer is OSA; for those weighing less than thirty-three pounds, only

40-50% of primary bone cancer is OSA.

The exact cause of OSA is unknown. One theory is that small "micro-fractures" occur in the long bones as they bear the weight of the dog's body. The multiple minor traumas and injuries, the thinking goes, stimulate excessive inflammation and bone growth; this may increase the chances that genetic mutations and malignancies will develop.

Radiation therapy (for other types of cancer) can cause OSA later in life (rarely, 3-5%). In these cases, OSA develops in a bone that was included in the original radiation therapy field, and usually happens a full three to five years after radiation treatments.

Dogs that have experienced a bone fracture, bone trauma or bone infection are at increased risk for OSA, as are those who have metallic implants in their bones (used to repair a fracture). Taller dogs also tend to be at increased risk.

Sex hormones may protect against OSA development; in one study, Rottweilers who were spayed or neutered before one year of age were four times more likely to develop OSA later in life.

A number of genes have been implicated in OSA development, including p53, retinoblastoma, PTEN, and possibly c-Kit. There are also several chemical factors involved in angiogenesis – new blood vessel formation – that seem to play a role in OSA development and progression.

What are the Signs of Osteosarcoma?

The first sign of OSA is usually limping or refusing to put weight on the involved leg. Bone tumors hurt, especially when the bone bears weight; they are painful enough to make even the most stoic of dogs flinch or limp.

Swelling may be visible in the area of the tumor, although if the tumor is high on the leg, beneath the shoulder or thigh muscles, or hidden under a lot of fur, this may be less obvious.

Many dogs are so unwilling to show pain that they hide these symptoms until very late; be sure to get X-rays early when your dog does not respond to pain medications and rest (especially important for large breeds). If there is significant bone destruction (lysis), the bone can weaken enough to cause a pathologic fracture. This happens rarely – in fewer than 3% of cases; when it does it causes sudden, severe pain.

Most dogs will feel well, other than the pain associated with the tumor, unless lung metastasis has occurred, when they may have a few other general signs, such as decreased appetite and low energy. It is uncommon for the dog with lung metastasis to cough or have difficulty breathing until it is advanced.

While OSA is not usually caught in routine blood work, sometimes elevated alkaline phosphatase (ALP) levels are detected. If this is the case, the prognosis is worsened. (Increased ALP is not specific for bone cancer; other conditions are also associated with it).

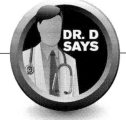

Fluoridated water may also be a risk factor for male dogs. I write about this at length on page 77.

How Is Osteosarcoma Diagnosed?

When OSA is suspected, X-rays can show classic bone changes associated with these tumors. The location of lesions and their typical "sunburst" appearance will warn the vet that the tumors may be OSA. When the dog is older, of a larger breed, or if pain cannot be controlled easily, suspicions rise even higher.

Normally, I recommend confirming a cancer diagnosis before performing a cancer surgery; I make an exception when the lesions are suspected to be OSA. Whatever their cause – OSA or an infection – bone lesions cannot be repaired, and they put the dog at risk for a serious and painful fracture. Aggressive surgery, usually amputation, is the immediate next step for severe bone lesions, because this removes the destructive process (whatever it may be) immediately, and the dog's bone-related pain ceases. A biopsy on the removed limb can confirm what caused the lesions, and appropriate post-surgery treatments can be planned after the results are in.

In other words, if OSA is suspected, the usual course of action is to skip an aspirate or biopsy and proceed immediately to staging the cancer, followed by an amputation.

Some owners and some vets don't want skip the aspirate or the biopsy, however. These owners may not want to treat if the lesion is confirmed to be OSA, or they may want to try a "limb spare" procedure (see below). Not every limb can be saved; either way, these owners want a confirmed diagnosis before deciding how and whether to treat the cancer, and certainly before they make a decision that cannot be reversed. To confirm OSA, a bone aspirate can be taken or a biopsy can be performed.

The advantage of a bone aspirate is that it

is done under sedation and is less likely to cause a fracture in the bone. Unfortunately, it is not always conclusive and can only confirm the presence of a sarcoma, not what type it is. One test that may help in this case is a special stain, recently developed, which can be applied to the aspirate to show if alkaline phosphatase is present. If it is, OSA is confirmed. However, alkaline phosphatase is not always present in the bones of dogs with OSA, so negative staining for alkaline phosphatase does not rule out OSA.

A bone biopsy can conclusively confirm OSA, but can also be problematic. Biopsies remove a small portion of bone for examination and this can increase the risk of fracture. The need to "know for sure" should be carefully weighed against the possibility of a serious break.

If a biopsy is done, an experienced surgeon should perform the procedure, because it is common to see biopsies taken from the edge, rather than the middle, of the lesion. This mistake leads to a misdiagnosis of OSA in 50% of cases. It is also important to make sure that the tract the bone aspirate created and/or the site of the bone biopsy are either removed in a later surgery or included in the radiation field, during later treatments.

Whether the limb is removed pre- or post-biopsy, it should also be submitted for analysis. The more tissue the pathologist has to look at, the more thorough his evaluation can be.

Whether you forgo an aspirate and biopsy or not, definitely run staging tests before starting chemotherapy, radiation treatments or even, an amputation. Three-view X-rays of the chest cavity should be taken, to look for lung metastasis. Ten to fifteen percent of dogs with OSA have detectable spread to the lungs when they are diagnosed and it is important to accurately assess the situation. The prognosis worsens significantly with detectable metastasis on the chest X-rays; then, you may reconsider putting your dog through an amputation.

As we've discussed, microscopic lesions – micrometastasis – are present in 90% of dogs with OSA. While chest CT scans can sometimes pick up these smaller lesions, the test requires anesthesia and is expensive. Also, current treatment recommendations and prognoses are based on results of chest X-rays, not CT scans, so if small and early metastasis is detected on CT, its effects on prognosis and survival are not known. Even if metastasis is not found, I recommend proceeding as if metastasis were likely and chemotherapy necessary.

Full blood panels, including a CBC and chemistry panel, should be run, and a urinalysis performed. Regional lymph nodes should be aspirated or biopsied to check for metastasis, even if they appear to be normal. Although lymph node spread is uncommon (occurring in fewer than 5% of dogs), its presence is a negative prognostic factor; treated dogs that also have lymph node involvement live only two months, compared to eleven months for those without. Knowing whether OSA has spread to the lymph nodes can help you make treatment decisions. (Make sure that your vet or surgeon requests the lymph node evaluation when submitting the amputation, because these are not routinely evaluated at all labs.)

Tumors spreading to other bones are the second most common site of metastasis, so if there are signs of pain or lameness in another area of the body, regional X-rays should be taken to look for lesions. I do not typically recommend whole body X-rays, because of the added cost (it takes a lot of X-rays in a big dog to get this done) and the overall low probability that a dog has bone metastasis at diagnosis (about 6%). However, when a dog is lame or hurting in more than one secondary area, whole body X-rays can be considered.

In a few cases, nuclear bone scans can be helpful, although they are not widely available and there is some conflict over their usefulness, because they detect any active bone growth. Growth can, of course, be bone metastasis, and it may also be evidence of osteoarthritis or infection. If a positive site is found on a nuclear bone scan, a bone biopsy will still be required to make an accurate diagnosis.

Although metastasis to the abdominal organs is uncommon, I still recommend an abdominal ultrasound for dogs confirmed for or suspected of OSA. It's not painful or invasive, and it can be used to evaluate the dog's overall state of health, before embarking on extensive and expensive treatments.

What Is the Prognosis for Osteosarcoma?

I provide a staging system for other cancers in this book, usually based on the World Health Organization's (WHO) official system. Unfortunately, the WHO's human-based staging system is not particularly useful for OSA, because most dogs are already in an advanced stage when we discover the cancer. For this reason, I have chosen not to include it.

In general, OSA is a fast-moving, aggressive dog cancer, with 95% eventually metastasizing. Without treatment, most dogs with OSA are euthanized within two months because of progressive pain, poor quality of life, a pathologic fracture, or the possibility of one.

Dogs treated with amputation alone have a median survival time of four to five months, with at least 90% succumbing by one year and only 2% surviving to two years.

Dogs treated with amputation *and* chemotherapy experience a lengthened median survival time of ten months to one year, with 20-25% of dogs still alive at two years.

Clearly, dogs who receive amputation and chemotherapy experience a better prognosis. There are also other well-established and reliable predictors to help you determine your dog's prognosis.

Dogs with smaller tumors; dogs with no lung, bone or lymph node metastasis at the time of diagnosis; dogs with normal alkaline phosphatase (ALP) levels and dogs whose biopsies indicate a low grade of cancer, all have a better prognosis.

A dog whose ALP level returns to normal within forty days of surgery has a better prognosis than a dog whose levels remain elevated.

Dogs who undergo limb-spare procedures (techniques which are designed to avoid amputation) *and* are treated with antibiotics for infections at the surgical site, actually experience improved survival rates. This is likely due to the activation of immune cells and their response to stimulated inflammatory chemicals.

What Are the Available Protocols for Osteosarcoma?

Conventional treatment for OSA targets the primary tumor with local treatment (surgery and/or radiation) and targets the likely micrometastasis with systemic treatment (chemotherapy).

The main goal of local treatment is to prevent recurrence and control the pain that dogs inevitably feel with OSA. Amputation, as radical as it may sound, is usually the best treatment option. The complete removal of the affected limb prevents a possibly sudden and painful fracture and effectively removes the source of deep, aching bone pain.

If it is hard for you to contemplate amputation, you are not alone – most owners simply cannot imagine how their dogs could live a good life without all four limbs. It's important to know that they are usually happy after having made the choice to amputate. Dogs typically adapt very well to the loss of a limb and can still run, play and even swim. Many dogs have already started bearing more weight on the unaffected limbs, so their recovery time post-amputation is often just a few days. You can purchase a harness or sling a towel under his belly to assist your dog during recovery.

Amputation is not right for every dog. Dogs with very severe arthritis and some neurological conditions may not be able to walk well after an amputation; older dogs with average, moderate arthritis, usually do well on three legs. In any case, it is worth checking the opposing limb carefully to make sure it seems capable of bearing the added weight. It's also worth noting that lesions confined to the scapula can often be removed by just removing the scapula, not the whole leg.

For dogs whose owners are reluctant to amputate, and for dogs with pre-existing conditions that preclude amputation, a limb-sparing procedure might be a good approach. These procedures vary, depending upon the case, and usually involve removing only the affected bone and then replacing it with a bone from a donor, or from the patient, himself (in these cases, the cancerous bone is removed, radiated with high doses, and replaced). The new implant should be plated and fused, which may not be possible in every location; the ends of the radius and ulna bones at the wrist are the best locations for limb-sparing procedures. To be a candidate, your dog should have less than 50% of the bone involved in OSA, no fractures, minimal soft tissue involvement and a lesion that does not wrap around the whole bone.

Limb-sparing surgeries are more involved than amputations, more expensive and require a specialty hospital with the ability and experience to perform the advanced techniques involved. Survival times remain the same and these dogs have higher recurrence rates (20-30%). Limb-sparing techniques also do not address metastasis or micrometastasis, so chemotherapy is still needed for longer survival times.

Complications, including fractures and infections, are more likely to occur in limb-sparing surgeries than in amputations. These may require additional surgeries or even the very amputation that we were trying to avoid. As an interesting aside, dogs who develop infections are more likely to have overall successful surgeries and live longer – this is likely because the immune system's response is strengthened by fighting the bacterial infection.

Some dogs are candidates for surgery to remove metastasized OSA lung tumors. When the primary tumor is under control and the metastasis is isolated and detected more than ten months after the original diagnosis, there is no other disease present, fewer than three or four metastatic lesions are visible and there are no new lesions after a month's time, your dog may be a candidate for surgery. In one study, the mean survival time after lung metastasis surgery was six months, with a range of one month to four years.

Radiation therapy may also be used to treat OSA. The most common use is palliative intent therapy, which is aimed at reducing pain and increasing quality of life in dogs that do not get an amputation. The palliative protocol usually involves two to four once-per-week treatments. Radiation can reduce inflammation, lessen pain, improve the dog's ability to walk and aid in the healing of micro-fractures. The majority of dogs do well on radiation: 75-90% ex-

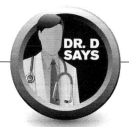

DR. D SAYS

The conventional treatments Dr. Ettinger recommends for osteosarcoma should be considered part of step one of Full Spectrum cancer care (Chapter 11). Please review that chapter for more general information about surgery, radiation and chemotherapy and how to handle their common side effects.

For more information on all other Full Spectrum steps, including nutraceuticals, immune boosters, dietary changes and brain chemistry modification strategies, review Full Spectrum cancer care, which begins on page 103.

You will also find information about specific chemotherapy agents in Chapter 41.

perience good effects, usually after one or two treatments. For some dogs, these effects last only months, while for others they last over a year. During this time these dogs need less pain medication or no pain medications at all; the reason is not completely understood: it seems that radiation therapy releases pain-killing endorphins. Chemotherapy treatments given in addition to palliative radiation have been associated with better results, also.

Radiosurgery can also be used as a limb-sparing technique – an alternative to the surgery described above – when amputation is not possible or not desirable. This is an advanced radiation therapy technique, available only at certain specialty hospitals (my hospital has the CyberKnife unit, which can focus high doses of radiation at very specific tumor sites with minimal radiation going to surrounding tissues). A CT scan is required to evaluate the extent of bone destruction from the OSA tumor and to carefully plan the radiosurgery, if it is indicated. Only one radiosurgery is required for limb OSA, and most dogs do well afterwards, with about 30% experiencing some form of complication. Complications depend upon the case (one is a bone fracture); the risk increases when the tumor has destroyed a lot of cortical bone (the very dense, hard outer shell of most bones). Radiosurgery is a fairly new technique; so far, the results at my hospital show that dogs receiving radiosurgery and chemotherapy to control metastasis have a median survival time of about one year, similar to the median survival time for dogs treated with amputation and chemotherapy. If you want to save your dog's limb, you can afford radiosurgery, you can get to a hospital which offers it and your dog is a good candidate, this may be a good option to consider.

Surgery and radiation techniques offer local control of the primary OSA tumor (and sometimes of isolated metastasized tumors); local therapy is not enough to keep OSA metastasis at bay. Because most dogs (90%) have micrometastasis at the time of diagnosis and 95% of dogs will develop detectable metastasis, you should use a systemic therapy – in other words, chemotherapy. Without it, dogs without amputation live only two months and dogs with amputations live four to five months (median survival times).

The most common chemotherapy drugs are doxorubicin, carboplatin, and cisplatin, which you can read about in Chapter 41. The published protocols vary on which drugs to use, frequency and number of treatments and, unfortunately, there is no single best protocol I can recommend. Consulting with an experienced oncologist, who can look at your dog's case and weigh the options, is your best bet. The best time to start chemotherapy is soon after surgery (ten to fourteen days) and before the likely metastasis is detectable.

Once metastasis has been detected, there are several ways to treat it. In addition to using surgery, there is additional chemotherapy, including aerosol chemotherapy, which delivers the drug via the inhaled breath, directly to the lungs, without being diluted in the bloodstream. Another option is metronomic chemotherapy: frequent and low doses of chemotherapy, which can help block angiogenesis (new blood vessel formation) and block or slow metastasis (see page 137). There has also been some success with immunotherapy (see below) and with a radioactive bone-seeking isotope, samarium, which literally seeks out the metastasis for targeted destruction.

Additional Considerations for Osteosarcoma

There are some other treatments that you may want to consider for your dog with OSA. For example, a class of drugs called bisphosphonates, used in humans with osteoporosis to stop bone resorption (bone loss, which happens when cells called osteoclasts break down the bones), is now being used in human cancer patients with bone metastasis. When used in dogs with OSA, bisphosphonates stop bone resorption and may have a direct toxic effect on OSA cancer cells. Treatments are usually given via

IV fluids, over a few hours and there is a low risk of kidney toxicity (the kidneys should be tested before each treatment). This treatment is still new; although we do not yet know how much time it buys, it may be worth inquiring. In addition to its possible anti-tumor benefits, I have found bisphosphonates helpful for reducing bone pain from the primary tumor when surgery is not elected or the tumor is inoperable.

Immunotherapy, which is the direct stimulation of the immune system to fight cancer cells, has also been shown to be helpful. Inhaling interleukin-2 liposomes, for example, has been shown to be both safe and effective in dogs with advanced lung metastasis. This aerosolized therapy stabilized and/or caused regression for their lung disease. Dogs also found it easy to take. Another immunotherapy, called L-MTP-PE, increased survival times to fifteen months, when combined with chemotherapy. While this option is exciting, unfortunately, it is not yet commercially available. Hopefully, this and other new immunotherapies will come on the market soon.

COX-2 inhibiting drugs such as NSAIDs (non-steroidal anti-inflammatory drugs) are being investigated as another approach to controlling metastasis in OSA. COX-2 is involved in inflammation and these drugs stop its mechanism and reduce inflammation. They also, however, seem to have an impact on angiogenesis, which means they slow or stop tumors from forming new blood vessels.

Oral pain medications may be needed when amputation is declined or when there is detectable metastasis, especially to the bone. NSAIDs can be helpful, though rarely sufficient by themselves; they pose an increased risk for negative gastrointestinal affects such as vomiting and stomach ulcers, also. When NSAIDs cannot be tolerated, prednisone can be used in anti-inflammatory doses. (Remember to never use prednisone, any other steroid, or any anti-inflammatory with NSAIDs, due to the risk of stomach ulceration.)

Additional pain medications that are useful are acetaminophen with codeine, Tramadol, sustained-release morphine, gabapentin and amantadine. Many of these drugs can be used in combinations for best effects: some of my patients are on four or more pain medications to control their pain.

Another good pain control option is a Fentanyl skin patch, which allows a continuous dose of pain medication to be absorbed through the skin. Because this patch needs to be changed by the vet every three to five days, you may find it too burdensome to use.

I Was Bent Every Day – So I Vented Every Day!

"I used the **Vent if You're Bent** exercise daily! I kept a journal where I could put all my feelings and emotions down on paper as a way to release them. Some days I said the same things, others, I was mad or emotional about different aspects of this disease that had affected the whole family. I also used the **Cheat Day** on occasion, because, knowing he had osteosarcoma, and realizing that it is the most aggressive and hard to treat cancer, I felt that he shouldn't be denied what he loved, however, I didn't want to "feed" the cancer either. The **Message Massage** also helped him immensely. I could feel him relax under the pressure of the massage and soothing words."

- Jill Stout, Medford, Oregon

As always, dogs on pain medications of any kind should be closely monitored for side effects and signs of toxicity.

The Bottom Line

While a diagnosis of OSA may be very scary, it is not an immediate death sentence. There is a wide variety of options available depending upon the underlying health of your dog, the extent of the disease at diagnosis and your ability to commit to extensive treatments.

Beyond Traditional Treatments

"It is beyond daunting when one first gets the news. Often there are some very hard decisions to make. One I had was - am I doing this for me or her? Especially with an amputation - will her life be as enjoyable? As much as I respect my Vet, he like many others does not have the knowledge and information to go beyond the traditional treatment. I am so happy I did my own research and found Dr. Dressler's book. It is very empowering and gave me some of the direction I needed to move forward. I believe every Vet should have this book as a resource to offer people when they are faced with this life-changing news."

- Keefer Irwin, Rochester, Vermont

Chapter 33: Hemangiosarcoma

Hemangiosarcoma is a cancer of the lining of the blood vessels, and it occurs more frequently in dogs than in any other species. Because blood vessels are everywhere, hemangiosarcoma can develop in any location. The most common site for a primary hemangiosarcoma tumor is the spleen, followed by the right atrium of the heart. Other primary locations include the skin, subcutis (a layer of tissue just under the skin), muscle tissue and liver. Hemangiosarcoma, also called angiosarcoma and malignant hemangioendothelioma, is often abbreviated as HSA.

HSA is an aggressive and highly metastatic malignancy. More than half of dogs already have detectable spread when they are diagnosed, and may feel sick or even experience internal bleeding.

The standard of care for HSA is surgery, followed by chemotherapy (usually doxorubicin). Depending upon the tumor's location, radiation may

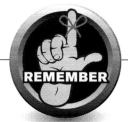

REMEMBER

When you need to look up the definition of a word or phrase, find it listed in Chapter 5, which begins on page 46.

also be used after surgery to avoid recurrence. Radiation is particularly indicated for skin or subdermal HSA with narrow or incomplete margins.

New approaches for care are being investigated, and we need them, because the long-term prognosis for dogs with HSA of the internal organs is poor: one to three months for dogs who receive surgery and six months for dogs who receive surgery and chemotherapy. Dogs with non-ruptured spleens (stage I) may live a few months longer. About ten percent of dogs who receive standard treatment live one year past the initial diagnosis.

Dogs with skin HSA generally have an improved median survival time, depending upon the stage of the cancer.

What Is Hemangiosarcoma?

HSA develops in the endothelial cells, which line the interior of the blood vessels. The blood vessels — arteries, veins, and capillaries — carry blood throughout the body, through their vast and complicated network. Nearly every tissue needs blood, so every cell is close to a blood vessel of some sort. The sheer enormity of the blood circulatory system is one reason why HSA tumors can develop anywhere in the body.

The spleen is the most common location for HSA; in fact, two-thirds of dogs who have splenic masses have cancer, and two-thirds of those cancers are HSA. This pattern is commonly referred to as the two-thirds rule.

The right atrium of the heart is the second most common site for HSA, accounting for 40% of all heart cancers and making HSA the most common heart tumor. Other common locations are the skin, under the skin (in the hypodermis or subcutis), the muscles and, rarely, the liver (liver lesions are more likely metastasis than primary tumors). HSA, which occurs in the spleen, the liver and/or in other internal organs, is referred to as visceral HSA.

Over half the number of dogs with HSA have detectable spread at the time of diagnosis, because HSA is so very aggressive and metastatic. It spreads both locally, into the tissues around the primary tumor site, and distantly, through the blood stream. Cancer cells can also spread directly into the abdomen if the tumor is bleeding or ruptures, which is called transabdominal transplantation. It's more common for HSA to metastasize through the bloodstream to the lungs, abdominal lymph nodes, omentum (a fatty organ found throughout the abdomen), brain, bone and muscle.

Which Dogs Are at Risk for Hemangiosarcoma?

HSA is usually seen in middle-aged and older dogs; its precise cause is not known.

Subcutaneous and visceral tumors inside the body occur most frequently in the Golden Retriever, German Shepherd and Labrador Retriever.

HSA heart tumors most frequently occur in the Golden Retriever, German Shepherd, Rottweiler, Greyhound and other large-breed dogs.

Skin HSA is associated with light exposure, specifically UV or ultraviolet light. Skin tumors typically develop in areas with no or very sparse hair, and more frequently in breeds with thin coats and light-colored skin, including Pit Bulls, Whippets, Boxers and Dalmatians.

In one study of over 1,300 dogs, neutering appeared to increase the risk of cardiac tumor in both sexes. Intact females were least likely to develop a cardiac tumor, whereas spayed females were most likely to develop one.

What are the Signs of Hemangiosarcoma?

Dogs often feel sick when they are first diagnosed with HSA. Owners usually bring them in for a variety of vague symptoms, such as a loss of appetite, decrease in energy, weight loss, vomiting or diarrhea. Upon examination (palpation, abdominal X-rays or abdominal ultrasound), the vet often finds an enlarged spleen, which is a red flag for visceral HSA. Occasionally, a mass is found during a routine physical exam, when the dog is otherwise asymptomatic. At other times, an ultrasound or X-ray, performed for other health issues, detects the masses.

Dogs with a more advanced splenic cancer may have much more dramatic symptoms, caused by a ruptured or bleeding tumor. If a tumor has ruptured, dogs may experience sudden and severe weakness or a total collapse, which is a potentially life-threatening situation. A splenic rupture causes anemia (low red blood cell counts) and internal bleeding into the abdomen, which is called hemoabdomen. A hemoabdomen can cause a distended belly, circulatory failure, uncontrolled internal bleeding, abnormal heart rhythms and a clotting problem, called disseminated intravascular coagulation (DIC). DIC is a serious blood disorder: first the proteins controlling blood clotting become abnormally active, creating small blood clots, and then abruptly stop clotting altogether, leading to uncontrollable bleeding.

If HSA has developed in the heart, the tumor may bleed into the pericardial cavity. The pericardium is a tough sac that completely encases the heart and protects it from internal damage by producing small amounts of pericardial fluid, which acts as a cushion. When a tumor bleeds, or effuses, into this sac, it can put excess pressure on the heart and actually impair its function. In this case, dogs may have vague signs like loss of appetite, weight loss and low energy – or more severe conditions, like an anemic collapse or even heart arrhythmias. When too much fluid builds up, it can cause a potentially fatal crisis, called tamponade: the pericardium has become so full that the heart no longer has room to beat – the chambers cannot fill with blood, or pump it out effectively. If your dog collapses or loses consciousness, prompt and dramatic intervention is required.

HSAs that develop in the skin are typically smooth, hairless, raised bumps ranging in color from dark red to purple. They are normally found on the belly or other areas with sparse hair, although both their location and appearance can vary. It's important to understand that while they are called "skin HSA," these tumors can be found in all skin layers, including the subcutaneous tissues and the muscle underneath.

How Is Hemangiosarcoma Diagnosed?

When HSA is suspected, a thorough physical examination must be performed. Your vet will certainly look for an enlarged spleen, which may be discovered during a routine palpation of the abdomen. When there is hemoabdomen (internal bleeding), a fluid wave may also be detected: a literal "wave" that moves across the belly when it is gently pressed.

An enlarged spleen found on abdominal X-rays should be confirmed with an abdominal ultrasound, which provides more information about the internal organs than do X-rays, including which organs have masses, possible metastatic lesions and the amount of abdominal fluid.

If abdominal fluid is seen, it should be sampled (aspirated) to determine whether it is blood. Cancer cells are rarely present in the aspirate, so, while it cannot typically confirm HSA, it can confirm potentially dangerous internal bleeding.

While it is standard to aspirate spleen, heart and liver masses discovered on ultrasound, these masses should not be aspirated when splenic HSA is suspected. Cancer cells are rarely present in aspirate, and because HSA is an inherently bloody cancer, aspirating masses can cause potentially dangerous bleeding and tumor rupture. As confirmation of HSA with aspiration of masses is rarely possible, this procedure is not worth the risk. The rare exception is when a suspicious lesion does not appear to have many blood vessels.

Superficial masses, such as skin and regional lymph nodes, suspected for HSA represent a low risk for life-threatening bleeding, so these masses should be aspirated to confirm the diagnosis.

Aspirates are rarely able to confirm the presence of splenic HSA, so the standard confirmation for this type of cancer is a surgical biopsy that removes the entire spleen.

If heart HSA is suspected, an echocardiogram (an ultrasound of the heart) is the best way to diagnose the mass. This produces the most detailed view of the heart and its structures, but masses in the right atrium, which is where HSA often occurs, are hard to see for the inexperienced eye. When it comes to these masses, your best bet is to get an experienced cardiologist to do the echocardiogram and interpret the results. When there is visible pericardial effusion on the echocardiogram, it should be aspirated and examined for cancer cells, even though the results of this test are often unreliable for confirming HSA – malignancies are not found at all in three out of four samples.

Why do I recommend a pericardial aspirate, if it doesn't usually help diagnose HSA? There are several good reasons. For one, it *can* diagnose lymphoma, another cancer likely to show up in the heart. Lymphoma is highly treatable with chemotherapy, so when found, treatments can be started immediately. Also, the pH level of the sample can be evaluated, which can help to predict whether cancer is present – although this is not definitive, in itself (its usefulness is debated amongst oncologists).

Furthermore, if the echocardiogram fails to confirm a mass, the aspirate of the pericardial fluid may reveal elevated levels of a protein called cardiac troponin I. This marker rises with the incidence of heart muscle ischemia (lack of blood) and necrosis (cell death), both of which occur with pericardial effusion, and even more so in dogs with cardiac hemangiosarcoma. Cardiac Tropin I tests are not routinely run in most hospitals; your vet may be able to get it through a specialized lab, if he thinks it will be useful.

Finally, removing the fluid from the pericardial sac will temporarily alleviate symptoms and stabilize your dog. This is often the most important reason to do this procedure.

Regardless of the site of the primary tumor, we typically look for spread right away, with the first X-rays and ultrasounds of the most common sites: the liver, lungs, mesentery and omentum (abdominal organs), heart, kidney, brain, muscles and lymph nodes. Half of the dogs suspected for HSA already have detectable spread at diagnosis, and knowing the

Singing Through the Pain

"While going through the experience of splenic hemangiosarcoma with my golden doodle Ellie, I sometimes felt overwhelmed with anger and sadness. I also felt uncomfortable about crying a lot in front of Ellie. Needing a safe place to vent my feelings led me to make a special connection with a song. I would get in my car, start to drive, put on the song and just let my emotions go. Sometimes I'd end up crying so hard I'd have to pull-over, but I always felt so much relief afterward. Having a safe place to release my emotional pain was a huge part of taking care of me so I could better take care of Ellie."

- *Sarah N. Bertsch, Hudson, Wisconsin*

stage of the cancer is helpful when making treatment decisions later.

Metastatic lung lesions can often be seen on chest X-rays, although CT scans are more sensitive and show smaller lesions more easily. The heart may appear round (called globoid) on chest X-rays; this appearance suggests bleeding into the pericardial fluid. X-rays rarely show the heart masses themselves, however, so whether the heart is globoid or normal, it is helpful to get an echocardiogram to rule out a heart mass. Not everyone agrees that dogs with splenic masses also get echocardiograms to look for spread to the heart; I mention it because one study determined that one out of four dogs with spleen HSA had a concurrent heart tumor.

Dogs suspected for heart HSA should have

both chest imaging (X-ray or CT scan) and abdominal ultrasounds to look for metastasis.

During the initial spleen removal, every lesion found in the abdomen suspected to be metastatic should be biopsied, and the liver will routinely be biopsied, even if its appearance is normal.

Even though not every oncologist agrees with me about this, I feel strongly that relying on an ultrasound to diagnose liver metastasis is a mistake. The liver is a rapidly regenerating organ, and we often see nodules – which are associated with rebuilding tissue – and mistake them for metastasis, even at surgery. Although dangerous to misinterpret an ultrasound in this way, it happens, especially with HSA cases. If a radiologist or vet thinks liver lesions are metastatic based solely on their appearance at surgery or on an ultrasound, ask for a biopsy to confirm the suspicion. I have seen many owners decide against surgery or even euthanize their dogs on the spot because they have been told (mistakenly) that HSA has already spread to the liver. Conversely, a liver that appears normal on ultrasound may still have metastasis, so it, too, should be biopsied.

In addition to imaging tests, a complete exam for HSA includes blood work – a complete blood count (CBC), chemistry panel, urinalysis and clotting profile are the bare minimum. When an abnormal heart rhythm is detected, an electrocardiogram should be run.

In addition to the aspirate used to confirm skin HSA, dogs with skin masses should have nearby lymph nodes aspirated to check for metastasis, plus chest images and abdominal ultrasounds to check for spread. They should also be carefully examined for masses, since skin HSA tends to spread to other areas of the skin.

Your vet may want to check the levels of vas-cular endothelial growth factor (VEGF), which is associated with cell division and the growth of new blood vessels (angiogenesis). VEGF can play a major role in tumor growth in humans, and for some cancers, its levels in the blood can help us understand whether the disease is very advanced, how it will progress and how it is likely to respond to therapy. A study of VEGF in dogs shows that while VEGF levels were higher in dogs with HSA, the levels couldn't tell us the stage of the cancer, whether it would respond to treatment, or how long the dog would live. For these reasons, VEGF levels are probably not useful to confirm HSA or formulate a treatment plan in dogs. This is also why it is not used as an early detection or screening test, and is not routinely run in most veterinary hospitals. Knowing your dog's VEGF levels might be helpful for your case and your vet may be able to get them from a specialized lab.

What Is the Prognosis for Hemangiosarcoma?

HSA is a fast-moving, aggressive cancer (half the number of afflicted dogs have already metastasized at the time of diagnosis). This is a tough disease for both oncologists and owners, because it is rarely caught early.

Here is the World Health Organization's staging system for hemangiosarcoma:

Visceral HSA

Stage I: A tumor smaller than 5 centimeter, confined to the primary site, with no regional or distant metastasis.

Stage II: A tumor greater than 5 centimeter or a ruptured tumor, or smaller than 5 centimeter with confined regional metastasis, but no distant metastasis.

Stage III: A tumor greater than 5 centimeter or a ruptured tumor, or a tumor that has invaded adjacent structures, with or without lymph node metastasis or distant metastasis.

Skin HSA

Stage I: A tumor confined to the skin.

Stage II: A tumor that involves the hypodermis or subcutis (the layers underneath the skin).

Stage III: A tumor with muscle involvement.

Dogs who do not receive any treatment for their visceral HSA have a very short life expectancy (days to weeks).

Dogs who receive surgery alone for their splenic HSA have a median survival time of one to three months, and those receiving both surgery and post-operative chemotherapy (see the treatment section, below) have median survival times of six months. A stage I (the spleen has not ruptured) prognosis improves by a few months when treated with chemotherapy after surgery.

Dogs with heart HSA who have the mass removed and get follow-up chemotherapy have six-month median survival times.

Even with treatment, one-year survival times for splenic and heart HSA are uncommon – roughly ten percent.

Dogs with stage I skin HSA fare better: they have a median survival time of twenty-six months (over two years); dogs with stage II and III skin HSA (subcutaneous and muscle tumors) have median survival times of six to ten months. According to one recent study, dogs with subcutaneous HSA can experience median survival times over four years in length with aggressive surgery (wide, clean margins), with or without radiation therapy and with a chemotherapy protocol that uses doxorubicin.

What Are the Available Protocols for Hemangiosarcoma?

The first treatment for HSA of any kind is surgery, followed by chemotherapy. Because so many dogs are unstable at the time of diagnosis – suffering from hemoabdomen or pericardial effusion – the very first priority is usually stabilization.

Surgery and Visceral HSA

When the anemia is severe (from bleeding into the abdomen or pericardium), a blood transfusion is often required to make your dog stable enough for anesthesia. A clotting test should be run and fresh frozen plasma may be needed to further stabilize a dog with clotting abnormalities.

Once your dog is stable, the goal of surgery for visceral HSA is to remove the tumor and prevent or minimize future bleeding episodes. This nearly always requires a complete removal of the spleen. About 25% of dogs develop temporary abnormal heart rhythms following a splenectomy, so an ECG should be used to monitor the heart during and after surgery. While heart arrhythmias occasionally require drugs to manage, most resolve within days.

Surgery and Heart HSA

When your dog has pericardial effusion, the fluid is usually removed or "tapped" in a procedure called pericardiocentesis, relieving pressure on the heart. Sometimes this procedure only increases comfort temporarily, because fluid can re-accumulate within a day or week without additional therapy. Once the excess fluid is removed and your dog is stabilized, a heart operation can be considered.

The first option is to remove part of the peri-

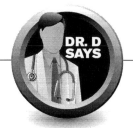

The conventional treatments Dr. Ettinger recommends for hemangiosarcoma should be considered part of step one of Full Spectrum cancer care (Chapter 11). Please review that chapter for more general information about surgery, radiation and chemotherapy and how to handle their common side effects.

For more information on all other Full Spectrum steps, including nutraceuticals, immune boosters, dietary changes and brain chemistry modification strategies, review Full Spectrum cancer care, which begins on page 103.

You will also find information about specific chemotherapy agents in Chapter 41.

cardium – the sac around the heart – to allow fluid to accumulate in the chest, around the lungs. Even though fluid around the lungs can cause difficulty in breathing, that space can hold more fluid than the pericardium, and this gives the heart more room to function properly for longer. This procedure is considered palliative.

The second option is to remove the heart mass itself, which has been shown to increase median survival times to one to four months (similar to the me-

dian survival times for other visceral surgeries). This option is out of reach for some owners, because it requires an experienced heart surgeon and twenty-four hour intensive care after surgery. It also has a relatively high mortality rate – about fifteen percent of dogs undergoing this procedure die during surgery or during hospitalization afterwards.

Chemotherapy for Visceral and Heart HSA

As I noted above, median survival times for dogs with visceral or heart HSA are only one to four months with surgery alone. Post-operative chemotherapy increases that survival time to six months, which is why I recommend chemotherapy for all dogs with HSA of the internal organs, the heart, subcutis or muscle HSA.

(I do *not* recommend chemotherapy as a stand-alone treatment, because survival times are very poor without surgery first.)

Doxorubicin is the most (and possibly the only) effective chemotherapy drug for HSA. Protocols vary and are evolving, so, there is no one best protocol to recommend. As you'll read in the section on chemotherapy, doxorubicin is a potent vesicant, which causes severe damage to skin and other tissues if it gets outside the vein. It must be handled very carefully and I strongly recommend you have an oncologist handle these treatments.

Most published protocols consist of five or six treatments, but I recommend a more extensive chemotherapy schedule. Chemotherapy treatments should be a regular event for the rest of your dog's life. This aggressive disease requires aggressive treatments, and in my experience dogs can live a good life while on chemotherapy. Of course, I recommend periodic imaging tests to see if the disease is progressing internally and evaluate whether the chemotherapy is having the desired effect. We typically stop using doxorubicin after six treatments due to its potentially toxic effects on the heart; past this point, consider transitioning to a metronomic protocol (see below).

When your dog has a ruptured spleen or hemoabdomen (free blood in the abdomen) at the time of diagnosis, I also consider adding intracavity chemotherapy to the protocol. You'll remember that HSA is capable of spreading throughout the abdomen, when released into the cavity by a rupture. In this strategy, we chase that transabdominal seeding by depositing chemotherapy drugs directly into the abdominal or chest cavities, rather than into a vein and the blood circulation. Doxorubicin must be injected directly into the vein to avoid tissue damage, so it cannot be used for this technique, but carboplatin or mitoxantrone may be used. The drugs are still absorbed and processed by the body, so side effects are similar to traditional IV chemotherapy. Since doxorubicin is the standard of care, I alternate IV doxorubicin with intracavity chemotherapy. It is unclear as of this writing whether this technique extends survival times; I only offer it as a possibility for inclusion in your treatment plan.

Skin HSA

As with visceral HSA, the primary treatment for dogs with skin and subdermal HSA is surgery. The goal is to remove the tumor completely with wide (two to three centimeter) margins, if possible. A recent study has shown that aggressive surgery and clean surgical margins are related to long survival times – over four years tumor-free for dogs with subcutaneous HSA treated with surgery and doxorubicin (with or without radiation).

When the tumor location forces the surgeon to use narrow margins or the biopsy shows dirty surgical margins, radiation may be needed to prevent recurrence at the surgical incision.

When the tumor is non-resectable, palliative radiation may help to reduce it, and stereotactic radiosurgery can also be considered.

I recommend chemotherapy for skin HSA, based on the stage of the cancer. Less than 30% of stage I HSA cases metastasize, so when the surgery achieves clean margins or radiation was done after surgery, the HSA may be cured. In these cases, I recommend rigorous, routine checks every three to four months without fail to check for new masses and for metastasis. In addition, I may recommend chemotherapy on a case-by-case basis for stage I dogs whose biopsies show an increased risk of metastasis.

Stage II and III HSA skin tumors, on the other hand, are highly metastatic, similar to HSA of the internal organs. Most dogs with subdermal HSA ultimately succumb to metastasis, so I recommend the chemotherapy protocols discussed for the internal organs, above.

Additional Considerations for Hemangiosarcoma

An exciting new approach to chemotherapy is called metronomic chemotherapy, which abandons the traditional technique (higher doses – the maximum tolerated dose – with longer breaks in between) in favor of low doses of oral chemotherapy agents, given daily or with few breaks. This therapy is technically not aimed at killing cancer cells – instead, it targets their blood supply and metastasis routes by inhibiting angiogenesis, or the growth of new blood vessels.

Because HSA is a tumor of the lining of the blood vessels, this approach is a logical route to try. Not only does it target and destroy endothelial cells in the blood vessels (the very cells involved in this cancer and also the vessels that carry blood and oxygen to these tumors), but also seems to enhance the immune system's response to tumors. A recent study showed that a metronomic approach is comparable to conventional chemotherapy, so it merits consideration, especially since the new class of drugs, called tyrosine kinase inhibitors (Palladia, for example), have anti-angiogenic effects. It is not yet clear whether metronomic chemotherapy will result in longer survival times for HSA patients, and there is still much to be learned. Nevertheless, I like the minimal side effects of these protocols and the fact that the owner can usually manage them at home. There may also be value to combining metronomic protocols with traditional doxorubicin, for example. Protocols are constantly evolving, and even though close supervision and routine visits to the vet are still necessary, I strongly recommend you consider metronomic chemotherapy with your vet or oncologist.

There is a lot of interesting research happening in the field of immunotherapy applied to HSA, however, the protocols being worked out are not yet available commercially. It is worth asking your vet or oncologist about this approach, as medicine is constantly evolving. Newer approaches are needed and are being investigated.

Don't Give Up

"Even though at first you may think the situation is insurmountable, please do not throw in the towel. You can, through help and guidance and understanding, help you and your friend through these tough times. It's normal to be confused, sad and angry at the same time. You need information from knowledgeable people. You need to become informed on everything dealing with the problem. You can then base your decision and plan of action based on what is best for your friend. The treatment is for them, so don't give up; do what is possible for them and for you."

- Jon Marshall, Norman, Oklahoma

The Bottom Line

While a diagnosis of HSA is very discouraging, there are treatments available that can extend your dog's life. I urge you to consider all of the options carefully and make a well-informed decision. It is important to remember that treated dogs can live longer and live well.

Chapter 34: Transitional Cell Carcinoma

Transitional cell carcinoma is a cancer of the urinary tract. Tumors are most often found in the bladder and they can also be found in the urethra, ureters and prostate gland. Transitional cell carcinoma is commonly referred to by its initials, TCC.

Bladder TCC moves very fast, spreading locally through the urinary tract and distantly to areas such as the lymph nodes, lung, liver and bone. About 15% of all afflicted dogs already have metastasis at the time of diagnosis, and another 50% will develop metastasis as the disease progresses.

Due to the complicated nature of the urinary tract, TCC is rarely curable. Although surgeries can debulk (reduce the size) of tumors, it is next to impossible to achieve complete removal. For this reason, surgery is considered palliative, and following it up with chemotherapy and Cox-2-inhibitor therapies is the standard of care. Dogs treated with surgery alone live three to four months; dogs treated with piroxicam alone live six to seven months; median survival times increase to one year when surgery and piroxicam are combined with the chemotherapy drug mitoxantrone.

While curing TCC is not likely, it is considered a very treatable cancer. Combining therapies can both extend life and make dogs much more comfortable.

What Is Transitional Cell Carcinoma?

TCC is a cancer of the urinary system, a system made up of several organs working together to remove metabolic wastes from the blood and flush them out of the body. The upper portion of the system consists of the two kidneys (one on each side of the body). The kidneys have several important bodily functions, not the least of which is filtering the blood for elimination of toxins and wastes. These bean-shaped organs create the fluid we call urine, which flows down to the lower urinary system through the ureters (tubes) into the bladder. The bladder is a hollow bag, which expands as it collects the urine. When your dog urinates, the bladder releases the urine through the urethra, a tube that traverses the genital area until it reaches the exterior. The prostate

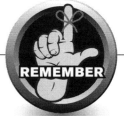

When you need to look up the definition of a word or phrase, find it listed in Chapter 5, which begins on page 46.

gland surrounds the urethra in male dogs and empties its fluids into the urethra through tiny ducts, or tubes.

The ureters, the bladder and the urethra are lined with special cells called transitional epithelial cells, unusual cells that can change shape – stretch or contract – and make it possible for these organs to accommodate the fluctuations in the amount of urine present in the system. Transitional cell carcinoma develops in, and is named for, these cells.

TCC most commonly develops in the trigone, the triangular area formed by the two ureters and the urethra on the inside of the bladder wall. In over half of TCC cases, tumors extend from the bladder down into the urethra. Thirty percent of male dogs with TCC also have it in their prostates, arising from where the urethra passes through the prostate.

TCC is the most common bladder and urethra cancer (squamous cell carcinoma, lieomyosarcoma, and lymphoma follow). While cancer of the lower urinary tract is relatively rare in dogs, the majority of cancers are malignant and metastatic. Bladder TCC in particular is both locally invasive and highly metastatic, spreading most commonly to the lymph nodes, lungs, liver and bone.

Which Dogs Are at Risk for Transitional Cell Carcinoma?

There are several environmental factors that can contribute to the development of TCC, but there also seems to be a genetic risk for some breeds. At high risk are Shetland Sheepdogs, Beagles, Collies, and many terriers (Scottish, West Highland White, Airedale, and Wirehaired Fox). The two breeds at highest risk are Scottish Terriers and Shetland Sheepdogs.

TCC development is associated with exposure to insecticides, including household insecticides,

the mosquito-killing compounds often sprayed on marshland, and topical flea and tick medications. For this reason, I recommend the new spot-on topical flea control products, which appear to be safer, especially for high-risk breeds. Exposure to herbicides, such as weed-control chemicals and other lawn chemicals, is also a risk factor.

Female dogs have a greater tendency to develop TCC than male dogs do, perhaps because male dogs urinate more frequently, as they mark their territory. As their urine spends less time in the bladder, the toxins from pesticides and herbicides and other carcinogens spend less time in contact with the urinary tract.

Obese dogs are at a higher risk for TCC, for a similar reason – cancer-causing toxins are often stored in fat cells, which contribute to the developing cancer.

Dogs treated with the chemotherapy drug cyclophosphamide are also at a higher risk for developing TCC, due to urinary tract damage.

A study has shown that Scotties, consuming vegetables at least three times a week, had a decreased risk of bladder cancer. The addition of vegetables to your dog's diet (such as those in Dr. Dressler's cancer diet) may be helpful.

What are the Signs of Transitional Cell Carcinoma?

Transitional cell carcinoma can be misdiagnosed as a urinary tract infection because the symptoms are so similar. The signs for each condition are identical: straining to urinate, blood in the urine, and frequent, small urinations. Some dogs may also strain when defecating. To complicate matters further, many dogs with TCC have a secondary bladder infection, too. If underlying cancer is not suspected, antibiotics may help to alleviate the symptoms, for a time. When symptoms recur, especially in older dogs, vets should check for TCC.

Urinary tract infections are irritating and painful because there is the constant urge to urinate, even when the bladder is not full. The location of the tumor can also result in partial or complete obstruction of the flow of urine. For example, the trigone region, where TCC most often develops, is very sensitive to pressure – when it's stretched we feel the urge to urinate – and a tumor here can be uncomfortable.

Urinary tract tumors can also be dangerous, because they can significantly alter the functioning of the whole system. If you think of the urinary system as a hose, and imagine putting a kink in that hose, you'll understand how this works: kinks "back up" the water and lead to a stretching above the obstruction. A partial obstruction of the urinary tract can cause a dilation (widening) of the ureters and fluid to back up into the kidneys, which can lead to kidney failure. A complete obstruction can quickly become a life-threatening emergency.

Sometimes dogs are diagnosed after they are brought in to the vet for lameness or difficulty walking. In these cases, X-ray examinations usually reveal bone lesions, which turn out to be metastatic TCC.

How Is Transitional Cell Carcinoma Diagnosed?

There is a screening test for TCC, called the Veterinary Bladder Tumor Antigen test (VBTA test). The test can be run at your vet's office, and requires a free-catch urine sample, which you can collect yourself, no more than 48 hours old. If this test is negative, it is very unlikely that the dog has TCC, and further

work-up is likely to be unnecessary. If the VBTA test is positive, however, TCC is suspected and further tests should be run to confirm the diagnosis. Positive results are not confirmation for TCC, because false-positives can occur if there is blood and protein in the urine, which happens during bladder infections. Because of this, the usefulness of the VBTA is limited when the dog is already sick; it is best used as an early screening test for normal, asymptomatic dogs at high risk for developing TCC.

If TCC is suspected, with or without VBTA tests, urinalysis is usually the first test. This can be a free catch sample or a sterile sample collected directly from the bladder. The urinalysis usually shows elevated white blood cell levels, elevated red blood cell levels, and proteins and bacteria in the urine. These results, unfortunately, are what would also be expected in the case of a urinary tract infection. Although the examination of the urine sediment reveals tumor cells in about one-third of cases – even this discovery does not confirm TCC, because normal transitional cells can appear unusual and cancerous if there is a lot of inflammation in the system (which there is, during an infection).

To get a sterile urine sample to confirm a bladder infection, a cystocentesis is performed. A needle is inserted through the abdomen, directly into the bladder, so that a urine sample can be drawn into a collecting syringe. This is often done with ultrasound guidance, and does not usually require sedation. Then this urine sample must be cultured at the lab to determine whether there is a urinary tract infection, and what are the appropriate antibiotics to treat it.

Cystocentesis has its risks for patients with TCC; there have been reports of tumor cells seeding the track of the needle as it is withdrawn from the body, effectively spreading the cancer. Also, seeding tumor cells can occur while handling the tumor during regular bladder surgery, so caution is recommended in general. Proper oncology surgery guidelines dictate that the surgeon change gloves and instruments after handling all tumors and before suturing the patient closed. While cystocentesis has its risks, it is debatable whether to avoid the procedure in all patients. Secondary UTIs are common at diagnosis and during treatment, and many of my patients recently had a cystocentesis as part of their bladder work-up. So, if your dog had a cystocentesis just before the diagnosis, don't worry. Getting a urinary tract infection diagnosed and properly treated is just as important.

Since the cytology of urine found during a routine urinalysis only confirms TCC in a third of cases, a biopsy is often required to confirm a diagnosis and initiate a treatment plan. The best biopsy samples come from cystoscopy (using a fiber-optic scope passed through the urethra into the bladder) or from a bladder surgery (both of these require general anesthesia), although an ultrasound may also show the tumor.

The tumor's size and location is important to know and a little tricky to discover, because the bladder's function as a constantly changing hollow organ means it looks different depending upon how much urine is inside. The ideal way to make sure that the size and location are fully understood is for the vet to pass sterile saline fluid through a catheter into the bladder to fill it. The bladder is first emptied of urine and then filled with the same amount of fluid volume every time an ultrasound is performed; this is the only way to be sure that measurements are consistent, from one test to the next. Since female dogs need to be sedated for catheterization, do discuss the pros and cons of this procedure with your vet.

Abdominal ultrasounds can also help look for metastasis within the abdomen. The liver is a common location for metastasis, as are the regional lymph nodes; fifteen percent of TCC infections have spread by the time of diagnosis. Looking for metastasis is important, because half of all dogs will experience spread as the disease advances. In addition to ultrasound, three-view chest X-rays or chest CT scans should be done to check the lungs for spread. I recommend that these images be reviewed by a board-certified radiologist, as chest X-rays are commonly misinterpreted in older dogs. For example, lung nodules may represent benign, age-related changes but appear cancerous to an untrained eye. If a qualified radiologist is not available, I recommend suspending judgment on lung nodules and checking them later for changes. If they change, they may indicate spread – if they stay the same, they may just be age-related. A chest CT scan is more sensitive and may show more details than an X-ray.

In addition to these imaging tests, I recommend running routine blood work to check the general health of your dog. If increased kidney markers or high potassium levels are found, this can indicate an obstruction of the urinary tract by the tumor, and emergency measures must be taken to unblock it. If a catheter cannot be used, stents placed surgically might be needed to allow the urine to flow while treatment is begun.

What Is the Prognosis for Transitional Cell Carcinoma?

The best way to determine the long-term prognosis is to look at the stage of TCC at the time of diagnosis.

- **Stage T1:** Superficial tumor.
- **Stage T2:** The tumor is in the wall of the

bladder.

- **Stage T3:** The tumor is invading the surrounding tissue or organs.

T1 tumors generally respond better to treatment, and dogs with no metastasis have a median survival time of six to seven months.

Dogs with lymph node metastasis or metastasis to distant locations (liver, lungs or bones, for example) have a median survival time of two to three months.

If the prostate gland is involved, the prognosis worsens. The prognosis also worsens if the dog is young.

If left untreated, TCC can cause significant pain and loss of quality of life; a urinary system obstruction is also possible. We do not have any statistics to tell us the median survival time for dogs left untreated; my guess would be that these factors would limit life to a couple of months. The irritation and pain of this illness is hard for your dog and his owner to bear.

What Are the Available Protocols for Transitional Cell Carcinoma?

There are three goals for treating TCC: to make the dog more comfortable, to control the primary mass, and to prevent or delay metastasis.

Surgery is usually the first treatment used, although not curative for bladder TCC because it is usually impossible to completely remove (excise) a bladder tumor that is not caught very early. The trigone, where most bladder tumors develop, is a complex area of urinary tubes and nerves, making it very difficult to perform an aggressive surgery and achieve clean margins. It can be hard for any surgeon to determine which tissue is normal and which is not, by sight alone. Many dogs also have microscopic multifocal lesions; these microscopic cancerous or precancerous cells can occur even in normal bladder tissue. For this reason TCC recurrence is very common, even when a biopsy indicates clean margins.

Why do surgery, if it doesn't help to cure TCC? Because surgery can debulk (reduce the size of) tumors that may otherwise cause an obstruction, and it can decrease the tumor burden in the bladder, giving your dog less pain and more time. Surgery also has the potential to make chemotherapy more effective.

Dogs treated with surgery alone live only three to four months, because TCC tends to recur and is highly metastatic. Adding post-surgical chemotherapy treatments can prevent recurrence, prevent or delay metastasis, and extend survival times.

The most common protocols use mitoxantrone combined with the NSAID piroxicam, which extends survival times to twelve to fourteen months. About twenty percent of afflicted dogs respond to protocols that use piroxicam alone; these dogs experience a six to seven month median survival time and an overall good quality of life. Piroxicam is an NSAID, so it can cause stomach ulceration when used over the long-term, which is why I recommend giving misoprostol throughout treatments to protect the stomach.

While mitoxantrone and piroxicam protocols are considered the standard of care, there are other chemotherapy protocols, which use doxorubicin and platinum-based drugs, such as carboplatin and cisplatin. Carboplatin is safer for the kidneys than cisplatin, and dogs respond better when it is combined with piroxicam. The opposite is true for cisplatin – all NSAIDs, including piroxicam, worsen kidney toxic-

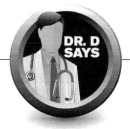

DR. D SAYS

The conventional treatments Dr. Ettinger recommends for transitional cell carcinoma should be considered part of step one of Full Spectrum cancer care (Chapter 11). Please review that chapter for more general information about surgery, radiation and chemotherapy and how to handle their common side effects.

For more information on all other Full Spectrum steps, including nutraceuticals, immune boosters, dietary changes and brain chemistry modification strategies, review Full Spectrum cancer care, which begins on page 103.

You will also find information about specific chemotherapy agents in Chapter 41.

ity when they are used with cisplatin, so, be careful not to give anti-inflammatories when your dog is on cisplatin (the use of any platinum-based drug requires careful monitoring). These protocols are likely to evolve as other chemotherapy drugs (such as vinblastine) are evaluated.

Some tumors are inoperable, so some owners simply decline surgery; in these cases, chemotherapy with piroxicam can be used as a solo treatment. Before completely declining surgery, however, I recommend you consult with your surgeon and weigh the pros and cons carefully.

If a urinary tract infection (UTI) is present at the time of diagnosis or during treatment, antibiotics may be prescribed to treat the infection and alleviate its symptoms.

Additional Considerations for Transitional Cell Carcinoma

When surgery is particularly difficult because of the tumor location, a type of laser surgery called carbon dioxide (CO_2) laser ablation may be helpful. The best outcomes happen when this surgery is combined with mitoxantrone and piroxicam protocols. Although survival times achieved with CO_2 laser ablation and treatment with mitoxantrone and piroxicam were similar to survival times associated with chemotherapy alone, resolution of symptoms was better with the combined treatment.

When there is a urinary tract obstruction, a cystostomy (the surgical implantation of a permanent catheter into the bladder) can be used to bypass the obstruction, drain the bladder and alleviate the pain. A urethral stent may also relieve obstructions in the urethra. In this case, a thin tube is inserted into the urethra to allow urine to flow past the obstruction. There can be complications from these procedures that may make them impossible for some dogs; your surgeon will have the best insight into your dog's case. I have managed patients who have undergone both of these procedures and they can be good options for the right dog and right owner.

Some owners want to try photodynamic therapy (PDT), which uses light of a specific wavelength to help kill tumor cells, as it is sometimes used for bladder cancer in humans. Unfortunately, this therapy is not currently effective for TCC in dogs, although it is still being investigated. Although not widely available, it is occasionally used for dogs with squamous cell carcinomas in the mouth.

Radiation therapy can be considered, although high doses have some severe side effects, including bladder fibrosis and scarring of the urethra. This can cause obstructions and severe complications, so the dose is limited to remain safe for the bladder.

CyberKnife radiosurgery can also be considered for prostatic TCC, and we have used it at my clinic. This palliative use of radiation combined with mitoxantrone and piroxicam seems to be safe and can stabilize the disease. It has not been used in many dogs, so its ultimate efficacy is still being explored.

The Bottom Line

TCC is a highly metastatic disease that is not likely to be cured. That said, I consider it a treatable cancer; combining therapies can both extend life and make dogs much more comfortable than they are at diagnosis.

Falsely Comforted By Surgery

"Shadow's experience has opened awareness and knowledge that we will use to help all of our dogs, and everyone we meet to both fight and prevent cancer. It's the number one cause of death in our beloved dogs, and the reasons are mostly man-made, from environment to food to attitude. One lesson I learned in both our dogs, is that they both had a minor cancer experience about 6 months before a major one was diagnosed. With Shadow, he had a malignant growth on his leg that was excised and the vet told us it had been taken out completely. With Keymos, at 12 years his testes got hard, a sign of cancer changes and he was castrated. About six months after each experience both dogs had a larger, life-threatening diagnosis of cancer. Had we realized that the earlier experience placed cancer cells in the body that we could start to fight instead of feeling comforted by surgery, we may have prevented further spread. The most important lesson we have learned is to get off our lazy butts and give our dogs the best natural diet possible, the second is to not take things for granted and to make sure every day they feel joy and play with us. It is good for us all."

- Susan Harper, High Wycombe, England

Chapter 35: Oral Cancer

Oral cancer is the fourth most common type of dog cancer. Several types of cancers can be found in the mouth, including melanomas, fibrosarcomas (FSA), squamous cell carcinomas (SCC) and the dental tumors known as epulides and ameloblastomas.

Oral tumors can occur in any location in the mouth: along the gums, the lips, the tongue, the palate (roof of the mouth) or pharynx (the upper part of the throat). Tumors that appear closer to the front of the mouth tend to have a better prognosis than those deeper in the oral cavity.

Early detection is critical, because the earlier these tumors are found and the smaller they are, the more responsive to treatment. Larger tumors found later may already have started to invade the local tissues, a common behavior. This progression can happen very slowly or very quickly. Distant spread, or metastasis, can also occur, usually much later in the disease.

Because these tumors can be so locally invasive, the goal of treatment is to control the primary tumor site with surgery and/or radiation. Surgery is the most economical, quick and curative treatment. Preventing tumor recurrence is very important because recurring tumors are much less likely to respond to later treatments. Finding an experienced surgeon who can do an aggressive first surgery is my highest recommendation.

The relative overall prognosis for oral cancer is usually good to excellent, with median survival times

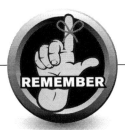

When you need to look up the definition of a word or phrase, find it listed in Chapter 5, which begins on page 46.

ranging from one year to over two years, depending upon the type of tumor.

What Is Oral Cancer?

Oral cancer, the fourth most common type of dog cancer, is typified by several types of tumors that can occur in the oral cavity. The most common is melanoma (discussed separately in Chapter 40) and the second most common are squamous cell carcinomas, or tumors that develop in squamous epithelial cells. The word squamous is Latin for "scale," as in scales on a fish, and describes the way these often-flat cells tend to overlap. Epithelial cells generally line the inside of the body, so there are many squamous epithelial cells in the oral cavity. Squamous cell carcinoma is often referred to by its initials, SCC. These tumors are locally invasive, spreading into the surrounding tissues, and they often involve the bone by the time of diagnosis. Depending upon where

SCC occurs, it may or may not spread distantly. SCC found deeper in the mouth (in the caudal region at the back), at the base of the tongue, or on or around the tonsils tends to be more metastatic.

A less common oral tumor, fibrosarcoma, accounts for 10-20% of cases. Sometimes called fibroblastic sarcoma, usually shortened to FSA, fibrosarcomas are tumors that develop in fibroblasts, specialized cells responsible for creating connective tissue. They are very invasive to local tissues, although less metastatic than SCC; metastasis occurs in less than 30% of all FSA cases. When it occurs, metastasis spreads to the lungs and occasionally regional lymph nodes in the head and neck.

Some tricky FSA tumors look benign under the biopsy microscope, then behave in the body like very aggressive malignancies. They grow extremely rapidly, recur often and invade the bone. These FSAs are given a mixed name to match their mixed appearance and behavior: Hi-Low FSA. They commonly occur on the upper jaw (maxilla) and the roof of the mouth (palate) of large breed dogs, especially the Golden Retriever. If your dog's FSA is called benign but behaves like an aggressive malignancy, it is probably a Hi-Low FSA, and should be treated like a malignancy.

The remaining oral tumors, about 5%, are benign tumors, called dental tumors, including epulides and ameloblastomas. Most of these tumors are easily controlled with surgery or radiation, do not metastasize and have a great prognosis when treated as outlined here. Please note that while classified as benign, these tumors can still have malignant effects, and should be treated.

Which Dogs Are at Risk for Oral Cancer?

While tobacco use, especially combined with alcohol use, has been proven to cause oral cancer in humans, the cause of most canine oral cancer is not known, with one exception. Oral carcinomas and sarcomas can occur years after radiation therapy is used to shrink benign dental tumors.

There are some risk factors associated with oral cancers: male dogs tend to develop more oral cancer of all kinds than females do, and white dogs seem to be predisposed to SCC of the tongue. SCC of the tonsils is ten times more likely to occur in dogs that live in urban areas. Oral FSA and SCC are more common in large breed dogs. Oral FSA also occurs more frequently in male dogs.

Some breeds are more likely to develop oral tumors: Doberman Pinschers, Golden Retrievers, Gordon and Irish Setters, Schnauzers, Cocker Spaniels, German Shepherds and Scottish Terriers. Oral FSA occurs more frequently in Golden Retrievers and Labrador Retrievers. Acanthomatous ameloblastoma, a benign dental tumor, occurs more commonly in Shetland and Old English Sheepdogs.

What are the Signs of Oral Cancer?

Dogs are usually brought in to the vet for symptoms such as bad breath, excessive drooling, difficulty in eating or swallowing, pain while eating, pawing at the mouth, bleeding teeth, bloody saliva, tooth loss, facial swelling or ulceration and weight loss.

Most oral tumors are not noticed until they are advanced, because most owners do not look in their dogs' mouths on a regular basis. Those who practice daily canine oral hygiene and make regular dental cleanings a priority tend to find oral tumors early, which is vital for an optimal outcome. The earlier a tumor is found, the smaller it is likely to be, and the less invasive to surrounding tissues.

Tumors located towards the front of the mouth (the rostral region) are usually noticed earlier, which means they are typically smaller at the time of diagnosis than those found in the back of the mouth (the caudal region).

Sometimes vets discover oral tumors during routine cleanings; loose teeth with little tartar or dental disease signal the possibility of cancer. In these cases, a tooth extraction and biopsy of the socket is in order.

How Is Oral Cancer Diagnosed?

Some dogs, especially if they are experiencing pain in the region of the mouth, need a short sedation for a thorough oral exam. The first test run is usually a fine needle aspirate, which can provide a preliminary diagnosis. (Dogs may not need sedation if their mass is rostral (towards the nose).) To get a more concrete picture of what type of tumor is present and what the prognosis is, a biopsy is recommended, and this is usually done during the oral exam, since the dog is already sedated.

Biopsies should be taken from inside the oral cavity (not from the outside of the body), to avoid contaminating normal tissues. Oral tumors are often infected or necrotic (filled with dying or dead tissue), so it is important to get a large enough sample to ensure that tumor tissue is included. The biopsy will determine whether the tumor is a melanoma, SCC, FSA or other dental tumor.

Most oral tumors are locally invasive into sur-rounding tissues, including bone; distant spread is less likely than with other cancers. Even so, I recommend more tests to discover how far the cancer has spread, because this knowledge can help you to understand your dog's prognosis and plan treatments accordingly.

Depending upon the case, your vet may want to run blood work, a urinalysis, three-view chest imaging or a chest CT scan, abdominal ultrasounds and lymph node aspirates.

Lymph nodes are particularly important to aspirate, because you cannot tell by their appearance whether they are metastatic. For example, in one study, 40% of dogs had normal-sized lymph nodes that had metastasized, while half of dogs with enlarged lymph nodes did not have metastasis. The bottom line is: lymph node size does not correlate to metastasis, so aspiration is indicated for both normal-sized and enlarged regional lymph nodes.

The head and mouth have many complicated structures and many lymph nodes, so there are several to check. For example, lymph nodes on the right side of the jaw may drain the left side of the jaw, and vice versa, which means a mass on the right side may metastasize to the left lymph node; both sides should be checked, as should the long chains of lymph nodes deeper in the head and neck.

Highly detailed CT scans or dental radiographs (X-rays) are often needed to really understand just how invasive and extensive an oral tumor has become. This information will help determine treatment decisions later.

What Is the Prognosis for Oral Cancer?

With the wide variety of tumor types, there is a wide variety of prognoses, plus some general prognostic factors to keep in mind.

The official staging system for canine oral tumors is as follows:

- **Stage I:** The tumor is smaller than 2 centimeter in diameter, with no metastasis to regional lymph nodes.
- **Stage II:** The tumor is 2-4 centimeter in diameter, with no metastasis to regional lymph nodes.
- **Stage III:** The tumor is over 4 centimeter in diameter, and/or there is metastasis in one or more regional lymph nodes.
- **Stage IV:** The tumor is any size, with distant metastasis.

The higher the stage is, the worse the prognosis. In general, tumors at the back of the oral cavity have a worse prognosis. Tumors that recur also worsen the dog's prognosis.

Oral tumors tend to progress locally, and most dogs die as a result of this local disease. If left untreated, symptoms tend to get worse, and dogs progressively and sometimes rapidly lose their quality of life. Watching their dogs experience progressively worsening pain, difficulty while eating or swallowing, oral bleeding, tumor infections and weight loss typically prompts owners to choose euthanasia.

What Are the Available Protocols for Oral Cancer?

Both SCC and FSA tumors have often involved the bone and invaded other local tissues by the time they are diagnosed, so the goal of treatment is to control the region with surgery and/or radiation.

The first treatment is usually surgery. Complete excision is essential, as second and third tumor surgeries are usually unsuccessful and recurring tu-

mors worsen your dog's prognosis. An aggressive surgeon, who will make wide excisions, is more likely to achieve complete tumor removal, so I recommend a specialist who is comfortable and experienced in oral surgeries. It is worth the added expense to get this surgery right the first time.

While it is hard to imagine your dog missing a large part of her jaw, I can report that owners are usually satisfied after the surgery. Radical surgeries are usually well tolerated by the dog, even when large

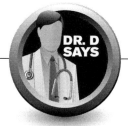

The conventional treatments Dr. Ettinger recommends for oral cancer should be considered part of step one of Full Spectrum cancer care (Chapter 11). Please review that chapter for more general information about surgery, radiation and chemotherapy and how to handle their common side effects.

For more information on all other Full Spectrum steps, including nutraceuticals, immune boosters, dietary changes and brain chemistry modification strategies, review Full Spectrum cancer care, which begins on page 103.

You will also find information about specific chemotherapy agents in Chapter 41.

portions of the jaw must be resected. They feel less pain, and they can still use their mouths well. Often surgeons can show you a picture of a dog with a similar procedure so you can visualize what your dog will look like after having healed from surgery.

Radiation therapy can, in some cases, dramatically improve the life expectancy of a dog with an oral tumor. As we discussed in Chapter 11, radiation has several side effects, some of which occur immediately and some, later. Early side effects include inflammation of the gums, hair loss, skin burning, difficulty eating and eye issues (such as conjunctivitis). Fewer than five percent of patients experience late-occurring side effects, such as an uncomfortable condition called dry eye, fistulas (holes between the nasal and/or oral cavities), bone damage (rarely), malignant bone tumors and, if the eyes were in the radiation field, cataracts. If you are near a CyberKnife or other radiosurgery device, it is well worth considering this type of conformational therapy, which can dramatically lessen the side effects of radiation.

While chemotherapy is sometimes considered, oral cancer rarely metastasizes to distant locations, so it is not usually indicated. Of course, all dogs are considered on a case-by-case basis, and if spread is found (especially to local lymph nodes), chemotherapy is recommended.

There are a few specific considerations for each tumor type.

SCC

The goal of SCC treatments is local tumor control, and surgical excision is usually the most economical, the quickest and most curative surgery. When feasible, this is my first choice of treatment. Seventy to ninety percent of dogs with SCC survive for one year with these surgeries, and survival times as long as eleven to twenty-six months have been reported. Rostral tumors (in the front of the mouth), may even be cured. Clean margins on the post-surgical biopsy offer even more hope, because recurrence is much less likely. Surgeries of the lower jaw are also less likely to recur (10%) than upper jaw surgeries (30%). If your dog has a caudal SCC tumor in the back of the mouth, at the base of the tongue, or on the tonsils, the prognosis worsens because these tumors are more likely to spread. After surgery, additional radiation therapy may be necessary, and, often, chemotherapy.

Carcinomas, and SCC in particular, are sensitive to radiation, so it is worth considering. In general, radiation therapy is best for treating microscopic disease after surgery removes the visible or measurable tumor. Also, radiation can treat regional lymph nodes. If used as a stand-alone therapy for SCC, median survival times of twelve to sixteen months are reported. Combined with surgery, however, those survival times lengthen to thirty-six months. The most important factor in predicting how responsive a tumor will be to radiation is its size – the smaller the tumor, the more radiation helps.

FSA

The first choice of treatment for FSA tumors is surgical excision. Wide margins of at least two centimeters are necessary, if possible, to completely remove the tumor. Even with these wide margins, however, FSA may leave microscopic cells behind. Local recurrence occurs in about half of FSA cases and this is the usual cause of death. The median survival time is approximately one year with aggressive therapy of surgery or radiation therapy alone. Combined, the use of surgery and radiation improves survival times to eighteen months. The high likelihood of recurrence is both frustrating and upsetting, which is why I advocate for aggressive approaches to FSA.

For that tricky Hi-Low FSA, surgery rarely achieves clean margins, so radiation is highly recommended after surgery. In general, oral Hi-Low FSA tumors are not as sensitive to radiation, so using it as a standalone therapy is not recommended.

Benign Dental Tumors

Even though benign dental tumors may not be malignancies, they can cause problems, and so surgery and radiation therapy are often recommended. They are usually well controlled with treatment, even when tumors are large. Over ninety percent of dogs are alive at one year, and the median survival time is two to five years.

Dental tumor surgery must be aggressive, because these tumors are likely to recur. For example, tumors that arise in the periodontal ligaments, the connective tissues that anchor teeth in their sockets, tend to recur. When such a tumor is found, the vet must remove not only the mass, but also the entire tooth, socket and ligament. If your dog has an acanthomatous ameloblastoma, aggressive, partial jaw removal with at least one centimeter margins is required and is usually curative.

Radiation therapy is useful for non-resectable dental tumors, incomplete resections and recurrent tumors. Acanthomatous ameloblastoma tumors are particularly sensitive to radiation, with 90% under control after treatment, especially smaller tumors of less than four centimeters. Larger tumors are more likely to recur, and radiation typically controls only about 30% of these tumors. It is worth noting that, while it is rare, three to twelve percent of dogs with acanthomatous ameloblastoma develop malignant tumors years later as a result of receiving radiation therapy.

Additional Considerations for Oral Cancer

If you decide against surgery, or if the tumor is non-resectable (for example, a tumor of the upper palate that crosses the midline), you might consider a course of palliative radiation. This decision will be based on how involved the tumor looks on the CT scan, not on the oral exam alone.

While chemotherapy can delay metastasis in many other cancers, metastatic rates in oral cancers are typically pretty low, so chemotherapy is usually not considered. The exception to this rule is SCC found at the back of the mouth, the base of the tongue or the tonsils. Tonsillar SCC has a metastatic rate of over 90% to the regional lymph nodes and 60-70% to the lungs, so chemotherapy is recommended to help control this spread. The best protocols are still being worked out; consult with your oncologist about the latest research. Chemotherapy is recommended after local control has been attempted with surgery and/or radiation, and may even provide some local response in these cases.

The NSAID piroxicam may help to slow tumor progression, due to its anti-inflammatory and anti-cancer properties, especially for carcinomas, and specifically for SCC. It can also help reduce the pain and inflammation associated with tumors, especially bone invasion.

While we are not yet sure how exactly piroxicam works against cancer, there is speculation that its inhibition of an enzyme called cyclooxygenase (COX-2) is at work. This enzyme blocks angiogenesis and therefore tumor growth, and piroxicam has a 20% response rate when used alone to treat SCC. A second, small study used carboplatin chemotherapy in addition to piroxicam, which bumped the response rate to almost 60%. Unfortunately, the study sample was too small to say for certain that these are typical results.

In addition to this specific anti-cancer effect for SCC, piroxicam has been effective at delaying the recurrence of soft tissue sarcomas when it's combined with chemotherapy. Metronomic protocols, which use low doses of oral chemotherapy to block new tumor blood vessel formation (rather than trying to kill cancer directly), show some promise, too. Since oral FSA is a type of soft tissue sarcoma, and with the recent arrival of the promising anti-angiogenic drug, Palladia, metronomic protocols may be an excellent alternative to post-surgical radiation therapy or as a palliative option for local tumor control.

The Bottom Line

Although aggressive surgeries may be required to control oral cancers, they are highly treatable, especially when detected early. Finding an experienced surgeon who can do an aggressive first surgery is my highest recommendation Most owners in my practice are satisfied with the outcome after surgery, radiation therapy and, less commonly, chemotherapy.

Don't Be Afraid

"This is one of the toughest things you will ever go through. Make sure you find the right vets, do your research, and double check your research. Not all vets are made the same. Be INVOLVED in your pets care. Research, research, research. Just like when a human goes to a doctor and you have to be your own advocate, you need to be your pet's advocate too. Don't be afraid to seek a specialist, don't be afraid to ask for your pets records to go see a specialist, and don't be afraid to seek a second opinion. Don't be afraid to ask questions, and don't be afraid to question anything that doesn't feel right in your gut. Stay positive around your dog. That's not to say, that you can't go hide in your car by yourself and bawl your eyes out. For me, I hid in the shower and cried my heart out, but as soon as I came out I had to put on a happy face and bring out that positive energy for Daisy. Do what you can to help stimulate your dog. You may not be able to do the things you used to do, but maybe just going for a ride, playing a game of paddy cake or hide the cookie, or sitting at a field, by the water, at a park, and just watching the world go by together. That can make a world of difference to your pup and give them something to look forward to every day."

- Chris Shoulet, Bethesda, Maryland

Chapter 36: Nasal Tumors

Nasal tumors develop in several tissue types found in the nasal and sinus cavities in the head. They tend to be very invasive locally, spreading into the neighboring tissues and often showing extensive bone involvement at the time of diagnosis. Despite their local aggression, they are not likely to have metastasized at the time of diagnosis.

Nasal tumors are typically not cured with treatment, although life can be extended with radiation therapy and sometimes, surgery. Most afflicted dogs live for about one year with treatment, and some live as long as two and a half years, depending upon the tumor type. While there are unavoidable side effects to radiation (see page 125), dogs generally tolerate the treatments.

What are Nasal Tumors?

Nasal tumors start inside the nose or sinus cavity, the tumor type varying, depending upon the tissue in which they occur. The vast majority of nasal tumors are malignancies that arise in the inside lining of the sinuses, cartilage, bone or lymphoid tissues.

About two-thirds of nasal cancers are carcinomas, or cancers of the epithelial cells. The many types of epithelial cells create the lining of the organs and structures in the body. The most common cancers are adenocarcinomas (ACA), which occur in cells that secrete fluids. Overlapping, fish-scale-shaped squamous cells develop squamous cell carcinoma (SCC). There are also undifferentiated carcinomas, whose specific cell of origin has not been determined.

Sarcomas, cancers that develop from connective tissues, account for the other one-third of nasal tumors. Fibrosarcomas develop from connective tissue, osteosarcomas develop from bone, and chondrosarcomas develop from cartilage. While the lymph tissues in the nasal and sinus cavities can also develop cancer (lymphoma), dogs suffer less often from nasal lymphoma than cats do.

Which Dogs Are at Risk for Nasal Tumors?

Environmental toxin exposure is a risk factor for developing nasal tumors. Substances like second-hand tobacco-smoke, topical insecticides (flea and tick control medications), and indoor coal and kerosene heaters have been associated with nasal tumors.

The nose and sinuses act as a filter for the lungs, removing these and other pollutants and irritants from the air before they reach the interior of

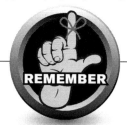

REMEMBER

When you need to look up the definition of a word or phrase, find it listed in Chapter 5, which begins on page 46.

the body. Dogs with long noses likely filter more of these pollutants, which is why they are at a higher risk for nasal cancer.

There is also a link between elevated levels of the enzyme called COX-2, which is involved with inflammation, and dogs with carcinomas. It's possible that inflammation and excess COX-2 expression plays a role in the development of nasal tumors.

Certain breeds are at a higher risk for developing nasal tumors, all having long noses: Airedale Terriers, Basset Hounds, Collies, German Shepherds, German Short-Haired Pointers, Keeshounds and Old English Sheepdogs.

What are the Signs of Nasal Tumors?

The first sign of a nasal tumor is nasal discharge; unfortunately, a runny nose is not always a red flag for owners, so, the average length of time between first noticing symptoms and getting a diagnosis is three months.

Nasal discharge from one or both nostrils (nares) can be clear, yellow, green, thick or runny. There may be blood in the discharge or your dog could even have a chronic bloody nose (called epistaxis). Some dogs will sneeze a lot. The first diagnosis is often a nasal or sinus infection, and antibiotics may be given. This often improves or even clears up the symptoms at first, but they usually return after the medications are stopped.

Eventually the tumor will fill up the airway and obstruct breathing. As this happens, dogs may breathe noisily or have difficulty breathing (some owners notice this most when their dogs are sleeping). The muzzle may become visibly deformed, and the eyes may bulge out of the skull as they are dis-

placed by the tumor.

A nasal tumor can sometimes affect the temporomandibular joint (TMJ), which is the joint that attaches the jawbone to the rest of the skull. When this happens, your dog can find it painful to open her mouth or chew her food.

In the rare cases when the tumor invades the bone and reaches the brain, there can be seizures or behavioral changes: running around in circles, barking for no reason or other odd behaviors.

How Are Nasal Tumors Diagnosed?

Nasal tumors are diagnosed through imaging tests and a biopsy. The first step is to get blood work and a urinalysis, so you can have an overall snapshot of the baseline health of your dog.

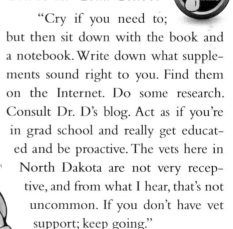

Keep Going – as if You're In Grad School

"Cry if you need to; but then sit down with the book and a notebook. Write down what supplements sound right to you. Find them on the Internet. Do some research. Consult Dr. D's blog. Act as if you're in grad school and really get educated and be proactive. The vets here in North Dakota are not very receptive, and from what I hear, that's not uncommon. If you don't have vet support; keep going."

- Kris Kitko, Bismarck, North Dakota

If your dog is suffering epistaxis (a bloody nose), the cause could be a tumor, and it could also be high blood pressure or blood clotting abnormalities. Make sure her blood pressure gets checked, and that the blood test called a coagulation panel is run to rule out other issues. High blood pressure and excessive bleeding tendencies can also cause problems during nasal tumor biopsy and treatment, so it's important to have this information in any case.

Imaging tests should be performed to measure the extent and severity of the tumor and to see if it has invaded the bone (many have). While it may seem logical to perform the less invasive and less expensive X-ray screening, it is not sensitive enough to pick up most of what is happening inside the skull, and does not help to diagnose nasal tumors. Good skull X-rays require heavy sedation or anesthesia, too, and do not provide enough information. I recommend saving money and time by skipping the X-ray and getting a CT (computed tomography) scan, instead. It provides much more detail and it is also a requirement for radiation therapy, the standard treatment for nasal tumors.

A CT scan helps the vet know where to look for tumors during a rhinoscopy, or nasal biopsy, also. During a rhinoscopy, a fiber-optic scope is passed up through the nostrils into the nasal cavity to visually inspect the passages for tumors, clumps of fungus (called fungal plaques) and other possible causes of nasal symptoms. Suspicious masses should be sampled this way – through the nose – rather than through the outer surface of the skin, so that cancer cells are not pulled into otherwise normal tissues. Multiple samples must be taken, both for biopsy and fungal cultures.

A recent study shows that a nasal hydropulsion technique, which collects pieces of nasal tumors for biopsy by pushing a large volume of water through the nasal cavity, can literally dislodge and "flush out" nasal tumors in 90% of cases. While this technique does not completely remove the entire tumor, especially a tumor that has invaded the deeper tissues and bones, it can dislodge large enough pieces of tumor to use for biopsy samples. It also can relieve some of the obstruction in the nasal and sinus cavities, making it easier for the dog to breathe for the time being. This technique is worth considering as a biopsy collection strategy because of its debulking and palliative effects (simple saline flushes do not provide large enough biopsy samples to have the same effect). This procedure is typically done under anesthesia.

Rhinoscopy, biopsy and CT scans all require general anesthesia, so they are best done together. The CT scan will be administered first, because rhinoscopy and biopsy can cause bleeding that will show up on the scan and could be misinterpreted as a tumor.

Metastasis at the time of diagnosis is uncommon, but it does happen, and 40% of all dogs with nasal tumors will experience metastasis as the disease progresses. For this reason, and because treatment strategies may alter, depending upon the extent of the metastasis, I recommend staging the cancer – finding out where it is in the body – before starting treatment.

The most common sites of spread are the regional lymph nodes and the lungs. About 10% of dogs have lymph node metastasis at diagnosis, so I typically aspirate the regional lymph nodes under the same anesthesia as the head CT scan, rhinoscopy and biopsy. Aspirate every accessible lymph node, even those of normal size. Three-view thoracic X-rays or a chest CT can show metastasis to the lungs.

What Is the Prognosis for Nasal Tumors?

It can be difficult to come up with a prognosis for nasal tumors, because while there are actually three separate staging systems, each of which measures the extent of the tumor and how much bone invasion is present, none actually helps us predict either the course of the disease or the prognosis. I don't find them helpful, so I have left them out of this book.

There is some evidence that tumors extending into the sinuses, eyes and their surrounding tissues, and/or the bone that separates the nose from the brain, are more serious than other nasal tumors. The factors have not been confirmed with enough studies, so at this point, one nasal tumor cannot yet be definitively labeled as "worse" than any other.

In general, if nasal tumors are left untreated, afflicted dogs have a median survival time of three months.

What Are the Available Protocols for Nasal Tumors?

For most cancers, we use surgery to remove the tumor, then follow up with radiation to kill microscopic local spread and/or chemotherapy to treat distant metastasis. Nasal cancer is different: by the time of diagnosis most tumors have invaded the bone, making clean margins nearly impossible. Removing bones in the skull can have a marked disfiguring effect on your dog, and surgeries are rarely effective as a standalone treatment (resulting in median survival times of only three to nine months).

Unless the tumor is a rare case – *very* small and well-defined – surgery is not the first course of treatment. It's not even used to debulk (reduce the size of)

tumors before other treatments. These surgeries tend to increase side effects and don't do anything to prolong life. Instead, to control the tumor, reduce pain and extend life, the standard of care is radiation therapy.

There are many published protocols for radiation therapy and most require multiple treatments. Using radiation therapy for sarcomas, especially chondrosarcomas, results in the best prognosis: median survival times of thirty months. Dogs with adenocarcinoma (ACA) live about twelve to eighteen months with radiation therapy. Undifferentiated

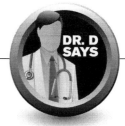

The conventional treatments Dr. Ettinger recommends for nasal tumors should be considered part of step one of Full Spectrum cancer care (Chapter 11). Please review that chapter for more general information about surgery, radiation and chemotherapy and how to handle their common side effects.

For more information on all other Full Spectrum steps, including nutraceuticals, immune boosters, dietary changes and brain chemistry modification strategies, review Full Spectrum cancer care, which begins on page 103.

You will also find information about specific chemotherapy agents in Chapter 41.

sarcomas and SCC (squamous cell carcinoma) fare worse, with survival times from eight to ten months with radiation therapy.

It is important to remember that radiation does not destroy cancer cells instantly: it damages their DNA and they die later, when they try to divide. As a result, radiation therapy does not show instant results – the tumor remains largely the same size immediately after treatment. The most reduction will be seen three to six months after treatments end. In the meantime, oral antibiotics, pain medications and eye medications may be needed, to manage side effects.

Radiation does carry undeniable and unavoidable side effects. Typically, during the second half of therapy and in the first few weeks after radiation, there is inflammation in the field of treatment. Because of the location of nasal tumors, this usually means inflammation of the nasal and oral mucous membranes, the skin and the eyes. This will go away over time, usually within a few weeks. Side effects that occur later (months to years later) are often permanent. Many dogs develop a condition called dry eye, in which the tear ducts are damaged and stop lubricating the eye. This condition requires daily, life-long administration of eye medications. Another side effect is eye cataracts, which can be surgically corrected. You will have to weigh the benefits of life extension, tumor control and pain management against the risks of these side effects. My opinion is that most dogs tolerate this treatment, live longer and have a good quality of life.

Additional Considerations for Nasal Tumors

Although surgery *prior* to radiation therapy is not generally helpful, using surgery *after* radiation, to remove residual or recurrent tumors, may significant-ly extend survival time. In a recent study, the median survival time with surgery increased to forty-eight months, compared to radiation therapy alone: twenty months in the study. Side effects did increase: nasal inflammation, bone inflammation and dead bone (osteonecrosis). This study was relatively small and is not yet the standard of care; it may be helpful for your dog.

If stereotactic radiosurgery, 3-D conformal radiation or intensity-modulated radiation (IMRT) is available to you, you might consider these exciting new forms of radiation therapy. These tools deliver higher doses more accurately, with less exposure of normal tissue than traditional radiation, which radically reduces side effects.

Fewer treatments are typically needed with stereotactic radiosurgery, as well. My radiation colleague and I have treated over fifty nasal tumors with our CyberKnife radiosurgery machine, so far. Although it is still too early to fully evaluate the outcome of these surgeries, average survival times are well over a year and significant side effects, like skin burns and mucositis, are dramatically reduced.

There are some drugs that act as radioprotectors (protecting normal tissue from radiation exposure) and radiosensitizers (enhancing tumor cell kill). Not yet fully explored for canine nasal radiation therapy, they have been helpful in people. For example, the radioprotector amifostine decreases early and late side effects in humans and allows treatments to be given without breaks. If using drugs like these in dogs can extend survival time or decrease toxicity, they may be worth future studies and your consideration.

Some chemotherapy drugs are known to increase the sensitivity of tumors to radiation in humans; the best protocols have not yet been worked out for dogs. We are also not sure if using chemotherapy drugs actually improves sensitivity in dogs or extends survival times.

Some dog owners want to know whether using chemotherapy as a standalone treatment is worthwhile. Unfortunately, it doesn't seem to be helpful for extending life. Platinum-based protocols (carboplatin and cisplatin) may be considered for symptom relief; they do not extend life.

Palliative radiation therapy is an option to consider if a full course of radiation does not appeal to you. Usually given in one to four treatments (rather than the fifteen to twenty used in conventional radiation), it is less expensive than conventional radiation or stereotactic radiosurgery and associated with fewer early side effects, too. However, the response does not last as long; in one study, 95% of dogs had symptom improvement, 40% had treatment-induced side effects and the median survival time was seven months.

Oral piroxicam or other NSAIDs may help nasal tumors, especially carcinomas, because of their anti-inflammatory and anti-cancer properties. Keep in mind that dogs should be on only one NSAID at a time, and they should not be combined with steroids. The use of more than one anti-inflammatory agent can increase the risk of stomach ulceration.

The Bottom Line

Nasal tumors are tough cancers to treat with any therapy other than radiation, and they are not likely to be cured. Even so, I consider them treatable cancers; radiation can extend life, control symptoms and make dogs much more comfortable than they are at diagnosis.

Chapter 37: Soft Tissue Sarcomas

Soft tissue sarcomas develop in a variety of connective tissues, muscles and fat. They can be found in sites all over the body, from head to trunk to paws, and can vary widely in their appearance and effect on the body. The majority of these tumors are usually aggressive locally, which means they invade the neighboring tissues. They are also prone to recur, although they typically don't metastasize.

Of all the malignant tumors, having soft tissue sarcomas is not the worst-case scenario for your dog. Low and intermediate grades of soft tissue sarcomas are very treatable and have excellent long-term survival rates (some up to five years). The recommended treatments include surgery and/or radiation for low and intermediate grades, and, occasionally, chemotherapy. Chemotherapy may also be recommended for higher grades, which tend to be more metastatic and have lower survival rates (up to eight months, once lung metastasis is confirmed).

Soft tissue sarcoma is often referred to by its initials, STS. Other names for STS are mesenchymal tumor, soft part tumor and soft part sarcoma.

What Is Soft Tissue Sarcoma?

Soft tissue sarcomas comprise a broad group of tumors that develop in many different locations and have similar behavior, cellular features, treatment recommendations and prognoses. They can occur in any site in the body and are named for the tissue with which they are associated. STS include: hemangio-

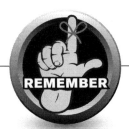

When you need to look up the definition of a word or phrase, find it listed in Chapter 5, which begins on page 46.

pericytomas, fibrosarcomas, peripheral nerve sheath tumors or neurofibrosarcomas, malignant fibrous histiocytomas, liposarcomas, myxosarcomas and undifferentiated sarcomas (sarcomas that cannot be specifically identified in a biopsy).

All of the above sarcomas occur in parts of the body that are on the outside – flesh, muscles, connective tissues, etc. Other sarcomas, those of the internal organs and the oral cavity, are considered separately because they are so different in metastatic rates, treatment and prognosis. The more common internal sarcomas include: oral tumors, nasal tumors, osteosarcoma and hemangiosarcoma, all of which are discussed in other chapters.

Locally invasive STS, on the other hand, have poorly defined margins and often infiltrate surrounding tissues with tentacles of cancer cells. In general, they tend to recur, especially if surgery is conservative, and especially if it features narrow margins.

When they metastasize, they generally do so through the bloodstream, typically to the lungs and liver. Regional lymph node metastasis is uncommon.

Low and intermediate grade STS tend to have a low metastasis rate of 10-20% and most commonly spread to the lungs. High grade STS is more metastatic, with 40-50% of these tumors spreading to the lungs and liver.

Which Dogs Are at Risk for Soft Tissue Sarcoma?

Genetic and environmental factors may be involved in STS; the cause of these tumors still remains poorly understood. (While cats can develop sarcomas at the site of injections, this is rare in dogs.)

STS tends to occur in larger breeds, without an apparent specific genetic cause. One study found that Rhodesian Ridgebacks and mixed breed dogs have a higher risk of STS, while another found that Flat-Coated Retrievers were more at risk, specifically for malignant fibrous histiocytoma. Older dogs tend to be more at risk, also.

What are the Signs of Soft Tissue Sarcoma?

Most dogs do not feel sick at the time of diagnosis and are brought in because their owners noticed masses that were getting larger. These masses tend to grow slowly and not be painful. They can occur anywhere on the body and, depending upon their location, may cause different symptoms. For example, a mass near a joint may cause pain when moving, or a mass on the ear might cause your dog to paw and scratch at his head.

Although STS are usually firm to the touch and fixed in place, they can also feel soft and have lobules (several rounded structures). STS can be confused with benign lipomas (fatty tumors).

The unknown origin of these tumors makes prevention unlikely, which is why it is so important to consistently and regularly monitor your dog for new skin or surface masses. The sooner a mass is found, the sooner it can be diagnosed and treated, if necessary.

How Is Soft Tissue Sarcoma Diagnosed?

Knowing the tumor type and the grade of STS is very important. It tells you what the likely prognosis is, and also makes treatment decisions easier. While some sarcomas, osteosarcoma, for example, do not need an aspirate or biopsy before starting treatment, STS always needs to be diagnosed by aspirate or biopsy, before surgery is performed.

All skin and subcutaneous masses need to be aspirated to make sure they are not mast cell tumors, benign fatty lipomas or abscesses (infections). When the aspirate confirms STS, a biopsy may not be needed before attempting surgery. Unfortunately, STS cells do not aspirate well – they can refuse to be drawn up the needle – so this test may not confirm STS. Sometimes dead tissue or inflamed tissue is drawn up, leading to a misdiagnosis of inflammation. If a tumor looks like STS and the aspirate only indicates inflammation, STS is still suspected and a biopsy is definitely in order.

Biopsies can be very useful, even if an aspirate confirms STS, and they are vital if it is not confirmed with an aspirate. A biopsy provides information that cytology/aspirates do not: tumor type and grade. STS tends to be locally invasive, and you don't want the biopsy to tract (or leave a path of) cancer cells through surrounding tissues, so the biopsy must be carefully planned, so as to take a sample from an area that will be removed later in a curative surgery or radiated during radiation surgery.

The temptation is strong to remove the entire visible tumor during the biopsy: such a surgery rarely "gets it all out." A second, curative surgery will likely be needed because STS generally requires aggressive surgeries with very wide margins in order to achieve clean margins. Knowing the tumor type (with a biopsy first) provides the best opportunity that only one curative-intent surgery will be needed.

In addition to the aspirate and/or biopsy, blood work and urinalysis are recommended to get information about your dog's general health.

To complete staging for STS, a lymph node aspirate should be performed on nodes that drain the tumor location. Even though lymph node metastasis is rare, it is not unheard of, and knowing your dog's status can help with prognosis and treatment planning. This is a minimally invasive test and it's worth doing. Keep in mind that you cannot tell if STS has spread to lymph nodes by noting their size or appearance.

To check for spread to the lungs, three-view thoracic X-rays should be taken prior to curative surgery. Because metastasis to the lungs significantly decreases survival time (in one study the median survival time with metastasis was about eight months), this knowledge can help you to plan your treatments.

Abdominal ultrasounds can be used for general health screening, and can also show spread to the lymph nodes, liver or other organs. This is especially important for STS that is on the abdomen or the back half of the body, because tumors in these locations often spread to internal organs.

When the mass is close to bone, X-rays should be taken of the area to see whether the bone has been invaded. Computer tomography (CT) scans or MRI scans can show details that help plan surgeries and radiation, helping the surgeon determine just how far the tumor extends into surrounding tissues. Tumors are rarely contained in the mass we feel with our fingers or see with the naked eye – knowing as much as possible about their spread can help plan a surgery and determine whether additional therapy (radiation or chemotherapy) will be needed.

Certain cellular markers in the tumor sample, when measured, can help predict your dog's prognosis when it comes to STS. I studied these markers during my oncology residency, and I bring them to your attention, because knowing your dog's levels can really help you make treatment decisions.

Our study demonstrated a link, between the marker Ki-67 (which rises when a lot of cells are dividing) and the grade of an STS tumor. For example, dogs with a low Ki-67 score had a median survival time of over forty months; dogs with a high Ki-67 score, on the other hand, have a median survival time of twenty-two months. Dogs with higher scores were also twelve times more likely to die, due to their STS, than dogs with low scores.

AgNOR, a type of protein, is another useful cell proliferation marker. Dogs with a high AgNOR were almost six times more likely to die due to their STS disease than dogs with low AgNOR values.

Another helpful test to use when trying to predict the behavior of a STS is the intratumoral microvessel density (IMD). This measures how much angiogenesis, or new blood vessel formation, characterizes the tumor. In a follow-up study, we found that the more angiogenesis is happening, the more aggressive the tumor is and the more likely it is to metastasize. The IMD is typically run as a panel with the proliferation markers, and is commercially available in only a few labs. If needed, your vet can contact a specialty lab.

Measuring these proliferation markers can help you to know whether your dog is in a high-risk category that might benefit from more aggressive treatments. These markers can be measured on a biopsy sample that is specially stained and examined at a laboratory. Biopsy tissue is typically kept for a year or more at most labs, so these tests do not need to be run right away. If needed, they can be run after the biopsy results are sent back and analyzed. I recommend you discuss these markers with your oncologist.

What Is the Prognosis for Soft Tissue Sarcoma?

The prognosis for STS tumors is variable, depending upon the tumor type, location, stage, grade and rate of cell division.

Here is the official staging for STS tumors:

Stage IA: The primary tumor is less than 5 centimeter, grade 1 or grade 2, with no lymph node or distant metastasis.

B: The primary tumor is larger than 5 centimeter, grade 1 or grade 2, with no lymph node or distant metastasis.

Stage IIA: The primary tumor is less than 5 centimeter, grade 3, with no lymph node or distant metastasis.

B: The primary tumor is greater than 5 centimeter, grade 3, with no lymph node or distant metastasis.

Stage IIIA: Any size and any grade of tumor, with lymph node metastasis.

B: Any size and any grade tumor with distant metastasis.

There is also a newer, modified staging system, which places less emphasis on tumor size and greater focus on the depth of invasion; I find it no more useful than the older system, however.

In general, the higher the stage is, the worse the prognosis. STS is highly treatable in low and intermediate grades, with survival times of up to five years with a combination of surgery and radiation.

Although not considered routine by most oncologists, measuring the proliferation and angiogenic markers listed in the previous section may also be helpful in assessing your dog's prognosis.

What Are the Available Protocols for Soft Tissue Sarcoma?

The most effective treatment for STS is a wide, surgical excision of the tumor. As I mentioned above, careful planning for this surgery can help ensure a complete removal the first time and prevent recurrence. Since STS tends to recur, achieving clean margins in the first surgery is vital.

A three-centimeter margin around the removed tumor, including a full tissue layer from underneath, is the minimum margin needed. In some cases an even wider margin may be needed, which is why knowing the tumor type and grade is so important. Your surgeon can plan the best surgery when he has CT scans or other detailed images to review. There is a 15% recurrence rate for STS overall, usually within one year; dogs with dirty margins have a recurrence rate of 30%, which is why a post-surgery biopsy of the removed tissue is critical to confirm complete excision.

It is very important your vet reads this biopsy

report closely and notes how wide the margins are. STS is very aggressive locally, and unless a wide, two or three-centimeter margin is clean, I am not confident that the procedure is a complete resection. (Tissue shrinks a little after it is removed from the body and before it is processed at the lab, which is one reason to err on the side of wider than necessary.) I mention this because I have personally seen biopsy reports call STS tumors clean even with very narrow one or two millimeter margins. This is careless medicine, and one of my pet peeves, because incomplete resections are ten times more likely to recur.

The biopsy will tell you the tumor's mitotic index rate and grade, also. The mitotic index rate – how fast the cells are multiplying – tends to be higher in tumors that are likely to metastasize. A high mitotic rate often correlates with a higher-grade tumor, and these worsen the prognosis, likelihood of metastasis and survival times.

Many STS tumors occur on limbs, which presents a particular problem for the surgeon: there may not be enough skin and tissue to get clean and wide margins. This means that recurrence is much more likely and later surgeries will be progressively more complicated and difficult. Some owners choose to amputate in these situations, because – although it is a radical surgery – amputation achieves the necessary wide margins and prevents recurrence.

Other owners choose a course of post-surgery radiation therapy to prevent recurrence. While this approach saves the limb and can be very effective, tumor recurrence is more likely than it is with amputation (and amputation may be necessary later, in any case). Even so, this is a popular option because it avoids amputation and offers the likelihood of long-term control.

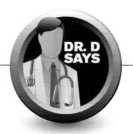

The conventional treatments Dr. Ettinger recommends for soft tissue sarcoma should be considered part of step one of Full Spectrum cancer care (Chapter 11). Please review that chapter for more general information about surgery, radiation and chemotherapy and how to handle their common side effects.

For more information on all other Full Spectrum steps, including nutraceuticals, immune boosters, dietary changes and brain chemistry modification strategies, review Full Spectrum cancer care, which begins on page 103.

You will also find information about specific chemotherapy agents in Chapter 41.

Other Considerations for Soft Tissue Sarcoma

Although surgery is clearly important, there is an increasing move toward a combined treatment of surgery and radiation therapy for narrow or incomplete margins. Most commonly, radiation therapy is started two to three weeks after surgery. A course of radiation therapy after surgery can help to control the tumor locally and prevent recurrence from microscopic cells. Low and intermediate grades of STS may really benefit from this combined approach: 75% of afflicted dogs are still alive, five years later, without tumor regrowth. STS is one of the few malignancies associated with five-year control rates, which justifies the extra expense and involvement of adding radiation treatments in the minds of owners who choose it. If your dog is a candidate for this approach, keep in mind the multiple anesthesia sessions (fifteen to twenty) and the early and late side effects (see page 125).

In some cases, radiation therapy may be recommended before surgery, to reduce the size of a tumor that is otherwise inoperable. There are no studies that prove whether pre- or post-operative radiation therapy has better response rates, better local control rates or fewer complications, so the decision is usually made on a case-by-case basis. I find the best outcomes are achieved when the team of specialists includes a surgeon, a medical oncologist and a radiation oncologist. Incidentally, radiation is not used as a sole treatment, because these tumors do not respond well to radiation alone.

STS does not respond well to chemotherapy, either, especially in the primary site. We may use chemotherapy to treat grade III and other high-risk tumors (those with high proliferation markers and microvessel scores) after surgery and/or radiation. In certain cases, the addition of chemotherapy may prevent or delay metastasis and possibly treat existing metastatic disease.

When chemotherapy is used to treat the primary STS tumor, for example a non-resectable tumor, it is considered palliative, not an attempt at a cure. It may shrink the mass a little, which can make the dog more comfortable.

Metronomic, or low-dose oral chemotherapy, has recently been reported to delay recurrence in dogs with incompletely removed low and intermediate grade tumors. Using chronic, low doses of oral cyclophosphamide and piroxicam may be an alternative to post-surgical radiation therapy. In studies, dogs who did not receive metronomic chemotherapy had a median recurrence at seven months, while dogs treated with metronomic chemotherapy reached about fourteen months. Clearly, these statistics are not as impressive as those associated with post-surgical radiation treatments; on the other hand, metronomic chemotherapy is less expensive and does not have the side effects associated with radiation, so therefore may be an attractive option.

The Bottom Line

Low or intermediate grade STS is treatable, with excellent long term control and survival rates associated with aggressive surgery or combined surgery and radiation treatments. The prospects are worse for a high-grade tumor, which is more likely to metastasize, but treatment and tumor control is still possible. Combining surgery, radiation and chemotherapy can extend life and enhance life quality.

Chapter 38: Brain Tumors

Brain tumors develop in the tissues of the brain, inside the head. Most grow slowly, and are often found long after becoming well established. While tumors invariably affect the brain's function, this adaptable organ can often compensate for the damage. This can go on for a long time, until decompensation occurs, which is when the brain can no longer cope. This often happens very quickly, and it may seem as if your dog is very sick "overnight." Brain tumors are relatively rare in dogs, and very serious. If left untreated, survival times range from one week to two months.

In most areas of the body, there is room for tumors to grow quite a bit before they start to squeeze out normal functioning tissue. In the confined space of the skull, however, tumors can rapidly take up space needed by the rest of the brain. The brain responds to compression with many different kinds of neurologic changes, from personality disorders to seizures.

What makes these tumors so difficult to treat is the lack of a firm diagnosis. Because the brain is hard to access, and biopsies are not commonly done, it is difficult to determine the type of tumor involved or the likely prognosis for your dog. The goal of treatment is to remove the tumor if possible, reduce its size, and relieve the symptoms associated with the mass, including brain inflammation and swelling. A combination of radiation, surgery and chemotherapy may be used, depending upon the tumor's size and location.

The inability to determine the tumor type, in the vast majority of cases, makes forming a prognosis quite difficult for your vet or oncologist. Left untreated, the prognosis is certainly poor: weeks to months. Brain tumors are named for the type of brain tissue they arise in; common tumors include: meningioma, glioma, choroid plexus tumor, ependymoma and medulloblastoma, to name a few.

What Is a Brain Tumor?

Brain tumors develop within normal cells found in the brain or the meninges (three layers that cover and protect the brain and spinal cord). The most common brain tumor is the meningioma, found in the meninges, which accounts for just under half of all cases. The second most common tumor is the glioma, which is found in the glial cells, which surround and protect the delicate neurons in the brain. These are followed by choroid plexus tumors, which develop in the space where cerebrospinal fluid

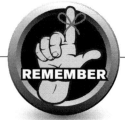

REMEMBER

When you need to look up the definition of a word or phrase, find it listed in Chapter 5, which begins on page 46.

is made; ependymomas, which occur in the lining of the ventricles of the brain; and medulloblastomas, which occur in the brain tissue in the cerebellum.

Other cancers, like pituitary tumors, nasal cancers and bone tumors, can invade the brain from their primary locations. Hemangiosarcoma, mammary carcinoma and lymphoma all metastasize to the brain. Although located in the brain, they are not primary brain cancers, and are not dealt with here.

We often classify tumors in other body locations as either malignant or benign, depending upon their cell characteristics when they are viewed under a microscope in a lab. Classifying brain tumors this way can be misleading: all brain tumors are malignant, in the sense that they are life-threatening and devastating, because they grow within the confined space of the skull. Their mass, and the associated inflammation and edema (swelling), compress the normal brain tissue, resulting in neurological changes. Whether symptoms stem from the tumor or the associated compression and/or inflammation, their overall effect is malignant.

Which Dogs Are at Risk for Brain Tumors?

There are no known risk factors for brain cancer, and only a few associations. Dogs with brain cancer are nearly always older than five years of age (95%). Studies have shown that dogs with meningioma, the most common brain cancer, have a high proportion of receptors in their cells for the hormone progesterone; both estrogen and progesterone can influence cancer development.

Certain breeds are also at increased risk: Golden Retrievers, Boxers, Doberman Pinschers, Scottish Terriers and Old English Sheepdogs.

Breeds with long, narrow heads, such as Collies and Greyhounds, may be at an increased risk for meningiomas, and dogs with a short snout or flat, pushed-in face, such as Boxers, Pugs and Boston Terriers may be at an increased risk for gliomas.

What are the Signs of a Brain Tumor?

Brain tumors are often first discovered when the dog starts having seizures, which happens in 45% of dogs with brain cancer. If your dog is four to five years or older and has a seizure, a brain tumor is the most likely cause.

Other owners may notice circling, drunk walking (ataxia), holding the head at a tilted angle, an altered mental status (your dog seems out of it), limb weakness or paralysis, or subtle behavior changes, including aggression. Sometimes the symptoms are much vaguer: increased lethargy or decreased appetite. The symptoms usually affect one side of the body more than the other side (are asymmetrical), because the lesion is usually on one side of the brain.

One of the difficulties with brain cancer is that some tumors develop so slowly that your dog's brain is able to compensate for the alterations, effectively masking the neurological symptoms or making them so subtle that they are hard to detect. Vague or subtle changes in behavior, happening over many months, for instance, can be easy to overlook by the owner and the vet.

In humans, the first symptom of a brain tumor is a severe, persistent headache, and it makes sense to think that dogs experience some sort of head pain, too. Since dogs cannot tell us directly if they have a headache, they may have other, more subtle ways of sending the message. When looking back, many owners realize that their dog has become less social, more depressed, more irritable or more sensitive to being handled.

How Is a Brain Tumor Diagnosed?

Brain cancer is suspected, based on your dog's age, breed, history of symptoms and neurological examination. The results of a neurological exam can vary based on where the lesion is located in the brain, how extensive it is and how quickly it is growing. A complete exam from a neurologist can usually reveal the area of the brain where the problem is located.

Confirmation of a brain tumor requires advanced brain imaging, preferably MRI (magnetic resonance imaging). MRIs are better for showing detail in soft tissues and highlighting subtle changes, making them ideal for brain scans. Computer tomography (CT) scans are adequate for brain tumors, and better for bone tumors that are compressing the brain from the skull. While CT is typically a little cheaper, both are expensive relative to X-rays. They also require anesthesia and a specialty hospital.

After the MRI (or CT) scans, your vet or oncologist may want to do a cerebrospinal fluid (CSF) tap. In this test, a needle is inserted into the spinal cord and the fluid that lubricates and cushions the brain and spinal cord, is drawn out to be examined. This test requires anesthesia, so it is usually scheduled immediately after the MRI, while your dog is still under.

Cancer cells are not usually detected in cerebrospinal fluid, even when cancer is present, but looking at it can help your oncologist to rule out other possible causes of your dog's symptoms, for example, an inflammatory condition. A study which measured the usefulness of the CSF tap found that 40% of the samples collected had protein and white blood cell counts that supported a diagnosis of cancer, 10% had completely normal fluid, and 50% had non-specific changes. If there is any doubt about your dog's diagnosis, this test may help.

In any other cancer, a biopsy would be necessary to confirm the diagnosis; brain cancer is very different. Biopsies are not usually done, because many tumors are just not accessible, and the expensive procedure is too risky. Unfortunately, without a confirmed diagnosis of the type of tumor, it is very difficult to make an accurate prognosis for your dog. If your vet or oncologist will not give you a specific prognosis, this is likely the reason.

Even though it is rare that brain cancer spreads to other organs, the rest of the body should still be checked for cancer, because meningioma has been reported to spread to the lungs and pancreas. It's also possible that the brain tumor is not a primary tumor, but a metastasis from another primary cancer, somewhere else in the body. In that case, treatment recommendations are likely to be very different than those for a primary brain cancer.

Staging tests I recommend include: blood work, urinalysis, chest imaging, such as three-view thoracic X-rays and abdominal imaging, typically ultrasound. These tests do not require anesthesia, so they are typically performed before a CT scan or MRI, which do.

What Is the Prognosis for Brain Tumors?

It is nearly impossible to give a specific prognosis for any given brain tumor, since so few offer reliable information from a biopsy. However, if left untreated, survival times usually range from one week to two months. If surgery, radiation and chemotherapy combinations outlined below are declined, palliative support can be given, using steroids and anti-convulsant medications. Some dogs show dramatic improvement on steroids alone, gaining weeks or months of life; adding anti-convulsant medications can extend survival times two to four months.

What Are the Available Protocols for Brain Tumors?

Because we so rarely know with certainty what type of tumor we're dealing with, brain tumors are often considered collectively for treatment and prognosis. The goals of treatment are to remove the tumor when possible, reduce the tumor's size and relieve the symptoms associated with the tumor: swelling and inflammation.

If possible, the tumor may be surgically removed or debulked (reduced in size). Whether this is possible or not will depend upon the location, size, invasiveness and extent of the tumor in question, so a good MRI scan is essential to plan the surgery. With recent advancements in surgical techniques, anesthesia and critical care, brain surgery is an option more and more often. Even a simple debulking of the mass can provide significant relief from the pressure and symptoms.

An advantage of surgery is that the tumor can be submitted for a biopsy, which will lead to a confirmed diagnosis and more information about the illness. Clearly, brain surgery requires an experienced and confident surgeon, typically a neurosurgeon. Intensive care and monitoring after surgery are also necessary. The median survival time for dogs with surgically removed brain tumors is seven to eight months, with a range of six to twenty-two months. Neurosurgeons can be found by using the "find a specialist" tool at www.AVCIM.org. Search for neu-

rologist, but check to see if they do brain surgery – the hospital should be able to confirm this before you book an appointment.

If a surgery is incomplete, traditional radiation may be used as a follow-up treatment. When used as an adjunct to surgery, radiation increases median survival times to about sixteen months, for all brain tumor types. Dogs with meningiomas can significantly extend their life expectancy, up to thirty months (two and a half years)!

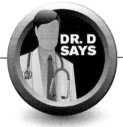

The conventional treatments Dr. Ettinger recommends for brain tumors should be considered part of step one of Full Spectrum cancer care (Chapter 11). Please review that chapter for more general information about surgery, radiation and chemotherapy and how to handle their common side effects.

For more information on all other Full Spectrum steps, including nutraceuticals, immune boosters, dietary changes and brain chemistry modification strategies, review Full Spectrum cancer care, which begins on page 103.

You will also find information about specific chemotherapy agents in Chapter 41.

Radiation therapy can be helpful for dogs with inoperable tumors, as well. The median survival time for brain tumors treated with traditional linear accelerators is about ten months, with a range of five to fifteen months. Of course, with radiation therapy, there are typically many treatments (sometimes as many as fifteen), all of which require anesthesia. Radiation side effects include (extremely rare, life-threatening) brain swelling, herniating (swelling so much that part of it is pushed out of the base of the skull), and brain death.

Radiosurgery, which is much more precise and has far fewer side effects, is proving ideal for brain tumors. My hospital has had the CyberKnife radiosurgery machine since 2008, and we have used it to treat more brain tumors than any other type. Human cancers have been treated with this machine for years; we are one of the first hospitals to use it to treat animals. It is too early to fully evaluate all of the data, but preliminary results for brain tumors offer your dog a median survival time of about fifteen months. This is about the same result as with traditional radiation therapy; far fewer treatments are required (one to three), however, and the side effects are less likely (although they still occur). So far, no herniations have occurred in dogs treated with radiosurgery, neither at our center nor at a veterinary school that also performs this technique.

Chemotherapy is typically not effective for brain tumors because of the physiological phenomena called the blood-brain barrier (BBB). Brain tissue can be damaged by coming into direct contact with blood, so there are some inherent protections built into the brain's structures to keep it from the blood supply. This barrier is semi-permeable: some materials can cross, while others can't. Most chemotherapy drugs cannot cross this barrier, but others can, including oral Lomustine and IV carmustine. These drugs seem to be the most effective therapies for gliomas and lymphoma (that involve the central nervous system). Oral hydoxyurea can also cross the BBB, which is effective for meningiomas. The median survival time for chemotherapy, as a standalone treatment, is seven months for dogs with all tumor types.

Don't Settle for the "C" Word

"... although everything seems so terrible and you're confused and feel helpless you have to try and firstly stay strong for one another. You have to see beyond the word cancer and take positive action immediately. Little steps at a time as there is so much information out there. Do your research, change the diet immediately. Remain high spirited and joyful as soon as you can in front of your dog as they can not only sense your pain but have to deal with theirs too. Remember there is positive guidance and great vets out there. Nothing is impossible: where there is a will there's a way! If it means trying everything then do, but make sure you spend your time researching the good not the bad. You're the driving force behind your dog's recovery. They need you just as you need them. It's not the end, don't settle for the C word – beat it as long as you can. At least you'll live to know that you tried everything in your power."

– *Margherita Ferlita, Surrey, England*

Additional Considerations for Brain Tumors

There are two state-of-the-art surgical techniques that may be of interest to some owners, because they allow for more complete tumor removal, crucial to delayed recurrence and longer survival times.

The first technique removes the tumor using endoscopy. This minimally invasive technique helps the surgeon to insert a camera into the brain, to see the tumor and make a more complete removal. There are minimal surgical complications with this technique, and in a study of thirty-three dogs, the results were notable. Dogs with meningiomas in the forebrain had a median survival time of 5.8 years, while dogs with meningioma in the caudal (back) area of the brain, in the brainstem or cerebellum, had median survival times of two years. Dogs with other types of tumors had a shorter survival time of six months. Not all neurosurgeons perform this specialized technique, but it may be worth inquiring.

The second cutting-edge technique to consider is the use of an ultrasonic aspirator. This advanced surgical device uses ultrasonic vibration to powerfully and precisely remove tumors. In a study on dogs with meningiomas who received this surgery, the median survival time was about forty-two months, or three and a half years, depending upon the subtype of the tumor.

Seizures are common for dogs with brain tumors, and should be managed as part of your dog's care. Cluster seizures – two or more seizures happening in a short period of time – require hospitalization and injectable anti-convulsants. If brain swelling or herniation is suspected, a medication called mannitol is administered via injection, and oral steroids such as prednisone, are given, to reduce the swelling. You

It's the Little Things

"In my line of work, I speak with dog lovers each and every day. Many of them have been through cancer with a dog or are facing that journey currently. There are a few things I would share with anyone watching their beloved pet struggle with cancer or any other disease for that matter: take every moment to be with your pet because nothing means more to them than your presence. Do the things that you can, and don't obsess over what you cannot. So often it is the very little things like a ten minute massage or hand feeding your dog or carrying them outside and standing over them in the cold night air or a meal you made yourself that really matter so much more than expensive treatments or heroic efforts. If and when the time comes when a difficult decision must be made, be thankful for the mercy that we as guardians can provide our pets."

- Lola Michelin, Shoreline, Washington

may need to continue these at home until instructed to taper off.

If your dog is having seizures more than every six to eight weeks, oral anti-convulsants you can administer at home will likely be prescribed. A consultation with a neurologist will be helpful, also.

Seizure management is not just a palliative measure; it can also extend life. When used alone, steroids can extend life by weeks or months, and steroids combined with anti-convulsants can extend life from two to four months.

The Bottom Line

Brain tumors are a devastating cancer to deal with, and there are treatment options that can be used to control the tumor, significantly extending life and making your dog more comfortable. Oral medications are often palliative, but may also help.

Chapter 39: Perianal and Anal Sac Tumors

Perianal and anal sac tumors develop in the glands near and around the anus, just under the tail. Some tumors, called adenomas, are completely benign and do not spread, while others, called adenocarcinomas, are malignant. Perianal sac adenocarcinomas grow quickly; anal sac adenocarcinomas both grow quickly and are more likely to spread – more than 50% of afflicted dogs already have metastasis at the time of diagnosis.

Adenomas are related to testosterone levels and often shrink on their own after an adult male dog is neutered. They can also be surgically removed. Adenocarcinomas require more aggressive surgery, because regrowth is common. Some may require a multi-modal approach combining surgery, chemotherapy and radiation in order to extend survival times and improve quality of life.

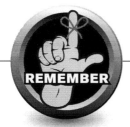

REMEMBER

When you need to look up the definition of a word or phrase, find it listed in Chapter 5, which begins on page 46.

The prognosis for these tumors varies widely depending upon the type of tumor and its own particular behavioral patterns.

Perianal adenomas are also known as hepatoid tumors and circumanal tumors, perianal adenocarcinomas as sebaceous adenocarcinomas, and anal sac adenocarcinoma as apocrine gland adenocarcinoma.

What Are Perianal and Anal Sac Tumors?

Any owner knows how dogs greet each other – by sniffing each other's rear. While this seems odd to us, it makes anatomical sense: dogs literally express themselves in this area. Their distinctive smells are not from the feces, alone, they're also coming from the anal sacs, two scent glands located on either side of the anus. These glands store secretions from apocrine (sweat) glands and sebaceous glands. Sebaceous glands secrete sebum, an oily, waxy substance that lubricates the skin and hair. They feed the anal sacs and surround the rest of the anus. These glands make it possible for the dog to defecate easily, and also provide a wealth of aromatic information for other dogs.

When the dog defecates, the anal glands secrete their stored sweat and oil, leaving that distinctive foul-smelling (to us) scent on the feces. Cancers that develop in these glands are called anal sac adenocarcinomas (ASACs). These account for 15–20%

of all perianal tumors and are the most aggressive. Because they specifically develop in the apocrine glands, or sweat glands, they are sometimes known as apocrine adenocarcinoma or apocrine gland anal sac adenocarcinomas (AGASACAs).

The many sebaceous glands in the anal region can also develop cancer. When testosterone levels elevate, these glands tend to enlarge and become noticeable. Benign tumors, called perianal adenomas, are very common in adult male dogs that are sexually intact or neutered late in life. Spayed females can also develop these tumors; this seems to be caused by elevated testosterone levels, which can happen with adrenal tumors and other testosterone-secreting tumors.

While most perianal tumors are benign, a few are malignant. When malignancies arise in the sebaceous glands of the anus, they're called perianal adenocarcinoma, and the role of testosterone in their development is less clear. They do occur most often in intact male dogs, and they also occur in neutered males and both intact and spayed females.

Other tumors can develop in the anal region, including squamous cell carcinoma in the lining of the anal sacs, lymphoma, mast cell tumors, skin melanoma, soft tissue sarcomas and transmissible venereal tumors (some of these are discussed in other chapters).

Which Dogs Are at Risk for Perianal and Anal Sac Tumors?

We used to think that females were more prone to anal sac adenocarcinoma than males; recently, reports show both males and females are equally affected.

Perianal tumors are one of the most common tumors in dogs, especially intact male dogs. Because testosterone influences the development of normal perianal glands and perianal tumors, neutering in early life can prevent perianal adenomas. Females that develop these tumors are typically spayed, and may have elevated testosterone levels, due to an adrenal tumor. There is also an association, in dogs, with testosterone-secreting testicular tumors.

Certain breeds are more prone to anal tumors than others. Those most likely to get perianal adenomas (benign tumors) are the arctic breeds such as Alaskan Malamutes, Siberian Huskies, Samoyeds and Norwegian Elkhounds. Other breeds predisposed to perianal adenomas are the Beagle, Cocker Spaniel, Shih Tzu and English Bulldog.

The more aggressive perianal adenocarcinoma shows up more often in large breeds, including German Shepherds and the arctic breeds: Alaskan Malamutes, Siberian Huskies, Samoyeds and Norwegian Elkhounds.

The following breeds are more likely to develop anal sac adenocarcinoma: Cocker Spaniels, English Springer Spaniels, German Shepherds and Golden Retrievers.

What are the Signs of Perianal and Anal Sac Tumors?

Vets find about one-third of the aggressive anal sac adenocarcinomas during a routine physical examination, which is why I urge you to request a rectal exam. A rectal exam can evaluate not only the anal sacs, but also lymph nodes and other glands in the anal region. This is important, because many times the primary tumor in the anal sac is very small, and there is much more extensive metastasis to the regional lymph nodes in the pelvic canal and under the lumbar spine, which may be palpable on an exam. A rectal exam can also reveal benign perianal adenomas.

If the tumor is not caught during a routine exam, owners often notice the mass itself swelling from underneath the tail. If the mass is not visible on the surface, the dog may show other symptoms, including straining to defecate, swelling in the area, licking or biting the region, or scooting along the ground in an attempt to relieve the associated itching or pain (or both).

Benign perianal adenomas usually develop over months or even years, and are mostly limited to one mass (although they can come in multiples).

Both perianal and anal sac adenocarcinomas grow more quickly, and these malignancies are more fixed (more attached to underlying tissues) and more likely to be ulcerated (open, raw, bleeding). If your dog is a female or a neutered male, the malignant perianal adenocarcinoma is more likely to occur than the benign perianal form.

Depending upon which study you look at, about 25-50% of dogs with anal sac adenocarcinoma have increased blood calcium levels at the time of diagnosis. These dogs may be drinking and urinating more often, vomiting, be physically weak and reluctant to eat or feel depressed.

How Are Perianal and Anal Sac Tumors Diagnosed?

A fine needle aspirate of the mass can usually help the vet to distinguish whether the tumor is an abscess (infection), a benign adenoma or a malignant carcinoma. The aspirate rarely requires sedation, and is an easy and quick test to run. The vet or the cy-

tologist at the lab will be able to tell what the mass is by looking at the cells under a microscope, and the malignancies are typically easy to tell from the benign tumors. Benign perianal adenomas contain cells shaped like liver cells, which is why they are often called "hepatoid" tumors (hepatocytes are liver cells).

If a carcinoma is confirmed by the aspirate, a surgery can be planned with a wide excision and submitted for biopsy to look at its margins. If the margins are not wide, a second surgery or radiation therapy may be recommended to prevent recurrence. (Wide margins are ideally two to three centimeters, but the location or size of the tumor may not allow for this. In most cases, we can get one to two centimeter margins in these tumors.)

If a malignancy is suspected, additional testing should be done before attempting a curative treatment. Urinalysis and blood work are recommended to get a general picture of the overall health of your dog. One of the important factors to look at on the

If I Had to Do It Over Again

"Be truly open-minded about alternative therapies. We used both traditional (radiation) and alternative (supplements, immune support etc.) at the same time. If I had it to do over again, I would have tried the alternatives first, and only done traditional if necessary. I think the traditional therapies really strained our twelve-year-old golden - I wish I had trusted the alternatives enough to really give them a go first."

- *Sheryl Poole, Andover, Massachusetts*

blood panel is the calcium levels.

About 25-50% of dogs with anal sac adeno-carcinoma have increased blood calcium levels at the time of diagnosis, because ASAC tumors produce PTHrp (parathyroid hormone-related peptide), a protein that causes blood calcium levels to rise. This marker is an indication that the tumor is particularly aggressive and requires prompt management. Dogs with elevated blood calcium have a worse prognosis.

One of the most common causes of elevated blood calcium is ASAC, but other diseases can also cause this condition. Lymphoma is the other most common cancer cause, followed by other non-cancer causes, such as kidney disease, Addison's disease, diseases that break down the bones such as hyperparathyroidism and vitamin D toxicity. Simple lab error can also be the culprit. All of these must be ruled out to make sure the elevated levels are associated with ASAC, and help you make treatment plans.

To confirm elevated blood calcium levels, a test that measures *ionized* calcium levels should be run. (Most chemistry panels measure total calcium, not ionized calcium.) This measures the active form, and if the levels are elevated, it's a sign that ASAC is the culprit. Even if total calcium levels are normal, check the ionized form, because knowing this number can be predictive for your dog's outcome. Your dog may need oral medications to lower these levels.

Metastasis occurs early in ASAC development, which is why looking for metastasis up front is important. More than 50% of dogs already have spread at the time of diagnosis. Up to 90% of these dogs will have regional lymph node metastasis, often in their sublumbar (under the lumbar spine) and intrapelvic (inside the pelvis) nodes. Metastasis can also spread to the liver, spleen, lungs and bone, so chest X-rays and abdominal ultrasounds should be run to check

these areas for suspicious lesions. If your dog is lame, regional X-rays should also be taken.

Perianal ACA is less aggressive in general, although 15% of dogs will have metastasis at the time of diagnosis, making checking for spread important. The same locations and tests are recommended as for ASAC.

What Is the Prognosis for Perianal and Anal Sac Tumors?

Here is the most recent staging system for these tumors published by Polton in 2007 for ASAC:

- **Stage 1:** The primary tumor is smaller than or equal to 2.5 centimeter in diameter, with no regional lymph node or distant metastasis.

- **Stage 2:** The primary tumor is greater than 2.5 centimeter in diameter, with no regional or distant metastasis.

- **Stage 3A:** The primary tumor is of any size, but there is regional lymph node involvement with tumors smaller than or equal to 4.5 centimeter in diameter, with no distant metastasis.

- **Stage 3B:** The primary tumor is of any size, but there is regional lymph node involvement with tumors greater than 4.5 centimeter in diameter, with no distant metastasis.

- **Stage 4:** The primary tumor is of any size, with or without lymph node involvement, and distant metastasis is present.

In general, the higher the stage is, the worse the prognosis. In general, the prognosis worsens when the primary tumor is large, when there is lymph node metastasis, when there is distant metastasis or an increase in ionized calcium levels.

The median survival time for dogs that have anal sac adenocarcinomas and are not treated is about eight months.

However, it's been shown that these tumors are truly variable from dog to dog. For example, one study looked at eleven dogs who did not receive treatment for their anal sac ACA, five of whom had bulky regional metastasis when they were diagnosed, and three of whom had both regional and lung metastasis. The median survival time for the group was about eight months, and the range of survival times was 0 days to 499 days (about sixteen months). While there were not many dogs in this study, it does illustrate that it's hard to say that these tumors have a "typical" behavior.

With full treatment (surgery, chemotherapy and radiation) as described below, studies show that dogs with anal sac adenocarcinoma have survival times approaching two to two and a half years.

With treatment for perianal ACA, the size of the primary tumor is very predictive of prognosis. Dogs with tumors smaller than 5 centimeters have a median survival time of two years, while those with tumors larger than 5 centimeter have a survival time of one year. Dogs with metastasis at time of diagnosis experience a median survival time of seven months.

The vast majority (90%) of perianal adenomas are cured completely with castration and surgical removal of the tumor.

What Are the Available Protocols for Perianal and Anal Sac Tumors?

Surgery is the first treatment for all perianal tu-mors, and may be the only treatment needed, depending upon the tumor type and the extent of the disease.

Perianal adenomas often resolve themselves when your dog is neutered, because the source of testosterone is removed with the surgery. Those that don't go away or shrink significantly can be surgically removed. Over 90% of these tumors will be cured with castration and tumor resection.

Perianal adenocarcinomas tend to recur, especially if they are larger than 5 centimeter in diameter at the time of diagnosis. For these tumors, a more aggressive surgery is required, with wide margins, and later surgeries may be necessary, if regrowth occurs. In these cases, the size of the tumor can predict the expected outcome: dogs with perianal ACA smaller than 5 centimeter live for two years, while those with perianal ACA over 5 centimeter live for one year. Dogs with metastasis at the time of diagnosis have median survival times of seven months, regardless of the size of the primary tumor.

Anal sac adenocarcinoma (ASAC) is even more aggressive, and may require a multi-modal approach. Controlling the disease locally with surgery and radiation is important, as is using chemotherapy to address the high probability of metastasis.

ASAC needs aggressive surgery with adequate margins; a poorly planned surgery (or biopsy) can actually spread the disease locally, compromising a successful outcome. For this reason, I strongly recommend running advanced imaging to thoroughly plan the biopsy or surgery ahead of time, especially for larger tumors. MRIs and CT scans can provide good detail about the primary tumor, the extent to which it has invaded local tissues and whether it has spread to regional lymph nodes (and which ones).

During the surgery, up to fifty percent of regional lymph nodes (typically the sublumbar lymph

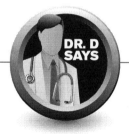

DR. D SAYS

The conventional treatments Dr. Ettinger recommends for perianal and anal sac tumors should be considered part of step one of Full Spectrum cancer care (Chapter 11). Please review that chapter for more general information about surgery, radiation and chemotherapy and how to handle their common side effects.

For more information on all other Full Spectrum steps, including nutraceuticals, immune boosters, dietary changes and brain chemistry modification strategies, review Full Spectrum cancer care, which begins on page 103.

You will also find information about specific chemotherapy agents in Chapter 41.

nodes) can usually be removed completely, although the surgeon will not know whether removal is possible until the surgery takes place. Removing metastatic lymph nodes can improve survival times, so this is important.

Sometimes, the anal sphincter must be partially removed during this surgery. This sphincter is the round muscle that literally keeps the anus closed between defecations, so removing it can make some owners worry that their dogs will become incontinent. This may be true for a little while after surgery, but dogs can lose up to 50% of the sphincter and still rehabilitate themselves, once they have healed. Fecal incontinence is usually not a concern for the long-term.

For ASAC treated only with surgery, median survival times are ten to eighteen months. Including surgery in your dog's treatment time is considered a must, because studies show that dogs who receive surgery fare better than those who do not.

If your dog has increased ionized calcium levels, survival times are shorter, usually six to nine months (note that some studies failed to show this was a negative predictor). The ionized calcium levels typically go back to normal levels after the surgery. Check them periodically to monitor for recurrence and/or spread.

If the surgery results in incomplete margins, radiation should be used to control microscopic disease and prevent recurrence and/or regional spread. Your radiation oncologist may also want to treat the sublumbar lymph nodes to prevent or delay metastasis. Keep in mind that there are side effects to radiation. In this area, the skin and the lining of the colon and rectum are affected, so your dog may have burning, irritation, inflammation and diarrhea for two to four weeks after treatment. Late side effects can also occur months or years later; in this area they tend to be chronic diarrhea, straining to defecate, scarring of the tissue or stricture (narrowing) of the anus.

Palliative radiation can be used for inoperable ASAC tumors, or for disease that is confined to the regional lymph nodes. This use of radiation may slow the progression of the disease, but is rarely curative. Early side effects are less common than with a full course of radiation therapy.

Because ASAC is so metastatic, chemotherapy

is recommended to delay the spread. The most effective drugs as of this writing are carboplatin, mitoxantrone, and Adriamycin, and others are being evaluated. Piroxicam and Palladia are also under evaluation; check with your oncologist.

Some recent studies show that survival times may approach two or even two and a half years when all three modalities are used to treat ASAC (surgery, radiation and chemotherapy). Another, smaller study of afflicted dogs with no distant metastasis, showed that surgery followed by daily, fractionated radiation therapy and mitoxantrone chemotherapy produced a survival time of thirty-one months or nearly three years. If your dog has ASAC with no distant metastasis and you can afford to use all three therapies, I strongly recommend considering it. (The exception is if clean margins are achieved surgically – in these radiation may not be recommended.)

Additional Considerations for Perianal and Anal Sac Tumors

Chemotherapy is sometimes used as a stand-alone therapy for inoperable ASAC tumors; this is considered palliative care and is associated with shorter survival times of seven months.

If your dog has elevated blood calcium levels, an injectable medication called pamidronate can be given intravenously to lower them and decrease associated symptoms. Prednisone can also be used.

Stool softeners may be helpful for dogs with intrapelvic masses that cause obstruction of the pelvic canal.

There Is Always Hope!

"There is always hope! You should learn everything you can about the type of cancer your fur baby has and then no matter how much or how little time you have, live each day for just that day. Yes, you will have 'down' days but don't brood on them, just know that they will happen. Look at the diet you are feeding your friend, and see where you can make it better, variety is very good for them too just as it is for you. Read and learn everything you can: the treatments, the medications, supplements and diets, because it is you who are the closest to your friend, and you know what is best for your dog."

- Shirley, Salem, Oregon

The Bottom Line

Perianal and anal sac tumors are extremely variable in their outcome – from curable to highly metastatic. Nevertheless, I consider even the aggressive ASAC a treatable cancer, when combined therapies are used. These can extend life and make dogs much more comfortable than they are at diagnosis.

Chapter 40: Melanoma

Melanoma is a common dog cancer that occurs in darkly pigmented skin. The most common forms are oral, digit, and skin, although melanomas can appear anywhere melanocytes, the cells they occur in, are located in the body.

Oral malignant melanoma (OMM) is the most common oral tumor in dogs, accounting for 30-40% of all oral tumors. It is highly metastatic and has often spread to distant sites away from the tumor by the time of diagnosis. Digit melanoma, which occurs on the toes, is also metastatic, although less so than the oral type. Although melanoma which occurs in the skin is very malignant in humans, it is typically benign in dogs.

Tumors treated aggressively and early are generally responsive to treatment. The smaller the tumor is when it is first found, the better the prognosis, which is why early detection is so important. Surgery is a must for oral melanomas, although radiation therapy can also be very helpful. Due to the high risk for metastasis, systemic therapy is also an important part of the treatment plan. A promising and exciting treatment option is immunotherapy, specifically the canine melanoma vaccine which is available through boarded oncologists. Chemotherapy used to be common for these tumors, and may still be considered to control distant metastasis if the vaccine is not used.

Digit melanomas also require an aggressive surgery, with chemotherapy to follow up on metastatic disease. Skin melanoma is usually benign and curable with surgery. For malignant forms, the melanoma vaccine is also recommended to control metastasis.

(I'll discuss the melanoma vaccine at length later in this chapter.)

If left untreated, oral malignant melanoma has a pretty grim prognosis of only two months survival time. With thorough treatment, dogs with oral tumors can survive one to two (plus) years. Dogs treated for digit tumors can survive two years, and dogs treated for benign skin tumors even longer.

Other names for melanoma include malignant melanoma, melanocytic tumor, and melanocytoma (benign melanomas).

What Is Melanoma?

Melanoma develops in the melanocytes, skin cells that are responsible for skin pigmentation. This is a common tumor in dogs, and can occur anywhere on the skin or inside the mouth, so we classify it by

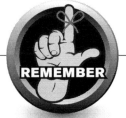

When you need to look up the definition of a word or phrase, find it listed in Chapter 5, which begins on page 46.

where it is located on the body. We'll discuss the most common types in this chapter.

Oral cancer is the fourth most common type of dog cancer, and oral malignant melanoma (OMM) is the most common oral tumor in dogs. OMM is highly malignant. These tumors are locally aggressive, often invading the bones of the jaw. They also metastasize to the local lymph nodes, liver, lungs and kidneys at rates greater than 60-80%. They appear along the gums, the lips, the palate (roof of the mouth), and the tongue. Oral melanoma should be assumed to be malignant even if the biopsy report suggests otherwise.

The highly pigmented nail bed on the toes is the next most common site for melanoma. Also called subungual melanoma, it is the second most common tumor of the digit in dogs. It is not as aggressive as oral melanoma, with metastasis rates of 30-60%.

Skin melanomas are generally benign in dogs, although malignant forms do develop, rarely. But even benign masses can cause problems, and should be treated.

Which Dogs Are at Risk for Melanoma?

We know quite a bit about the causes of oral cancer in people – tobacco and alcohol use in particular, and possibly persistent viral infections such as HPV. But when it comes to dogs, we don't know the cause of oral melanoma. We do know that male dogs get more oral tumors of any kind than females do, including oral melanoma.

Skin melanoma in humans is caused by sun exposure, but the same is not true for dogs. There are some breeds predisposed to skin melanoma, but we're not sure yet exactly why this is true.

Black dogs with more active melanocytes may be predisposed to melanoma, but dogs of any color can develop the illness. Melanomas are definitely more common in purebred dogs. The benign skin form of melanoma is most likely to occur in Doberman Pinschers and Miniature Schnauzers, while Miniature Poodles are more likely to have the malignant form of skin melanoma.

Poodles, Dachshunds, Scottish Terriers, Cocker Spaniels, and Retriever breeds tend to get more OMM than other breeds. Chow Chows get more melanomas of the tongue. OMM also tends to occur in smaller dogs (of lower weight) than the other oral tumors, and, in one study, German Shepherds and Boxers were at decreased risk for OMM.

What are the Signs of Melanoma?

Owners usually find melanoma of the skin and the toe by noticing the tumors, which sometimes look inflamed or ulcerated (open and possibly bleeding). They may be very pigmented, or dark, or they may have very little pigment, in which case they are called amelanotic (this is determined by a biopsy).

Much like other oral tumors, the oral melanomas located in the front of the mouth (also known as rostral) are more likely to be noticed by the owner. This early detection means they are often found when they're smaller, and therefore have a better general prognosis than those located in the rear of the mouth (also known as caudal). Because most owners do not spend much time looking in their dog's mouth, many tumors are not noticed early. More and more general practice vets are emphasizing the importance of regular home dental care for dogs, which gives me hope for more early detections for oral melanomas.

Symptoms owners notice at home are bad breath, excessive drooling, difficulty in eating or swallowing, pain while eating, pawing at the mouth, bleeding or bloody saliva, loss of teeth, facial swellings or deformities, and weight loss.

If the vet finds the oral tumor during a dental exam or cleaning, he will perform an immediate biopsy. One sign of trouble is if teeth are loose but there is not a lot of tartar or dental disease, for example. In this case, he should biopsy the socket after pulling the tooth, even if there is no visible mass. Most dogs need sedation for thorough oral exams or cleanings, so this is usually done during the same anesthesia used for the dental procedure.

How Is Melanoma Diagnosed?

Wherever the melanoma is located in the body, a fine needle aspirate will usually provide a preliminary diagnosis. A biopsy, however, will provide a definitive diagnosis and very important information for the prognosis.

For example, benign skin melanomas are distinguished from malignant skin melanomas by examining how many cells are dividing. This evaluation, called the mitotic index, can be seen in a biopsy sample, and will be very helpful in devising your treatment plan. Note that all oral melanomas are considered malignant, regardless of their mitotic index.

The biopsy sample must be taken carefully because the sample must be large, from the center of the mass, and not from areas filled with dead (necrotic) cells, inflammation, or pus – otherwise the biopsy sample might not represent the whole tumor well, which could lead to a misdiagnosis. Later, it is vital that the biopsy site be included in the surgery or in the radiation field.

In the case of oral melanoma, the biopsy nee-dle can track cancer cells, so it is important to take a sample from inside the mouth, not through normal tissue of the cheek or nasal cavity (for upper jaw tumors). Melanoma can also mimic other oral tumors, making confirming a diagnosis challenging for the pathologist. When this is the case, your oncologist may want to use a special stain for the biopsy, or get a biopsy second opinion.

Because melanoma is so likely to spread, full staging is recommended before treatments are begun. Blood work and urinalysis can tell you how healthy your dog is, in general. Chest imaging (three-view X-rays or a CT scan) can be used to check for lung metastasis, while abdominal ultrasounds can

Cancer Is Not a Death Sentence

"To Others Who are Experiencing What I am Going Through ... It is a breath of fresh air, learning from Dr. Dressler, that Cancer is NOT a death sentence. Every time I see my little one scratching her bed to make it, every time I see her prancing her little girly prance, every time I see her running along the beach, and most of all, every time I look into her loving, adoring eyes, I know without a doubt that nothing that I do for her is ever too much. Everything counts. Every day counts. And when the time comes for us to part, whether it be from cancer, or from age, I know that it will be she that tells me that it is time (but only for a short while, for hope is eternal)."

- *Joyce Parham, Julian, North Carolina*

check for spread to the liver, spleen and other organs. Lymph nodes in the region of the tumor should all be checked (aspirated), even if they appear normal, because metastasis is not correlated with normal or enlarged sizes.

In the case of an oral tumor, both the left and right mandibular (lower jaw) lymph nodes should be aspirated, because lymphatic draining can cross to the opposite side of the jaw. In other words, a mass on the right side of the mouth can metastasize to the left lymph nodes. There are also chains of lymph nodes in the head and the neck that should be checked. These cannot typically be felt on an exam, but they can be detected on a CT scan.

I strongly recommend a CT scan for oral mela-noma. The amount of detail you can see in a CT scan (or in dental X-rays, if need be) is extremely helpful in planning treatments. The tumor may be much more invasive and extensive than it seems on examination, and this information can inform treat-ment decisions later.

What Is the Prognosis for Melanoma?

Melanoma behaves differently, depending upon the location (more specifics are discussed in the treatment section); the most malignant form is oral malignant melanoma.

This is the official clinical staging system for canine oral malignant melanoma:

- **Stage I:** The primary tumor is smaller than 2 centimeter in diameter, with no lymph node involvement.
- **Stage II:** The primary tumor is between 2 and 4 centimeter in diameter, with no lymph node involvement.

- **Stage III:** The primary tumor is larger than 4 centimeter in diameter, with or without lymph node involvement.
- **Stage IV:** The primary tumor is of any size, with distant metastatic disease.

Dogs with oral melanoma who do not receive treatment have a median survival time of about two months. In general, the prognosis is better for dogs with a tumor under 2 centimeters in diameter, with no lymph node metastasis, no bony invasion, and a low mitotic index, as revealed under the microscope (a low mitotic index is anything less than 3/10 high-powered field).

What Are the Available Protocols for Melanoma?

The first course of action with any melanoma is surgery to remove the primary tumor. Radiation may be necessary to control local microscopic dis-ease, and the melanoma vaccine (or chemotherapy) is recommended to control distant metastasis. Let's look at each of these melanoma types separately, to get a more detailed picture.

Oral Malignant Melanoma

If there is no evidence of metastasis in distant body locations, and if wide (wider than two centime-ters) margins, including underlying bone, can be ob-tained, surgery is recommended for oral melanomas. Lymph nodes that drain the region of the tumor that test positive should also be removed surgically.

These surgeries are easier if the tumor is small, forward (rostral), and involve the lower jaw (man-dible). Surgeries on the mandible also tend to have lower recurrence rates. Sometimes the surgery must be quite radical, even removing half of the lower or upper jaw. Even so, owners report high satisfaction with these aggressive surgeries because they feel the mouth is less painful and still retains functionality. The median survival time for these resections is eight to ten months.

Of all the prognostic factors, the two most predictive factors in formulating a prognosis for your dog are the size of the primary tumor and the ability of the first treatment (usually surgery) to control the disease. When the tumor is smaller than two centimeters in diameter with no metastasis, and is treated with aggressive surgery resulting in clean, wide margins, the median survival time is seventeen months. Boarded surgeons tend to be more aggressive in their surgeries, which is why I recommend using one, if you can.

When the primary tumor is greater than two centimeters in diameter, or there is already lymph node metastasis, the median survival time with aggressive surgery is much shorter: four months. Dogs that get a conservative surgery (margins less than two centimeters wide and/or with dirty margins) have a 70% chance of recurrence and survival times of three to four months. These statistics explain the importance of early detection and an aggressive surgery.

Radiation therapy can be used as an alternative to surgery when the tumor is inoperable or you do not want to use surgery. In these cases, over 80% of dogs can achieve long-term local control over the disease, with complete response rates of 50-70% (which means the tumor disappears for a time) and median survival times of five to nine months.

There are fewer early side effects with melanoma radiation protocols, because they are not the same as traditional protocols. Called coarse-fractionation protocols, they feature fewer total treatments and higher doses per treatment. Higher doses at each

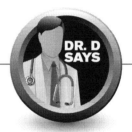

DR. D SAYS

The conventional treatments Dr. Ettinger recommends for melanoma should be considered part of step one of Full Spectrum cancer care (Chapter 11). Please review that chapter for more general information about surgery, radiation and chemotherapy and how to handle their common side effects.

For more information on all other Full Spectrum steps, including nutraceuticals, immune boosters, dietary changes and brain chemistry modification strategies, review Full Spectrum cancer care, which begins on page 103.

You will also find information about specific chemotherapy agents in Chapter 41.

treatment are required because melanoma cells are unique in their ability to repair radiation-induced damage. While there is an advantage to these protocols – fewer treatments, less anesthesia, fewer early side effects, less expense – there is a trade-off, too: your dog is more likely to have late side effects like bone damage, muscle damage and central nervous system damage, for example. I recommend close consultation with a radiation oncologist to determine whether the standard melanoma protocols are appropriate for your dog. If there is a good overall prognosis and an expectation of a longer survival time, she might recommend your dog receive standard doses over more sessions to minimize the late-occurring side effects.

Just as tumor size is predictive for surgery outcome, it's predictive for radiation therapy outcome. Dogs with tumors smaller than two centimeters often have a survival time of fifteen to twenty months, whereas, dogs with larger tumors and more advanced disease, metastasized to distant locations, typically live only five to six months.

Dogs with oral melanoma typically die because of their distant metastasis, which is more likely to occur in dogs with larger tumors or dogs that have already metastasized at the time of diagnosis. Because of melanoma's high rate of metastasis in general, following up surgery or radiation with systemic therapy (melanoma vaccine or chemotherapy) is an important part of the treatment plan for dogs with any stage of oral melanoma.

Carboplatin is the standard chemotherapy drug used for oral (and digit) melanoma, and it extends survival time to approximately one year after surgery. Its use, however, has dropped since the approval of the melanoma vaccine (see below), which is more effective. (Some oncologists use both.)

Fewer than 30% of dogs respond to chemotherapy when used as a standalone therapy in place of surgery or radiation, so it is not generally used on its own.

Digit Melanomas

Like oral melanomas, digit melanomas require an aggressive surgery to control the local disease. The best-case scenario is usually toe amputation, which can be done if there is no detectable local or dis-

> ### Don't Panic!
>
> "We humans, when we hear cancer, we automatically think - imminent death and that is not always the case. Don't panic. Make sure you seek as much information as possible about the cancer and treatment options because depending on the type of cancer there could be many treatment plans available. Do not rely on one medical opinion; I work with an oncologist and a holistic vet and they have been instrumental in helping my dog have the best possible immune system and therefore fight the cancer. Also, I am part of a few cancer groups. These groups can provide vital information for your pet because they have been there and done it. They also help you realize that there a lot of other people/dogs out there going through the same thing and can provide support."
>
> *- Marian Beeman,*
> *Fairfax Station, Virginia*

tant metastasis and wide margins (greater than two centimeters) can be obtained in the surgery. If these wide margins are not possible, leg amputation is considered. Median survival times of twelve months are typical with these surgeries.

If the owners decline limb amputation and the surgeon can't get two centimeter wide margins with a toe amputation, radiation therapy should be used to try to clean up the dirty margins (kill the remaining microscopic cancer cells). Radiation should also be given to any regional lymph nodes that test positive for metastasis.

Dogs with digit melanoma usually die due to distant metastasis, especially those with larger tumors or metastasis at the time of diagnosis. To combat or delay metastasis, which occurs in 30-60% of dogs with digit melanoma, the melanoma vaccine should be used following surgery and/or radiation. As with oral melanoma, chemotherapy, specifically carboplatin, may be considered. Also as with oral melanoma, the melanoma vaccine is more routinely recommended instead of chemotherapy (see below). In a recent study, dogs treated with both locoregional control (surgery and/or radiation) and the melanoma vaccine had a median survival time of about sixteen months, with 63% still alive after one year. In the same study, metastasis at the time of diagnosis reduced median survival times – dogs with metastasis had a median survival time of three and a half months, while treated dogs without metastasis had a median survival time of almost eighteen months.

Chemotherapy used as a standalone treatment for a primary digital melanoma is not recommended, as it is not effective enough.

Skin Melanoma

While benign skin melanomas are not malignant in general, some can have malignant potential and characteristics. For this reason, they should be treated. Surgery is the first therapy given to dogs with benign skin melanomas, affording them a median survival time of twenty-four months. Some dogs can be cured with this surgery alone.

Malignant skin melanomas must be treated with aggressive surgeries, with wide (greater than 2 cm) margins. These surgeries generally result in median survival times of seven to eleven months. If wide margins cannot be or are not obtained, a scar revision (second surgery) can be done. If that's not feasible,

radiation therapy may be used to delay recurrence at the surgery site.

Systemic therapy is also recommended for malignant skin melanomas (melanoma vaccine, or the chemotherapy drug carboplatin, see digital melanoma section above), although we do not yet know whether survival times are lengthened with this therapy.

Melanoma Vaccine

A new and exciting treatment option for all melanoma types is immunotherapy; a new vaccine is available that can be used to stimulate the immune system to fight the cancer cells. It can be used with all stages of melanoma, although it is less effective for stage IV melanoma with distant metastasis, or for dogs with measurable local disease (a tumor which has spread and can be seen and measured).

Traditionally, vaccines are used to prevent infections; this vaccine is very different. The canine melanoma vaccine (which is USDA-approved for dog melanoma) is a therapeutic vaccine, used not to prevent, but to treat the illness. I am excited about this vaccine, not only because it helps dogs with melanoma, but also because I was involved in the clinical trials. Here's how the vaccine works.

There is a normal body protein called tyrosinase, present on the outside of some cells in the body. Melanoma cells happen to manufacture a great deal of this protein. Because the immune system does not normally attack its own cells, the immune system does not recognize or attack either melanoma cells or regular cells when they have tyrosinase present.

This vaccine cleverly uses tyrosinase, created from another animal's DNA (humans, actually), to stimulate the immune system to target cells with a lot of this protein. The human version of tyrosinase is just different enough from dog tyrosinase to raise an alert in the immune system. The system mobilizes to destroy the new tyrosinase and anything similar to it. Melanoma cells are targeted because of their large amounts of tyrosinase, while normal cells, which have much less, are largely unaffected.

My mentor, Dr. Philip Bergman, led the studies of the DNA melanoma vaccines that led to the development of this vaccine, and I participated in the ongoing trials during my residency at Animal Medical Center (AMC) in New York City. The hospital partnered with Memorial Sloan-Kettering Cancer Center, also in New York City, to test a human melanoma vaccine. The studies produced significant and exciting results.

(Dogs and humans are similar physiologically, so dogs are often involved in human cancer research.)

Early studies involving dogs with advanced melanoma (stage II, III and IV) showed a median survival time of thirteen months for dogs on the trial vaccine, compared to five months for dogs on standard therapies. Importantly, the vaccine was demonstrated to be safe and active.

Further studies involved about 350 dogs at AMC. In these trials, dogs with minimal residual disease (MRD) remaining after local control (surgery and/or radiation), that were also treated with the vaccine, had increased survival time, over thirty-three months, versus dogs without the local control, who experienced eighteen months. To maximize the vaccine's effectiveness, we must achieve minimal residual disease: the primary tumor must be completely resected and/or treated with radiation (for incomplete margins). Non-resectable tumors should be treated with radiation therapy. The vaccine is also more effective when local lymph nodes are either negative for metastasis or, if positive, are surgically removed or treated with radiation. This does not apply to stage IV dogs with distant metastasis.

It can take months to develop significant immune response, so I advise starting to use the vaccine as soon as possible. There is some evidence that starting the vaccine before radiation treatments is helpful. This is because tumor cells release tyrosinase as they are killed by radiation, which can enhance the immune system's response.

The vaccine is administered through a transdermal device that goes into the muscle of the inner thigh. There is no needle involved, which allows the device to distribute the vaccine evenly into the muscles. The initial treatment consists of four doses of vaccine given at two-week intervals. After that, booster doses are administered every six months. Some dogs develop a low-grade fever, which doesn't last long. Mild skin reactions were noted in 5% of dogs in the studies, usually some skin redness that resolved quickly without the need for treatment. In some rare cases, dogs lost some pigment in their coats – in other words, some of their black coat turned white. There has been very little evidence of toxicity due to the vaccine.

In 2007, the USDA gave a conditional license to the vaccine, which allows a new treatment to be used, while still being monitored for safety and efficacy. In January of 2010, a full license was issued to Merial, the manufacturer, and Merial started selling Oncept, the commercial version of the vaccine. This is the first and only vaccine approved for the treatment of cancer, in any species, and is available only through medical oncologists.

As an interesting side note, human clinical trials are being conducted at Memorial Sloan-Kettering for a melanoma vaccine very similar to the canine version. I highly recommend using this vaccine, in conjunction with surgery and radiation; consult with an oncologist to determine whether it is appropriate for your dog's case.

Also, please note that while it may be tempting to think this vaccine can be used to prevent melanoma, this is not the case. It has only been tested in dogs with a diagnosis of melanoma, and the overall incidence of canine melanoma is too low to justify giving this vaccine to all dogs to attempt to prevent the disease.

The Bottom Line

While melanoma can be a distressing disease, there are many options for treatment. Treated dogs live longer and enjoy a good quality of life.

Find a Network

"Love your dog and give her the best you have, understand that this is an important and difficult time for both of you. Find a network of people who have been through it to support you, and get as much info as you can beyond what your own vet is telling you."

- *Ellen Slater, Redmond, Oregon*

Chapter 41: Common Veterinary Chemotherapy Drugs

Chemotherapy is an emotionally charged word for many people, because it has a reputation for terrible side effects, when used in human cancer. As we've pointed out before, using chemotherapy drugs to treat dogs is a different situation. It's true that most chemotherapy drugs have some side effects for dogs, though they are usually manageable and worth the effect of the drug. Unlike people, most dogs do not become seriously ill on chemotherapy, because we do not use high, curative doses. Most dog owners who choose chemotherapy are happy with the results and pleasantly surprised that their worst fears didn't come true. Oncologists are experts at managing side effects, and newer treatments often minimize side effects even more.

As Dr. Dressler pointed out in Chapter 1, our brains can create "rules of thumb" about stressful or painful events. If you're finding yourself breathing a little harder, or resistant to finding out more about the chemotherapy drugs that are recommended for your dog's cancer treatments, try his Three Deep Breaths exercise. If you've got a rule of thumb about chemotherapy, this chapter will likely trigger it.

Alkylating Agents

Alkylating Agents target DNA in several ways: they cross-link, or bind, strands of DNA together; create breaks in the DNA that cannot be repaired and alter the actual function of DNA. As a result, the cell cannot divide, and dies. These agents are most active in the resting phase of the cell cycle.

Cyclophosphamide

Cyclophosphamide (brand name Cytoxan) is the most common alkylating agent. It is used most commonly for lymphoma, and also for lymphoid leukemias, carcinomas, sarcomas and some autoimmune disorders. While most chemotherapy drugs come in just one form, cyclophosphamide comes in both an injection and a pill form.

Cyclophosphamide needs liver enzymes to "turn it on" before it becomes an active chemotherapy agent. If your dog has severe liver disease, she may not activate enough of the drug to produce an effective dose, which is a factor your vet or oncologist will likely take into account, when including it in your protocol and choosing a dosage.

Common side effects of cyclophosphamide include hair loss, nausea, vomiting, diarrhea and bone marrow suppression. Dogs on cyclophosphamide must be encouraged to urinate frequently for the three days after treatment, in order to clear the by-products from their urinary system. For this reason, it's commonly given in the morning (if you're using the oral form at home, make sure to give it early in the day) to allow for daytime urinations. Dogs will not necessarily feel the urge to urinate, so you should encourage your dog to relieve himself frequently, especially right before bedtime, for the next three days.

These frequent walks are necessary to prevent sterile hemorrhagic cystitis (SHC), which develops when one of the by-products of cyclophosphamide, acrolein, irritates the bladder, and 9% of dogs develop this condition. SHC is irritating and causes your dog to void small amounts, much more often than usual and sometimes pass blood in the urine. When your dog develops these symptoms, a urine test and urine culture must be run to rule out a possible bladder infection. When a bladder infection is present, the culture will show which antibiotic is needed; when there is no bladder infection, the irritation is probably due to the cyclophosphamide, which should no longer be used (chlorambucil is the typical replacement).

To further reduce the risk of developing SHC, I recommend pre-treating with a diuretic to help increase the output of urine. For example, an injection of furosemide (Lasix) decreases the risk of SHC to only 1.2%.

It is also important to keep your dog from dehydrating from urinating so often. Give your dog extra water and keep the bowl full. Also, be particularly careful to clean up urine, if your dog has an accident in the house.

Chlorambucil

Chlorambucil (brand name Leukeran), another alkylating agent, is most commonly given for small cell (low grade) lymphoma, chronic lymphocytic leukemia and, occasionally, mast cell tumors. It is also used as a replacement for cyclophosphamide, when SHC develops. This is an oral medication, typically given regularly (daily or every other day), at home, by owners.

Compared to other drugs, chlorambucil is minimally toxic. Most chemotherapy drugs cause bone marrow suppression within seven to fourteen days; chlorambucil has a much slower effect – it often takes months for symptoms to show up, and then the bone marrow can take weeks or even months to return to normal function. Because of this slow effect, routine follow up (usually every other week for the first two months, and then every four to six weeks) is important: to monitor for bone marrow suppression and to correct problems as they arise. These follow-ups must include a blood draw for a complete blood count (CBC).

Chlorambucil comes in tablets and is given by owners at home, every day or every other day, depending upon the prescription. In addition to bone marrow suppression, it can cause hair loss and, sometimes, nausea, vomiting and diarrhea.

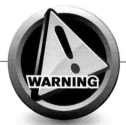

Not Safe for Pregnancy

No chemotherapy drug is safe for use in pregnant dogs. This is because the developing fetus in the womb is full of rapidly dividing cells – which are vulnerable to the chemotherapy.

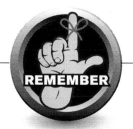

Side effects and Blood Tests

There are several common and expected side effects associated with chemotherapy drugs. Most dogs will experience mild digestive upset (vomiting, nausea or diarrhea), at least once or twice during the course of a typical chemotherapy protocol. This usually clears up easily on its own or with supportive at-home medications. In fewer than 5% of dogs, these symptoms may be so severe that dogs will require hospitalization for IV fluids, antibiotics and injectable anti-nausea drugs. Detailed information on how to manage these side effects is included in Chapter 11.

Remember: many chemotherapy drugs lower the levels of white blood cells, thereby suppressing immunity. Unless this suppression is very severe, most dogs do not have any symptoms associated with immunosuppression. Even so, it is important that your dog's blood be checked before every chemotherapy session and sometimes during follow-up visits. A complete blood count will show your oncologist how your dog is doing and help him calculate the best dosage of chemotherapy. See Chapter 11 for more details on chemotherapy.

In addition to a CBC, depending upon the drug involved, your oncologist may need to run other tests (for example, for liver or kidney values), before starting a chemotherapy treatment.

Lomustine

Lomustine (also called CCNU) is an alkylating agent used to treat mast cell tumors, some brain tumors, and lymphoma that has relapsed. It belongs to a unique group of drugs which can cross the brain's barrier (called the blood brain barrier) and get directly to the nervous tissue. Because of this ability, it may also be useful for lymphomas involving the brain and spinal cord.

This potent drug can cause vomiting, nausea and diarrhea. It can also cause severe bone marrow suppression, including very low white blood cell counts, usually seven to fourteen days after administration (these may not occur until after multiple doses, so blood counts must be monitored as treatments progress).

High doses of lomustine have led to liver damage in a small number of dogs, so I always check liver values before I administer a dose. Signs of liver damage are typically non-specific or vague, and can be similar to other chemotherapy side effects, including lethargy, loss of appetite, vomiting and diarrhea. (Call your vet immediately if you notice severe symptoms.) Most dogs recover from the liver toxicity, but the drug will typically need to be discontinued. Recent preliminary research suggests that using Denamarin (a liver supplement that combines Denosyl, also known as SAM-e, with milk thistle) may decrease the issue of elevated liver values and allow for more Lomustine doses. I use this supplement with my patients.

In a recent report, Lomustine used in a metronomic protocol (frequent, daily small doses given with no extended rest periods), was shown to avoid the SHC associated with chronic cyclophosphamide use. This protocol was generally well tolerated, with 27% needing to stop due to side effects. Fifteen percent developed elevated kidney values, and 21% developed elevated liver values, so these organs need to be closely monitored with blood work. Complete blood counts are also important, as is monitoring for gastro-intestinal side effects. Specific metronomic protocols, including tumor types, doses, and schedules, are still being developed.

Lomustine comes in capsule form only, and can be given at home, with the blood work checked and approved just before each dosing. Its potency makes it very dangerous, so be sure to follow the side effect management advice, detailed in Chapter 11. Give lomustine on an empty stomach, several hours after a meal, to reduce nausea and vomiting.

Mechlorethamine

Mechlorethamine (brand name Mustargen) is an alkylating agent and one of the original chemotherapy drugs. It's derived from mustard gas and often used in combination with several other drugs in the MOPP and MVPP protocols used to treat lymphoma (typically relapsed lymphomas).

Mustargen must be handled with great care, because it is a severe vesicant, which means that it has an extreme damaging effect on tissues, when it gets outside the vein during administration. It comes as an injection only, and must be given at the vet hospital by staff experienced in handling and using this specific drug. A carefully placed catheter must go directly into a vein, and great care must be taken to inject mechlorethamine directly into the vein, so that it does not damage other tissues. When it comes in contact with other tissues, there can be serious irritation. Other side effects include nausea, vomiting, diarrhea and low white blood cell counts.

Antimetabolites

A group of drugs, called antimetabolites, can be useful in treating cancer because of their ability to masquerade as part of the cancer cell. These plant alkaloids mimic the building blocks of DNA; when the cancer cell uses them to build new DNA, its structure is permanently weakened and the cell dies.

Cytosine arabinoside

One of the most popular of the antimetabolites is cytosine arabinoside. Used in leukemia and some lymphoma protocols, it interferes with the ability of the cancer cell to repair DNA or replicate. Cytosine arabinoside can cross the blood-brain barrier, which means that it can enter the nervous tissue in the brain and spinal cord. This makes it useful for lymphomas that are "hiding" in those tissues.

Cytosine arabinoside attacks cancer during the replication phase of the cell cycle (the S-phase or synthesis phase), only. To make sure the drug kills as many cancer cells as possible, it is dripped from an IV continuously over a long period of time, sometimes twelve or even twenty-four hours. Your dog is in the hospital during the entire course of treatment. Some oncologists avoid hospitalizing dogs, by dividing the dose into two to four fractions, which are given by subcutaneous injection over two days.

Some vomiting and diarrhea occur with cytosine arabinoside, and the main side effect is bone marrow suppression, which must be monitored with follow up CBCs.

Methotrexate

Another antimetabolite is methotrexate, which is used in some lymphoma protocols. Methotrexate works by blocking folic acid, an important nutrient, needed to build new cancer cell DNA. The most common side effects are gastrointestinal; it may cause

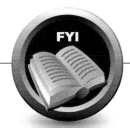

Chemotherapy and Dividing Cancer Cells

When a cell reproduces, it copies itself and divides in two. All cells, including cancer cells, go through the same series of steps when they do this. These steps, taken together, are called the cell cycle.

Each step in the cell cycle builds on the one before. If something goes wrong at any step along the way, reproduction may halt completely or, depending upon when the problem occurs, there may be permanent damage to the cell's DNA, preventing later replication or even causing cell death. Chemotherapy drugs, by and large, work by interrupting the cell cycle at one of these steps. Because actively dividing cells are more sensitive to DNA damage, chemotherapy is most effective against rapidly dividing tumors.

To vastly over-simplify the cell cycle for our purposes, the basic steps are these:

- The cell takes in nutrition and grows, accumulating the enzymes, ribonucleic acid (RNA), and proteins necessary for division. This phase is called the Gap 1 or G_1 phase.

- The cell uses proteins to duplicate its DNA, using a substance called ribonucleic acid (RNA), which is similar in form and function to DNA. The process of DNA replication is complex and involves many steps, each of which must be performed perfectly. This is called the Synthesis or S phase.

- The cell continues to grow and readies itself for the cell division. This is called the Gap 2 or G_2 phase and is the second period of RNA and protein synthesis.

- The cell stops growing and splits itself into two separate cells. These are sometimes called "daughter" cells, and each has (ideally) its own identical copy of the original cell's DNA. This is called the Mitosis or M phase.

- The cell stops dividing and enters a resting phase, during which it is relatively quiet and inactive. This is called the Gap 0 or G_0 phase, and it lasts until the cell must divide again, when the cycle starts over.

continued on next page

Chemotherapy and Dividing Cancer Cells, *continued*

Most chemotherapy drugs work by attacking the cell, while it prepares for mitosis, by damaging the DNA and/or RNA. Depending upon the drug's actions and where in the cell cycle it has its affect, chemotherapy can stop cell division, kill the cell directly and/or induce apoptosis (natural cell suicide). As you'll find out, some of the common chemotherapy drugs work only during very specific phases of the cell cycle. Thus, they may be given to your dog over a long period of time – 12 to 24 hours – so that the drug has a chance to kill as many cancer cells as possible as they pass through the sensitive phase of the cell cycle.

You'll remember that cancer cells have a survival advantage over normal cells because they divide without regulation, becoming more susceptible to chemotherapy drugs. That's why oncologists typically turn to chemotherapy when a tumor is rapidly dividing or at a high risk for metastasis. This is also an explanation for chemotherapy's expected side effects: rapidly dividing cells, including the hair follicle, the lining of the gastro-intestinal tract and the white blood cells, are often affected by chemotherapy drugs.

Tumors are typically found when they are about one centimeter in diameter, and this does not seem large to most owners or vets. But realize: a one-centimeter tumor contains about one billion cancer cells!

There's another problem with these one-centimeter tumors. By the time a tumor reaches this size, a significant number of its cells have entered the G_0 or resting phase, and are therefore resistant to chemotherapy. Of course, those cells usually rejoin the cell cycle and become sensitive to chemotherapy again, which is why we give chemotherapy treatments over time.

---

severe nausea, vomiting and diarrhea.

Methotrexate can also cause low red blood cell counts (anemia) and, with high doses, liver toxicity and kidney damage.

Antitumor Metabolites

The antitumor metabolites are another class of drugs, which include a type called anthracyclines. Anthracyclines work in several phases of the cell cycle, to cross-link DNA strands and alter the function of the enzyme topoisomerase type II, which winds and unwinds DNA during replication. Some anthracyclines,

such as doxorubicin, can also produce free radicals, which damage DNA and the cell's membrane.

Doxorubicin

Doxorubicin (brand name Adriamycin) is an extremely powerful chemotherapy drug that is used in many protocols. Used alone or in combination with other drugs, it's the basis of protocols for lymphoma, osteosarcoma, hemangiosarcoma, mammary cancer and a wide variety of carcinomas.

One of the ways doxorubicin kills cancer cells is by generating free radicals. Those free radicals create oxidation, which harms cancer cells, so you do not want to counteract that oxidation with mega-doses of antioxidants. As Dr. Dressler has discussed throughout this book, antioxidants sometimes interfere with chemotherapy drugs, and doxorubicin is the classic example of this phenomenon. If your dog is on doxorubicin, do not give antioxidants or substances that act like antioxidants; stop them one week before and one week after doxorubicin.

Doxorubicin is a fluid, administered by IV, directly into a vein through an indwelling catheter. Like Mustargen, it is a potent vesicant and causes severe damage to skin and other tissues. These injuries, in some severe cases, can require surgery to repair, and the tissue is typically slow to heal. For this reason, the drug must be directly injected into a vein and always through an indwelling IV catheter that is carefully placed for proper and safe administration.

Doxorubicin can cause expected side effects, such as hair loss, nausea, vomiting, diarrhea and bone marrow suppression (all discussed in Chapter 11). It can also cause an acute (sudden) allergic reaction in the body called anaphylaxis. During anaphylaxis, the immune system reacts to the drug by releasing histamines (the same thing can happen to people or dogs with "allergies," when an environmental allergen like pollen is encountered).

Rarely, anaphylaxis occurs during administration. Symptoms include vomiting, red skin, itchiness and difficulty breathing. Anaphylaxis can be treated with antihistamines, like diphenhydramine (brand name Benadryl) or corticosteroids. Symptoms usually reverse in the treatment room, and do not recur at home.

To avoid anaphylaxis, I recommend giving antihistamines before administering doxorubicin. Slow administration of the drug over twenty to thirty minutes also helps lower the chances that your dog will have an allergic reaction. In addition, I use Adriamy-

cin, rather than the generic form of doxorubicin, because published data show that it causes less anaphylaxis. In one study, thirty-four dogs were given both Adriamycin and the generic form. While Adriamycin caused zero side effects, the generic form caused itchiness, head-shaking, red skin, vocalization, vomiting, and high heart and breathing rates in thirteen out of the thirty-four afflicted dogs (44%). If you are going to use this potent drug, I strongly recommend using Adriamycin rather than the generic.

There is a risk for heart problems on doxorubicin. In the short term, abnormal heart rhythms (arrhythmias) can develop. These usually only occur during the actual administration of the drug, and cease when the treatment is over. The slow administration I recommend helps to reduce the likelihood of arrhythmias.

Chronic heart problems can also develop from using multiple doses of doxorubicin (more than six to eight doses) and sometimes these are long term, showing up months or years after treatments have ended. For example, dilated cardiomyopathy (DCM) can occur, a serious condition in which the heart grows enlarged and weakened and cannot pump blood effectively. As the body gets less blood supply, heart failure can occur or shortness of breath, coughing, swelling and lethargy can be experienced. Obviously, the quality of life can really plummet as a result of this condition.

DCM and other heart problems rarely occur as a result of just one dose of doxorubicin, and they are usually not seen, if the doses are limited. For this reason, I recommend no more than six to eight doses of doxorubicin. I also check for pre-existing heart problems before using doxorubicin, and weigh the decision carefully, when such a history exists. I also take extra care with deep-chested or giant breeds, because some are predisposed to heart disease (Dobermans and Boxers, for example).

Some oncologists recommend administering dexrazoxane (an iron chelator) just before administering doxorubicin because it can reduce the risk of heart toxicity. This combination is generally well tolerated, with minimal side effects, so I use this drug, also, when I suspect heart toxicity might be a problem. However, I decide on a case-by-case basis, because it is not yet known whether dexrazoxane's antioxidant properties interfere with doxorubicin's efficacy.

To protect your dog from infection, due to possible bone marrow suppression, I consider the use of preventative antibiotics. A recent study revealed that dogs with lymphoma and osteosarcoma, who received preventative antibiotics to help with bone marrow suppression, had lower hospitalization rates, lower toxicity and performed better overall.

Doxorubicin is more likely than some other chemotherapy drugs to affect appetite and/or cause nausea, vomiting or diarrhea. For this reason, I routinely recommend preventative oral medications (maropitant, brand name Cerenia) for the four days after treatment. This decision is validated by a recent placebo-controlled study in which dogs on the placebo experienced more and more severe vomiting and diarrhea than the dogs on Cerenia.

Doxorubicin is a powerful chemotherapy agent, and it's used in quite a few protocols because it can be very effective. The decision to use it is a complicated one, and must be considered carefully and in deep consultation with your vet or oncologist.

Also, keep in mind that it is broken down in the liver and excreted in the feces – so take extra care when you clean up after your dog (as outlined on page 134).

Mitoxantrone

Mitoxantrone is another anthracycline. It's used alone or in combination protocols to treat lymphoma, some sarcomas and some carcinomas, including anal sac adenocarcinoma and transitional cell carcinoma (TCC). Mitoxantrone is not as effective for lympho-

mas as doxorubicin; however, it is sometimes used as a replacement because it is not as toxic to the heart. For other cancers, like TCC, it is the drug of choice.

The most common side effect of mitoxantrone is bone marrow suppression. It usually lowers white blood cell counts, sometimes to severe levels. Other expected side effects, like nausea, vomiting and diarrhea, are typically mild.

Because it does not form free radicals, it is all right to use antioxidants with mitoxantrone.

Mitoxantrone is an irritant and must be injected directly into a vein. If it does contact other tissues, however, it is not as damaging as Mustargen and doxorubicin, and the damage can usually be treated topically.

Mitoxantrone is a distinctive blue liquid, so you may see a bluish hue to your dog's urine, or you may see the whites of his eyes turn a light shade of blue. This is normal and not considered toxic.

Enzymes

There is a type of chemotherapy drug that uses enzymes to battle cancer. One that I use in dogs with cancer is L-asparaginase (also called Elspar).

L-asparaginase

Instead of directly killing cancer cells, L-asparaginase breaks down asparagine, an amino acid and a building block for proteins. When asparagine breaks down, the cancer cell cannot create the necessary proteins to make DNA and RNA, so it cannot replicate. Healthy body cells can manufacture their own asparagine; tumor cells cannot. Because of this, L-asparaginase preferentially targets tumors without damaging other body cells.

L-asparaginase is used to treat lymphoma and lymphoid leukemia. It is given as an injection, typically into the muscles or under the skin (not as an IV injection). Dogs tolerate Elspar very well. It does not cause low cell counts, unless it is given with vincristine, and side effects, such as nausea, vomiting and diarrhea, are uncommon and usually mild.

There are a few important side effects to consider when using L-asparaginase. The first is anaphylaxis (allergic reaction). When an allergic reaction occurs, it usually happens after repeated treatments, and within thirty minutes after the treatment has ended, so your dog must be monitored for swelling, red skin and itchiness after receiving L-asparaginase. I keep my patients for observation for 30 minutes after treatment and also give antihistamines and/or steroids before treatment to counteract allergic effects. Anaphylaxis is rare, but the risk increases with repeated doses. (I use this agent often, and I have never had an episode.)

Pancreatitis, or inflammation of the pancreas, is another rare side effect to watch for. Your dog may be at risk if he has ever had pancreatitis before, so monitor your dog at home for symptoms such as abdominal pain, nausea, vomiting and fever. Call your vet immediately when any of these signs develop.

In a few cases, abnormal blood clotting (too much or too little, depending upon the case) can be a problem with L-asparaginase, particularly if your pet has clotting issues related to lymphoma.

Plant Alkaloids

Plant alkaloids are often used in chemotherapy treatments. They are sometimes referred to as vinca drugs because they are commonly derived from the periwinkle plant (vinca is the Latin name for periwinkle). Plant alkaloids disrupt the cell's ability to divide by interfering with the mitosis phase of the cell cycle.

Vincristine

Vincristine is the most commonly used plant alkaloid. Lymphoma and some sarcoma protocols combine it with other drugs, while transmissible venereal tumor protocols use it as a single agent.

Side effects like nausea, vomiting and diarrhea are usually mild, as is constipation, and vincristine is typically tolerated well. Bone marrow suppression and hair loss are not common side effects, although they can occur.

Vincristine is metabolized in the liver and excreted in the bile, which exits the body in the feces, so make sure you clean up after your dog carefully, according to the safety instructions on page 134. If your dog has a liver condition or disease, the dose of vincristine may need to be significantly lower, so check with your vet or oncologist, if this is true for your dog.

Like doxorubicin, vincristine is toxic to tissues when not injected directly into a vein. Though the damage it causes is typically not as severe as that of doxorubicin, it can still be severe enough to warrant extreme caution on the part of your vet or oncologist.

Vincristine occasionally damages the nerves, causing a condition called peripheral neuropathy, or temporary weakness and wobbliness when trying to move or stand.

Vinblastine

Another commonly used plant alkaloid is vinblastine, which is often used in lymphoma and mast cell tumor protocols. Much like vincristine, vinblastine can cause tissue damage when not injected directly into the vein.

Unlike vincristine, vinblastine can suppress the bone marrow, so follow up appointments to draw blood and run a CBC are very important. Other side effects include nausea, vomiting, diarrhea, loss of appetite and hair loss. Because vinblastine is metabolized by the liver and excreted in the feces, be very careful cleaning up after your dog and follow the safety instructions in Chapter 11. Your vet or oncologist may need to reduce your dog's dose if she has a liver condition.

Vinorelbine

Vinorelbine (brand name Navelbine) is another plant alkaloid from the vinca family. It's a newer drug, a "second generation" vinca drug (which means that it is a refinement of the first generation drugs like vincristine and vinblastine), and is particularly useful for lung tumors. It is metabolized in the liver, so your dog's doses may need to be reduced if he has a liver condition, and you must be extra careful when cleaning up after him.

Like its older sister drugs, vinorelbine is a severe vesicant, which must be injected directly into the vein to avoid tissue damage. Other side effects can include hair loss, nausea, vomiting, diarrhea and bone marrow suppression.

Platinum-based Chemotherapy

Another group of chemotherapy drugs is platinum-based. The beautiful white metal can be compounded (mixed) and administered as a fluid, directly into the vein. These drugs create cross-links, or bind strands of DNA together, so that they cannot separate from each other later during cell division. The two most common platinum compounds are cisplatin and carboplatin.

Cisplatin

Cisplatin can be used to treat osteosarcoma, some carcinomas (including squamous cell carcinoma), bladder tumors, and nasal cancers. This is a very toxic chemotherapy drug, and I personally do not use it in my practice because of its severe toxic side effects,

the complexity of its administration protocol, and my worries about staff safety.

Administering cisplatin is a daylong process. Beforehand, a CBC will be performed to check for normal blood cell counts. Cisplatin is hard on the kidneys, so the oncologist will also check the kidney markers and get a urine sample to see its concentration. If the bone marrow and kidneys seem able to handle the treatment, IV fluids are given at very high rates in order to cause diuresis, or increased urine production through the kidneys. Cisplatin is excreted in the urine, so these extra fluids (given both before and after treatment) keep the drug from resting in the kidneys and causing irreversible kidney damage, which is one of cisplatin's worst side effects.

Both because of the diuresis and the cisplatin, dogs urinate a great deal during and after treatment, which is why hospitals must keep the dog in a special cage that drains urine away. Staff must be very careful not to touch this urine directly, as it is toxic.

Cisplatin is not a particularly expensive drug, but the intensive procedures and the other medications needed to administer it can make it expensive to use.

In addition to the need to void large fluid volumes for hours on end, dogs also experience nausea and vomiting during treatment. Anti-nausea and anti-vomiting drugs are a required part of the protocol to counteract these side effects.

In addition to these side effects, some dogs experience severe bone marrow suppression. Hair loss may also occur, and nerve damage in the ear may (rarely), too, which results in permanent hearing loss and/or loss of balance and wobbliness while walking.

For all of these reasons, I prefer carboplatin when a platinum-based chemotherapy drug is needed.

Carboplatin

Carboplatin is used to treat sarcomas, including osteosarcoma, and some carcinomas. It's a newer platinum-based drug with fewer and much less severe side effects than cisplatin. It is expensive (although not as expensive as it once was); on the other hand, it doesn't require daylong hospitalization, extra staff or extra IV fluids.

Carboplatin is an IV drug. It can also be injected straight into the chest or abdominal cavity, which is sometimes helpful for dogs with large effusions accumulating in either cavity.

Unlike cisplatin, carboplatin does not directly damage the kidneys, does not cause vomiting during administration and does not require an extensive diuresis procedure. It takes ten to fifteen minutes to inject the drug, making it a much less intense than cisplatin.

The main side effect is bone marrow suppression, especially the white blood cells and platelets. While most chemotherapy drugs show bone marrow suppression after seven days, carboplatin takes ten to fourteen days. Checking on the bone marrow with a CBC is a standard follow up, as is monitoring your dog at home for easy bruising or bleeding problems. Your oncologist may also recommend antibiotics (see the doxorubicin section for details).

While carboplatin does not directly damage the kidneys like cisplatin does, it is ultimately cleared from the body through the kidneys and the urine. If your dog has kidney problems, your oncologist will likely reduce the dose to decrease the chance of side effects.

Tyrosine kinase inhibitors

Tyrosine kinase inhibitors, also known as TKIs or c-Kit inhibitors, are a relatively new class of drugs that offer targeted therapy. While most of the drugs we've talked about so far kill all rapidly dividing cells – including normal cells – TKIs target cells with specific mutations, or with abnormal proteins found only in some cancer cells. They leave most normal cells alone.

There are variations among TKI drugs and, therefore, differences in their effect on different patients' tumors. Three TKIs have been successfully used in dogs: imatinib (brand name Gleevec), masitinib (brand name Kinavet CA-1) and toceranib (brand name Palladia).

We are starting to use TKIs in combination with more traditional chemotherapy drugs. The hope is that, by giving them at the same time, or in alternating rounds of therapies, the more specific actions taken by TKIs will kill more tumor cells, help inhibit new blood vessel formation and increase the length of remissions. Of course, more drugs mean more potential toxic side effects, so this decision must be made carefully and on a case-by-case basis.

Palladia

Palladia is the first chemotherapy drug approved by the FDA specifically for use in dogs (all other chemotherapy drugs are human drugs that we have learned how to use effectively in dogs). Palladia is approved for mast cell tumors, specifically those of grade II and III, with or without regional lymph node involvement. Any other use of Palladia is technically off-label (but as always, vets can prescribe any medication for any condition they judge safe and appropriate).

Palladia targets mast cell tumors in two ways: it kills them directly by targeting the mutation, and also inhibits their ability to build new blood vessels. When looking at all of the original safety and efficacy trials as a whole, about 60% of the dogs experienced their mast cell tumors disappearing, regressing or stabilizing. Their overall health was also improved.

It is unlikely that one drug is all a dog needs to fight cancer. We must attack from different angles, using drugs with different mechanisms. For most MCT patients, I recommend a protocol that uses Palladia with other MCT drugs. These protocols are now being developed, evaluated, and optimized.

Palladia comes in pill form and is administered at home, usually every other day; it is still a powerful chemotherapy agent. Its use requires office visits, so your vet or oncologist can monitor your dog for problems. Regular visits, particularly for the first six to eight weeks will include full physical examinations, monitoring of body weight changes, blood work including CBCs and chemistry panels, and a fecal test for blood in the stool.

The most common side effects dogs experience on Palladia are nausea, vomiting and diarrhea. Lack of appetite, lethargy, lameness, weight loss and perforations (ulcers) in the stomach or intestines have also been reported. To detect a perforation, look for black or tarry feces and/or blood in the feces or vomit. Side effects can be serious, and when this or any other symptom is experienced, stop Palladia immediately and call your vet for advice.

It should be noted that most side effects occur within the first six weeks, and your oncologist may need to make dose adjustments, or even take a break for a week or two. In my own practice, I can find the right dose for the majority of dogs. Dogs are usually on Palladia for a minimum of six months, but I have managed some patients on the drug for greater than a year.

While Dr. Dressler has heard some real horror stories from readers about Palladia, I have found it to be no more problematic than other chemotherapy drugs, especially when handled by an experienced oncologist. I recommend watching your dog closely for side effects, committing to regular office visits, and asking your vet for advice on how to manage your dog proactively. It's a good idea to discuss possible side effects before you start Palladia, so you can really understand what to look for. Palladia must be handled very carefully according to the safe handling instructions in Chapter 11.

I am very excited by the addition of this drug to

our arsenal. Although it was approved specifically for MCT, oncologists including myself have used Palladia to treat other cancers, with promising results. Palladia's anti-angiogenic effects make it an excellent candidate for metronomic chemotherapy (see page 137). Data presented recently at the annual Veterinary Cancer Society meeting demonstrated its efficacy in OSA, anal sac carcinoma and thyroid carcinoma. As we continue to use this drug, we'll find out more about its potential for both traditional and metronomic chemotherapy.

Masitinib

Another tyrokinase inhibitor is masitinib (brand name Kinavet CA-1). Masitinib is a new drug in the United States (conditionally approved by the FDA in December of 2010), which had already been approved in Europe for mast cell tumors. Masitinib targets some of the same tyrosine kinase receptors (c-Kit) Palladia does, and also some cell structures involved in angiogenesis. Masitinib has been safely combined with other traditional chemotherapy drugs, when used in Europe (or in the U.S. through the FDA's compassionate use program). It has similar side effects to Palladia, including vomiting, diarrhea, low blood cell counts, low blood proteins and increased liver markers. Dogs sometimes develop resistance or intolerance to Palladia, in which case they may be helped by masitinib.

Gleevec

You may have heard of Gleevec, the brand name version of imatinib; in 2001 it was approved for use in humans for chronic myeloid leukemia (CML), a cancer of the white blood cells. This TKI targets an abnormal cellular protein, present in nearly all CML patients, called BCR-ABL. When normal, BCR-ABL is much less active than in the mutated form found in CML patients. This mutation seems to be involved in CML, and blocking its activity helps kill the leukemia cells. In 2002, Gleevec was also approved to treat a rare form of stomach cancer in humans, called gastrointestinal stromal tumor (GIST). Gleevec can also be used to treat mast cell tumors in dogs. It has similar side effects to Palladia, including vomiting, diarrhea, low blood cell counts, low blood proteins and increased liver markers.

Other Drugs

Corticosteroids (cortisol-based hormones) are often used in chemotherapy protocols. Many protocols use them in combination with other drugs.

Prednisone/Prednisolone

The steroid prednisone is converted to prednisolone in the liver. It can be used alone for lymphoma treatments, or in combination with other drugs in chemotherapy protocols.

Prednisone/prednisolone is an anti-inflammatory, which is why it can be so effective in treating cancer. As cancer creates inflammation in and around the tumor, reducing it often makes your dog more comfortable.

Prednisone is inexpensive, especially compared to other chemotherapy drugs, and it is used to treat many other diseases and conditions, so it feels familiar to many owners. Unlike other chemotherapy agents, prednisone can be handled with bare hands and does not make your dog's leavings toxic. It can be given at home in pill form. Prednisone does have a lot of side effects, which are usually mild, in comparison to other drugs used for cancer.

The most common and expected side effects include excessive thirst, urination and appetite. There can also be dark or black stools from stomach ulcers, loss of muscle, and immune suppression, which can leave your dog open to infections. Some dogs also experience increased panting. Long-term use can cause thinning of the hair and coat, changes in the skin color, and a "pot-belly." Other problems that can happen over time include diabetes, liver problems, kidney problems, and muscle loss or wasting, so it is best to limit its chronic use.

Prednisone should never be combined with other anti-inflammatory drugs like aspirin, ibuprofen, any other NSAIDs (non-steroidal anti-inflammatory drugs), carprofen (brand name Rimadyl), meloxicam (brand name Metacam), deracoxib (brand name Deramaxx), Tylenol with codeine, other corticosteroids like methylprednisolone or budesonide, or piroxicam (brand name Feldene). This is because all of these drugs have a potential to cause stomach ulcers, and combining any of them with prednisone can increase that risk. Using Apocaps with prednisone warrants special instructions, which can be found on page 169.

Another consideration, when using prednisone, is the potential necessity to taper off usage. After seven days of using prednisone, the body significantly decreases its own corticosteroid production. If prednisone is stopped abruptly, the body can be thrown into a kind of shock, with symptoms like nausea, vomiting, weakness, pain and fever. Tapering the use of prednisone, however, allows the adrenal glands (which produce corticosteroids) to gradually increase steroid production. This helps your dog's hormones to stay in balance. The longer you have used prednisone, the longer the tapering period, so check with your vet or oncologist.

Prednisone can be a very good, inexpensive option for some owners, although its use is complicated by many factors. Make sure you and your vet take all of your dog's health conditions into account as you decide whether to use prednisone.

Piroxicam

Piroxicam (brand name Feldene) is a non-steroidal anti-inflammatory drug (NSAID) that is commonly used in vet practices as an anti-inflammatory, for pain relief and to reduce fever. It is prescribed as an anti-cancer agent for transitional cell carcinoma and oral squamous cell carcinoma.

Piroxicam inhibits the growth of some tumors, apparently by shutting down an important enzyme called cyclooxygenase (COX-2). COX-2 converts certain acids into prostaglandins, which are known to promote tumor cell growth. They also promote the development of new blood vessels and immune suppression, which allows tumors to thrive. By inhibiting COX-2, prostaglandins are inhibited, so tumor growth can be slowed.

Piroxicam can be given at home in pill form and is not toxic to handle.

When piroxicam is used, it's important to monitor your dog for ulcers and gastro-intestinal bleeding. These symptoms include decreased appetite, vomiting (with or without blood), black and tarry stools, and diarrhea. If any of these symptoms crop up, stop giving piroxicam and call your vet or oncologist. The problems usually end soon after medication is stopped, but some temporary medications may be prescribed to help the ulcers heal.

To reduce the risk of ulcers, give piroxicam with food. You should also follow the dosing instructions exactly; even a small overdose can result in severe toxicity. If your dog is smaller than 70 pounds, your vet will need to get you compounded pills to accurately dose her. I often prescribe misoprostol to take along with piroxicam, because it can help prevent ulcers.

Some dogs, receiving high doses of piroxicam, have developed kidney toxicity, and long-term administration can cause irreversible damage. The kidney values and urine must be regularly monitored (every four to six weeks) while on this drug, and if your dog develops kidney issues, the dose must be lowered or the drug stopped. The medication must not be used at all, if your dog has pre-existing kidney disease.

Piroxicam can sometimes affect the function of the platelets, which leads to a lack of coagulation in the blood. This can cause bleeding that is difficult to stop, so make sure you report any history of a bleeding disorder to your vet before using piroxicam. It's also a good idea to stop piroxicam a few days before surgery to prevent bleeding issues on the operating table, but check with your veterinarian or surgeon for specific recommendations.

Piroxicam must not be used with any other anti-inflammatory or NSAID, including aspirin, ibuprofen, carprofen (brand name Rimadyl), meloxicam (brand name Metacam), deracoxib (brand name Deramaxx), Tylenol with codeine, prednisone, methylprednisolone or budesonide. All of these drugs potentially cause stomach ulcers, and combining any with prednisone can really increase this risk. Using Apocaps with piroxicam warrants special instructions, which can be found on page 169. If your dog has ever been sensitive to or allergic to any of these medications, do not use piroxicam.

Human in a Dog Suit

"Angus is a nine year-old Golden Doodle. He's the best dog we have ever had. We've always said he's like a human in a dog suit. He's always been there for us, always attentive, always ready to put his head on your lap, always ready to give love. Plus, he was fast. He looked like a thoroughbred when he ran. In June of 2010, my wife, Barb, was down at our house on the beach helping our daughter start up a restaurant and noticed him limping and staying off his rear leg. She drove him down to our "beach vet" to be checked and was diagnosed with osteosarcoma. He was one of the favorites at the vet's office and all of the "girls" who worked there were bawling along with my wife. When Barb got him back to the house, she called me and told me to sit down and laid it out -- the vet had said that, without treatment, Angus' prognosis was 6 -8 weeks as this was an extremely aggressive and lethal cancer. We must have cried on the phone for two hours. At the time, it was one of the most gut-wrenching things we had been through. It paled, however, compared to the death of our son, Dave, 5-months later (for which there is no comparison). Barb's someone that springs to action. She got on the phone and made an appointment with a leading veterinary oncologist in the Raleigh area (where we live), wrapped up a bunch of restaurant-related details, found Dr. Dresser's book on the internet and sent me the link, packed up her truck and got him back for a consultation. After consultation with the specialist, we signed up for amputation and a 4-week course of carboplatin, hearing that it could extend his life by 6 months and, maybe if we were lucky, a year. I printed out Dr. Dresser's book, put it in a 3-ring binder, and started reading. I had always been big into supplements, so was drawn to the chapters on alternative therapies. I probably read those chapters about 10 times before it started sinking in and we started off adding just a couple supplements to his meals and giving him purified water instead of tap water. Angus went in for amputation surgery on July 1, 2010 and we spent a long 4th of July weekend lying on the floor with him to reassure him and keep him from chewing his stiches out. Obviously, the wound was pretty gross. Like all good dogs, he kept licking our faces after we had just brought him in to have a leg chopped off. Cancer mechanisms and alternative treatments became our new obsession; I spent hours researching after work every night, reading Dr. Andrew Weill, Dr. Russell Blaylock, internet blog after internet blog, and as many clinical studies and papers I could find on medicinal mushrooms and artemisinin. Surprisingly, I found

continued on next page

Human in a Dog Suit, continued

Suzanne Somers' book Knockout to be superb. The more research we did, the more we fine-tuned Angus' regimen. I'm now a big believer in the theory of dogs self-medicating. We've never had to force pills down Angus' throat. He either eats them with his dinner or out of our hand...I persuade myself that he does this because he senses it will help cure his cancer. It's now 10 months since Angus was diagnosed. He has had to survive the stress of our grieving the loss of our son. And the stress of that event on him -- he knows...But, we have doubled our efforts to support Angus in dealing with his cancer. We aren't willing to lose two of our "boys" in the same year. Angus has been back to the oncologist twice for scans to see whether the cancer has spread (most dogs with osteosarcoma die when it spreads to their lungs). On both earlier visits, nothing showed on the scans and his blood counts were phenomenally good. He's still bright eyed and has a good appetite. We want to get him another summer at the beach. He's a great dog, a great friend. He deserves it."

- Al Marzetti, Raleigh, North Carolina

Part VI: Appendices

In this section you will find several helpful appendices. Appendix A contains all of the supplements Dr. Dressler recommends, in the general order of their importance. Appendix B describes supplements which are not included in Full Spectrum cancer care, for various reasons. Appendix C contains the resources Dr. Dressler recommends for purchasing supplements, finding out more information, or doing further research. Appendix D contains some advice for guardians curious about cancer prevention, and Appendix E lists the scientific and medical research citations used to write this book.

Appendix A:
The Supplement Hierarchy

by Dr. Demian Dressler, DVM

If you are working within a budget, or if your dog doesn't love taking pills, you may have to select supplements carefully. This appendix answers the common question "Which supplement or supplements are most important for my dog?" I've listed each supplement I recommend below, in their order of priority.

Just because a supplement is lower on the hierarchy, doesn't mean it is unimportant, however. To get my recommendation, supplements must have credible evidence for benefitting the majority of dogs with cancer. If you look at Appendix B, you'll see many supplements, which were excluded from Full Spectrum cancer care, even some generally beneficial supplements, and some which may be helpful for a small number of dogs. I excluded these because I don't like to overuse supplements, unnecessarily duplicate their actions and, most importantly, because most guardians just want to give the best, most helpful agents. Also, I excluded many supplements which are antioxidants with no or little evidence for direct anti-cancer benefits because they can interfere with more important pro-oxidant therapeutics, as discussed in Chapter 8.

The highest priority supplements in the Full Spectrum hierarchy are those which manage the common and expected side effects of chemotherapy and radiation treatments. If you are not using these treatments, or if your dog is not experiencing the named side effects, you can skip those supplements.

Carefully consider each of these supplements for interactions with other medications, conditions and cancer treatments, and, as always, I recommend checking with your veterinarian or oncologist to get her advice.

The Full Spectrum Supplement Hierarchy

Here are the supplements I recommend, in order of importance.

First Priority: Full Spectrum Side Effect Management

Guardians can use these supplements to help manage the side effects from chemotherapy or radiation, which is priority number one. If your dog is not suffering these symptoms or is not receiving these treatments, skip to Full Spectrum Nutraceuticals.

Fresh ginger root, useful for nausea and vomiting, see page 144 for details and precautions

Cimetidine, useful for nausea and vomiting, see page 145 for details and precautions

Glutamine, useful for healing after vomiting and diarrhea, also for weight loss due to cancer cachexia, see page 146 for details and precautions

Cordyceps, useful for protecting the kidneys and liver when using chemotherapy drugs known to adversely affect these organs, see page 148 for details and precautions

Coenzyme Q10, useful for protecting the heart when using chemotherapy drugs known to adversely affect this organ, see page 149 for details and precautions

Second Priority: Full Spectrum Nutraceuticals

Here are the recommended nutraceuticals, listed in order of their importance.

Apocaps, useful for most dogs, see Chapter 12 for details and precautions

Artemisinin, useful for some dogs, may be rotated with Apocaps, see Chapter 12 for details and precautions

Neoplasene, may be useful as a salvage technique, may be used along with Apocaps, see Chapter 12 for details and precautions

Third Priority: Other Full Spectrum Supplements

Here are the other recommended supplements, listed in their order of importance.

Mushroom-derived polysaccharides, useful for most dogs, especially when used with the product called Transfer Factor, see page 181 for details and precautions

Krill oil and/or fish oil, useful for most dogs, see page 202 for details and precautions

Dietary enzymes (used to pre-digest food), useful for most dogs, see page 207 for details and precautions

Modified citrus pectin, useful for most dogs, see page 190 for details and precautions

General Multivitamin, useful for most dogs (and strongly recommended if you are feeding a completely home-cooked diet), see page 186 for details and precautions

Doxycycline, useful for most dogs, see page 192 for details and precautions

Open Your Eyes and Mind

"Do not listen to the conventional wisdom of most vets. Open your eyes and your mind to alternatives that you and your dog are comfortable with. After all, this is your life and your dog's life and we should all be free to choose our own paths. Most importantly never let your dog suffer. In the end the result is the same and we learn to deal with the loss. First a day at a time and then a week and then a month. Eventually you will look back and know that for all those years your dog was your faithful companion and best friend you were able to give back by helping your dog live life to the fullest to the very end."

- Roxanna Davis, Apopka, Florida

Appendix B:
Excluded Supplements

by Dr. Demian Dressler, DVM

Many dog lovers are willing to try just about anything when their dogs have cancer, and there are many supplements purported to be good for cancer that I have assessed but decided to exclude from this book.

To make my Full Spectrum recommendations, I've spent a lot of time getting past the hype, the marketing, and the often-passionate online discussions. My recommendations are for foods and supplements you can manage at home, which have the biggest impact on dogs with cancer, and which are helpful for most dogs and most dog cancers.

Even so, I know you may have heard about supplements that aren't included in my recommendations. To keep you informed and let you know more about the way I think, here is a list of some of the major supplements I rejected for inclusion.

The reasons for rejection vary, and may include one or more of the following:

- **Might interfere with more important therapies.** As I stated in the sidebar on page 249, the first priority in Full Spectrum care is targeting cancer cells, followed by boosting the immune system. For example, supplements with strong antioxidant properties may interfere with important pro-oxidant therapies (such as chemotherapy, radiation, Apocaps and other apoptogens). If a supplement with antioxidant benefits does not have an anti-cancer effect, or if it has evidence for interfering with primary therapies that have known benefits, I rejected it.

- **Unconvincing evidence.** The supplement needs more than anecdotal evidence that it helps cancer. If it has only anecdotal evidence, it must have many reported successes. If not, the supplement was rejected.

- **Not effective when given by mouth.** Some supplements are effective when given by injection, but not by mouth. If the sup-

plement cannot be given by mouth and be effective, it was rejected.

- **Bioavailability issues when taken by mouth.** If the supplement is not absorbed into the bloodstream, or if the intestines and/or the liver break down the active ingredient before it gets into the bloodstream, the supplement was rejected.

- **Questionable safety.** I will not recommend a supplement unless my extensive research has demonstrated its safety. If a supplement did not have a healthy margin of safety based on known data, I rejected it.

- **Batch variability.** The supplement must have a uniform amount of active ingredient in each batch. Some supplements are cut with fillers, or may not have uniform amounts of the active ingredient in each batch or pill due to seasonal or regional differences. Depending upon many factors, this variability could reduce efficacy or even create a danger to the dog. Such supplements were rejected.

- **Unsafe with commonplace treatments.** Some supplements can cause more serious problems, when combined with other medications or treatments. These were excluded.

- **Impractical dosing requirements.** If a supplement requires a mega-dose to be effective, most guardians will not be able to get their dogs to take the required amount by mouth. These were excluded.

- **Unreasonable pricing.** Every supplement has a price tag, but some supplements are priced so unreasonably high that they were excluded.

- **Research not available in English.** Many supplements from Traditional Chinese Medicine, Ayurvedic Medicine, and aboriginal medicine systems were excluded because original research and medical textbooks are written in languages I cannot read. Because I can't accurately assess their evidence, I did not include them in Full Spectrum care. My hope is that with accelerating global communications I'll learn more in the future. I recommend consulting directly with practitioners from those systems if you are interested in their medicine, so you can get their expert advice.

The following list is not comprehensive; it contains the most popular supplements I rejected. As always, I reserve the right to change my mind and my recommendations as new data emerges.

Here are the most common supplements I considered for inclusion, and the reason(s) I rejected them:

Acai (Euterpe oleracea)

This trendy palm berry has some anti-inflammatory effects, due to the presence of anthocyanins. It also has antioxidant benefits, but those do not outweigh the possibility of interfering with the pro-oxidant supplement Apocaps and pro-oxidant chemotherapy and radiation treatments. Because of this, and because its safety in dogs is not yet known, I do not recommend it. *Not recommended; may not be safe.*

Algae Supplements (various, including Spirulina)

Blue-green algae has some evidence for use in detoxifying carcinogens, but not a huge amount. It is also high in omega-3 fatty acids, but not nearly as high as krill oil and high quality fish oils, which makes the dosing requirements impractical for use in dogs. If your dog does not tolerate fish or krill oil, you might consider using blue-green algae, but otherwise, this is a low-priority supplement. *Low priority supplement; impractical doses.*

Aloe Vera

There is some evidence that aloe vera stimulates the immune system, and it also has some antioxidant effects. There is some evidence for anti-cancer effects, but not enough to convince me to recommend it for that purpose. There is also a bioavailability issue with one of the most promising active ingredients, acemannan, which is difficult to absorb when taken by mouth. Aloe's antioxidant benefits do not outweigh its interfering effects with Apocaps and the pro-oxidant chemotherapy and radiation treatments. *Low priority supplement; antioxidant that may interfere with more important therapeutics; bioavailability issues.*

Antioxidants (Potent Commercial formulations such as MaxGL, Poly MVA)

We've discussed the complicated role pro-oxidants and anti-oxidants play in cancer throughout this book. To restate, Apocaps, pro-oxidant chemotherapy drugs, and radiation therapy may have lower success rates if strong antioxidants are used. For this reason, I do not recommend potent commercial antioxidants that deliver mega-doses. Instead, I recommend offering food rich in naturally occurring antioxidants, and supplemental dietary levels of antioxidants. At these levels, antioxidants have been shown to benefit life quality and increase success. Poly MVA is also very expensive, which is a secondary reason for my excluding it from Full Spectrum cancer care. *Antioxidants may interfere with more important therapeutics; cost-prohibitive.*

Artichoke extracts (Cynara cardunculus)

While components in artichoke extract have demonstrated anti-cancer effects, the number of pills needed is an impractical dose for dogs. Artichoke's active ingredients are included in Apocaps, making a separate supplement redundant. *Redundant as a supplement if taking Apocaps; impractical doses.*

Astralagus (Astralagus membranaceous)

The herb astralagus stimulates the immune system and has an antioxidant effect in the body (so it could interfere with pro-oxidant supplements like Apocaps, chemotherapy and radiation treatments). While there is some evidence that it has direct anti-cancer effects, it is not strong. For these reasons, I consider it a low-priority supplement. The exception would be if your dog does not tolerate medicinal mushrooms, and is not on Apocaps, pro-oxidant chemotherapy drugs, or radiation therapy. *Low-priority supplement.*

Baical Skullcap (Scuttelaria baicalensis)

This herb has a long historical record of use in Traditional Chinese Medicine. Its anti-cancer effects are promising and currently being substantiated in Western medicine. I am excited about the possibilities, but there is not enough data yet to start recommending it across the board. *May recommend in the future.*

Beres Drops

Beres Drops were created as an immune booster, but their efficacy was diminished when the product was reformulated without zinc. Zinc is included in Apocaps, which makes the Beres Drops a low priority. *Efficacy issues as formulated; redundant as a supplement if taking Apocaps.*

Black Tea Supplements

Please see my comments about EGCG and green tea supplements.

Cat's Claw (Uncaria tomentosa)

Cat's Claw is an herb with many reported uses, including as an anti-inflammatory; but the direct anti-cancer evidence is not strong. Because we don't know much about Cat's Claw, including what its active ingredients are, it is difficult to recommend a dosage. Also, published studies show the composition of its compounds can vary from batch to batch, because the plant grows in a variety of places at different times of year. It has antioxidant effects, but they do not outweigh its interfering effects on Apocaps and the pro-oxidant chemotherapy and radiation treatments. These reasons make it a low priority supplement. *Low priority supplement; batch variability; antioxidant that may interfere with more important therapeutics.*

Chamomile (Marticaria)

Components of chamomile have demonstrated anti-cancer effects, but the number of pills needed is impractical for dogs. Chamomile's active ingredients are also included in Apocaps, making the separate supplement redundant. *Redundant as a supplement if taking Apocaps; impractical doses on its own.*

Co Q-10 (Coenzyme Q10, ubiquinone)

This powerful antioxidant, which is found mainly in meat, is recommended on page 149 for dogs with heart-related side effects. For any other case, its antioxidant effects can interfere with the effects of Apocaps, pro-oxidant chemotherapy and radiation treatments. It also has some bioavailability issues, so unless your dog is at risk for cardiac side effects, I do not recommend Co Q-10. *Low priority supplement; antioxidant that may interfere with more important therapeutics; bioavailability issues.*

Cod Liver Oil

As I noted in the omega-3 discussion on page

204, cod liver oil has known toxicity issues in large doses. The dose required to offer meaningful support to dogs with cancer is very high. Using it could overdose dogs with fat-soluble vitamins, leading to toxicity. *Not safe.*

Colloidal Silver

Colloidal silver has antimicrobial effects and may be safe when used in small amounts, but there is little evidence of direct anticancer effects. Large amounts of this product are toxic to several body systems. *Not recommended; not safe.*

Curcumin (Curcuma longa)

I used to recommend the spice curcumin as a separate supplement because of its strong anti-cancer effects. Unfortunately, guardians had to jump through a lot of (rather messy) hoops in their kitchen to overcome bioavailability problems so the curcuminoids, the active ingredients in the spice, could be absorbed into the bloodstream. This difficulty in administration was one of the main reasons I created Apocaps. Curcumin is a primary ingredient in Apocaps, and absorption issues have been resolved. Giving curcumin separately is redundant and difficult. *Redundant as a supplement if taking Apocaps; bioavailability issues.*

Echinacea

This popular herb stimulates natural killer cells in lab animals, but the evidence for direct benefit in actual cancer patients is flimsy. In fact, the real-life evidence of actual immune efficacy when used for infection is also flimsy. Mushroom-derived polysaccharides, or medicinal mushrooms, are a much better choice. If your dog does not tolerate medicinal mushrooms, consider echinacea's use, but keep in mind that it is an antioxidant and may interfere with Apocaps, chemotherapy and radiation treatments. *Low priority supplement.*

EGCG and Green Tea Supplements

I used to recommend EGCG, the active ingredient in green tea, because of its cancer-fighting properties. However, I have since seen what I believe was EGCG interacting with other supplements in toxic ways, which leads me to make it a lower-priority supplement, which in some cases should be avoided altogether. I am cautious about taking EGCG with quercetin (page 422), for example, because clinically my experience is that this combination may have caused anemia in dogs. I do not have any studies to refute or support my experience, but it's a red flag for me. Quercetin is included in Apocaps, so if you are using them, I would avoid EGCG. I also do not recommend unrefined green tea extracts at all, because the stimulants in green tea may be unsafe for some dogs. *Low priority supplement; may not be safe in all dogs.*

Eleuthero (Siberian Ginseng, Eluetherococcus senticosus)

Eleuthero was named Siberian ginseng and has similar effects to ginseng, but it is not actually part of the ginseng family. This herb has a long history of use in Traditional Chinese Medicine for its anti-inflammatory and antioxidant effects; it also helps the body resist stress. While these effects may be helpful for your dog, evidence for direct anti-cancer effects is not as strong as in other supplements I recommend. Because of this, and because of its potential for interfering with pro-oxidant therapies, I give eleuthero a lower priority than other supplements. *Low priority supplement.*

Essiac

Essiac, or Essiac tea, is an herbal blend purported to cure cancer. After in-depth review by several authorities, it does not appear to have any beneficial effects on cancer. In fact, a form of Essiac was found to stimulate the growth of breast cancer cells in vitro.

I do not recommend Essiac in any form. *Not recommended; may not be safe.*

Flax Seed (Linum usitatissimum)

There are published studies demonstrating the anti-cancer effects of flax seeds, but the doses dogs need are huge. This makes it impractical to use for cancer treatments. Omega-3 fatty acids from krill and fish oil are a better choice. *Low priority supplement; impractical doses.*

Garlic (Allium sativim) capsules

Constituents in garlic have demonstrated anti-cancer benefits, which is why it is recommended for use in your dog's diet (see Chapter 14). However, garlic capsules may not be as useful as the actual food, because the active organosulfur compounds can become unstable when processed into a supplement. For this reason, I recommend using garlic in its natural state only, not in capsule form. *May be ineffective in capsule form; instead use natural food as outlined in Dog Cancer Diet.*

(Note: Although it does have antioxidant effects, its anti-cancer effects are more important. I recommend using garlic even if you are also using Apocaps, pro-oxidant chemotherapy, or radiation treatments, under veterinary supervision.)

Ginger supplements (Zingiber officinale)

Constituents in ginger have demonstrated anti-cancer benefits, and ginger is also helpful in managing nausea. For these reasons, I recommend using ginger as an anti-nausea treatment, in your dog's diet, and I have also added gingerols, the active ingredients, to Apocaps. Using pill forms of ginger in addition would be redundant. *Redundant as a supplement if taking Apocaps; use natural food as outlined in Dog Cancer Diet.*

(Note: Although it does have antioxidant effects, ginger's anti-cancer and anti-nausea effects are more important. I recommend using ginger even if you are also using Apocaps, pro-oxidant chemotherapy, or radiation treatments.)

Gingko (Gingko biloba)

There is some evidence that gingko biloba may help some oral tumors, but the overall evidence for direct anti-cancer activity is flimsy. I consider this a very low-priority supplement for most dogs with cancer. *Very low priority supplement.*

Ginseng (Panax ginseng, Panax)

Ginseng is an herb that has a wide variety of uses in Traditional Chinese medicine. It has some direct anti-cancer effects, but the evidence is not as strong as for other supplements I recommend. It also has an antioxidant effect in the body, which makes it a lower-priority supplement due to its interference with pro-oxidant chemotherapy, radiation, and Apocaps. *Low priority supplement.*

Grape Seed Extract (Vitis)

Grape seed extract is sometimes recommended as a cancer supplement, but the data for actual anti-cancer benefits are very limited when compared to other supplements I recommend. Grapes are toxic for dogs, sometimes fatally so, and we do not yet know which specific compound causes that toxicity. For this reason, I recommend avoiding all products containing or extracted from grapes. Grape seed extract also has an antioxidant effect, which makes it less helpful for dogs on pro-oxidant chemotherapy, radiation, or Apocaps. *Low priority supplement; may not be safe for dogs.*

Grapefruit Seed Extracts

There is evidence for grapefruit seed extract being an antimicrobial agent, but naringin and related compounds can affect the metabolism of some pharmaceuticals, including some chemotherapy drugs. There is little evidence for anti-cancer benefits. In addition, the antioxidant benefits do not outweigh its interfering effects on Apocaps and the pro-oxidant therapies, chemotherapy and radiation. For these reasons, I do not recommend grapefruit seed extracts. *Not recommended; unsafe interactions are possible.*

Hoxsey

Hoxsey is a mixture of herbs created by an insurance salesman in the 1920's and promoted as a cure for cancer. It has been found ineffective by several reviewing authorities, including the U.S. Food and Drug Administration (FDA) and the National Cancer Institute. The FDA banned its sale in the United States in 1960, but it is still talked about in online forums. Even Hoxsey didn't believe in the Hoxsey Treatment or Hoxsey Method – he treated his own prostate cancer with conventional medicine. I do not recommend this treatment at all. *Not recommended.*

Indole-3-Carbinol (I3C)

Indole-3-carbinol is a naturally occurring compound found in many vegetables, but especially cruciferous vegetables like brussels sprouts, cabbage and broccoli. Studies have shown it has both anti-carcinogenic and antioxidant effects. However, there is also some evidence that taking indole-3-carbinol as an oral supplement is toxic for dogs. It is for these safety concerns that I have excluded it, as well as the possibility that its antioxidant properties could interfere with important supplements like Apocaps, pro-oxidant chemotherapy and radiation treatments. Instead of using oral supplement forms, I recommend adding cruciferous vegetables to your dog's diet as outlined in Chapter 14. *May not be safe; use natural food sources as outlined in dog cancer diet*

IP-3 and IP-6
(inositol hexaphosphate)

These antioxidants may have some benefits for cancer patients, but they don't outweigh the interfering effects with Apocaps, and the pro-oxidant therapies chemotherapy and radiation. *Antioxidant that may interfere with more important therapeutics.*

Laetrile (Vitamin B 17, amygdalin)

Laetrile is usually made from apricot seeds or similar seeds, and has a complicated history of use and regulation. The evidence for laetrile's actual effect on cancer is controversial, and there is some concern that hydrogen cyanide is released when it is metabolized. This concern is validated by literature reporting serious cyanide poisoning in children after ingesting apricot pits. Laetrile's safety has never been assessed in dogs, and I do not recommend its use. *Not recommended; safety issues.*

Lutimax

I used to recommend Lutimax because it is one of the only supplements featuring luteolin, which has strong anti-cancer effects in the body (discussed in Chapter 12). Unfortunately, it also contains xylitol, which has been shown to cause liver injury and hypoglycemia in dogs when given in large amounts. I used to recommend Lutimax because of its main ingredient, but the possible xylitol issue remained. Given the large number of guardians using Lutimax according to the Full Spectrum plan, I was concerned that a dog with low-dose xylitol sensitivity might show up. Safety is critical, so I included luteolin as a main ingredient in Apocaps. Taking Lutimax at the same time as Apocaps is redundant. *Redundant as a supplement if taking Apocaps; safety issues in large amounts.*

Maritime Pine Bark Supplements

The anti-inflammatory effects of Maritime Pine Bark are well documented, but evidence for its direct anti-cancer effects is flimsy when compared to other supplements I recommend. Its antioxidant benefits do not outweigh its interfering effects on

Apocaps and the pro-oxidant therapies chemotherapy and radiation. *Low priority supplement; antioxidant which may interfere with more important therapeutics.*

Milk Thistle (Silybum marinarum)

In addition to other beneficial effects, constituents in milk thistle have demonstrated strong anti-cancer effects. However, the active compounds with anti-cancer properties (silymarin A and B and silybinin), are not easily absorbed by the body. To address this for dogs, I included silymarin and silybinin in Apocaps, and addressed the bioavailability issues with these ingredients. Using a separate milk thistle supplement would be redundant and much less effective due to the bioavailability problems when taken by mouth. *Redundant as a supplement if taking Apocaps; bioavailability issues.*

Mistletoe (Viscum album)

Mistletoe may increase the life quality of cancer patients, but evidence for its direct anti-cancer benefits is flimsy. Its antioxidant benefits do not outweigh its interfering effects on Apocaps, pro-oxidant chemotherapy and radiation. *Low priority supplement; antioxidant that may interfere with more important therapeutics.*

MMS (methyl methanesulfonate)

I am definitely interested in this relatively new substance, which clearly has a biologically active effect. However, systematic safety studies are lacking, and there is some evidence that it may be carcinogenic. I'm not comfortable recommending MMS at this time, but I may recommend it in the future if its safety is established. *May recommend in the future; safety not established.*

Onco Support

The antioxidant effects of Onco Support don't outweigh its interfering effects with Apocaps, pro-oxidant chemotherapy, and radiation. *Antioxidant that may interfere with more important therapeutics.*

Pau d'arco (Tabebuia avellanedae)

Pau d'arco is a South American tree reputed to be helpful for a variety of conditions. However, the tree itself is becoming scarcer every year, and imitation products are starting to hit the market. Pau d'arco contains hydroxyquinone, a known carcinogen, and, like Cat's Claw, there is no standardization of the supplement. The batch variability and possibility of unsafe or synthetic ingredients makes me uncomfortable with recommending this supplement. *Not recommended; batch variability; may not be safe.*

Prebiotics

Prebiotics stimulate the growth and activity of the healthy bacteria in the digestive system. While they can be useful for digestive upset and general health, they do not have direct anti-cancer benefits, so I consider them a low-priority supplement. Please see the probiotics discussion for more information. *Low priority supplement.*

Probiotics

Probiotics are live bacteria taken by mouth to promote a healthy digestive system. They can be useful in managing diarrhea and in some cases involving allergies or inflammatory gastro-intestinal diseases. They also have some nutritional benefit. However, probiotics lack specific anti-cancer actions in the body. Their lack of critical support for dogs with cancer makes them a low-priority supplement. *Low priority supplement.*

Quercetin

Quercetin has good evidence for anti-cancer effects, but when taken by mouth has low absorption in the body. I like quercetin enough to include it in Apocaps, where its bioavailability issues are addressed. For this reason, taking a separate supplement is redundant. *Redundant as a supplement if taking Apocaps.*

Red Clover (Trifolium pratense L.)

Red clover may have some use in bone tumor cases, because it may help with maintaining the bone's integrity. Otherwise, its overall anti-cancer evidence is very flimsy. It has antioxidant effects, but they do not outweigh its interfering effects on Apocaps and the pro-oxidant therapies chemotherapy and radiation. *Very low priority supplement.*

Resveratrol

Resveratrol has good anti-cancer effects in vitro, but the bioavailability of the anti-cancer compounds in vivo is low. It has some application for cancers in the lining of the digestive tract, (where the substance can contact tumors directly), but otherwise I do not recommend it because its antioxidant effects in even low doses may interfere with treatments like Apocaps, pro-oxidant chemotherapy and radiation. *Low priority supplement, bioavailability issues.*

SAM-e (s-adenosyl methionine)

This supplement may help with depression, which could affect survival times in human cancer patients. It also has benefit in cases of liver injury, as I mention on page 107 and Dr. Ettinger explains on page 397.

However, its benefits are not strong enough to recommend it across the board, because of its possible interference with Apocaps, pro-oxidant chemotherapy, and radiation. For these reasons, it is a low-priority supplement unless used to specifically protect the liver from potential toxicity. *Low priority supplement.*

Shark Cartilage

Shark cartilage has some isolated evidence for preventing angiogenesis, but the data is not strong. In

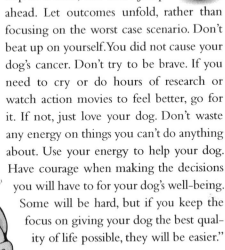

Let Outcomes Unfold

"Deal with it one day/step at a time, and don't jump ahead. Let outcomes unfold, rather than focusing on the worst case scenario. Don't beat up on yourself. You did not cause your dog's cancer. Don't try to be brave. If you need to cry or do hours of research or watch action movies to feel better, go for it. If not, just love your dog. Don't waste any energy on things you can't do anything about. Use your energy to help your dog. Have courage when making the decisions you will have to for your dog's well-being. Some will be hard, but if you keep the focus on giving your dog the best quality of life possible, they will be easier."

- *Susan McKay, Winnipeg, Manitoba*

addition to this, I am personally concerned because the harvesting of shark cartilage is a brutal process and may be threatening shark populations. For all of these reasons, I do not recommend shark cartilage. *Not recommended.*

Appendix C:
Helpful Resources

There are many websites listed in this book; the most important are compiled here for your easy reference. These were all active as of publication.

Full Spectrum Resources

DogCancerBlog.com: Visit my blog for my latest thoughts on dog cancer.

Apocaps.com: Visit this site to find out more about Apocaps. You will find the product label, Frequently Asked Questions section for guardians, and a wealth of more technical information for vets.

DogCancerShop.com: All of the supplements, books, and other items I have found useful for dogs with cancer can be found at this website.

Veterinary Websites

ACVIM.org: The website for the American College of Veterinary Internal Medicine has a "find a specialist" feature which can be used to find oncologists, neurologists, surgeons, or any other board-certified veterinary specialist.

VetCancerSociety.org: The Vet Cancer Society is a professional organization for vets who specialize in oncology. You can also find out about active clinical research trials.

AHVMA.org: The American Holistic Veterinary Medical Association is a professional organization for holistic and alternative veterinarians. You can use the "find a holistic veterinarian" feature to find a vet in your area. You can also go directly to their search feature at HolisticVetList.com.

AAVA.org: The American Academy of Veterinary Acupuncture is an association for U.S. vets and licensed vets from other countries who have been trained in approved acupuncture/TCM programs. You can use their "find an acupuncturist" feature to find one in your area.

VIIM.org: The Veterinary Institute of Integrative Medicine is a veterinary association similar to AHVMA. Their searchable index is handy for locating an alternative vet in your region.

OncuraPartners.com: Oncura Partners is a site that provides oncology consultation and treatments for veterinarians.

Health Websites and Hotlines

Environmental Protection Agency: The agency's website, www.epa.gov, has a great deal of information about known carcinogens. It's well organized and worth exploring. Specifically, find out about the safety of your drinking water at www.epa.gov/safewater/faq/faq.html or by calling 1-800-426-4791. You can find out if you're near a superfund site by visiting www.epa.gov/superfund/sites.

You can also call the Right to Know Hotline: 1-800-424-9346

Department of Health: Each state has a department of health, which will have information about possible carcinogens found in your area.

Financial Aid Websites

Magic Bullet Fund: For dogs with cancer whose treatment may extend life a year or more: www.themagicbulletfund.org

Angels for Animals: General financial help: www.angels4animals.org

United Animal Nations Lifeline: General financial help: www.uan.org

Canine Cancer Awareness: Help for dogs in need of cancer treatment: www.caninecancerawareness.org

Cody's Club: Financial help for dogs in need of radiation treatment: codysclub.bravehost.com

Riedel & Cody Fund: Provides an online community site where you can raise funds, apply for a grant, and network with others. www.cancerpets.org

Help-a-Pet: General financial help: www.help-a-pet.org/apply.html

In Memory of Magic: General financial help: www.imom.org

Pet Fund: Non-emergency financial help: www.thepetfund.com

Pigger's Pals: Financial help for owners seeking oncologists or surgical specialist services: www.piggerspals.org

AAHA Helping Pets Fund: General help for sick pets if your veterinarian is a member of AAHA (American Animal Hospital Association): www.aahahelpingpets.org

Helping Harley Working Dog Cancer Treatment Grants: For working dogs with cancer (service dogs, assistance dogs, etc.): www.grants.landofpuregold.com

OSLF Fund for Orthopedic Cases: Financial help for pets needing amputations or treatment for help in movement: www.oslf.org

Labrador Lifeline: Financial help for labs: www.labradorlifeline.org

Save Us Pets: Financial help for pets in New Jersey: www.saveuspets.org

Animal Cancer Therapy Subsidization Society: For pets with cancer in Alberta, Canada: www.actssalberta.org/application/

Greedy or Needy: A make-a-wish site: www.greedyorneedy.com

CareCredit: a healthcare credit card accepted by some veterinarians. Find out more at CareCredit.com

Appendix D:
Cancer Prevention & Longevity for Healthy Dogs

"How can I prevent cancer in my healthy dog?" is a very common question guardians ask after they finish this book. If your dog with cancer has a healthy brother or sister, or if you plan on having another dog in the future, you might wonder this, too.

Cancer prevention is an entirely different topic from cancer treatment, and is beyond the scope of this book. While it might seem logical to think that the dog cancer diet is good for healthy dogs, too, or that the supplements I recommend should be used to prevent cancer, this is not necessarily true. My recommendations in this book are designed to counteract cancer's tremendous force, not to keep an otherwise healthy dog from getting cancer.

On the other hand, we do know that certain lifestyle choices can make a dog's body a more hostile environment for cancer initiation and progression. Let's look at a few common-sense steps you can take:

- Seven or eight hours of sleep every night in a dark sleeping environment.
- Avoid obesity; ask your vet for help determining your dog's ideal body condition and weight, and then take steps to get him there.
- Isolation and depression have strong links to cancer in humans; spend time with your dog and enhance his joys of life any way you can.
- Increase healthy exercise.
- Add the brightly colored vegetables listed in Chapter 14 to your dog's diet.
- Lowering the amounts of red meat in your dog's diet in favor of leaner white meats and fish may help.
- Limit high carbohydrate foods like corn, wheat, and sugar.
- Choose dog foods that have not been processed at high temperatures. Some commercial foods I consider to be of better quality include Honest Kitchen, Orijen, Blue Buffalo, Halo Spot Stew, Taste of the Wild and Solid Gold.
- Avoid carcinogen exposure when you can; use glass or ceramic food and water bowls, avoid pesticides, lawn chemicals, car exhaust and tobacco smoke.

When getting a new puppy, consider the following:

- Avoid higher risk bloodlines; it is an unfortunate but unavoidable fact that some of our favorite breeds have such high cancer rates.
- Consider holding off on the starting the series of three puppy vaccinations until the eighth, or even tenth, week of life. A booster shot can be given at one year of age, and then not again until three years later: age four. Another booster can be given at age seven. Do not vaccinate

for diseases that are not present in your area, and run blood tests (titers) to see if vaccines are needed, if you have any doubts. Starting at age eight, run blood titers on an annual basis, and only give vaccines if they show a need.

- Weigh the pros and cons of sterilization carefully with your vet. Consider my general recommendation: spay females sometime between the third and fourth heat, and neuter males sometime between the ages of eighteen and twenty-four months.

There Is No Wrong Decision

"Take a breath! There is no wrong decision in this journey. It is really about the relationship between you and you dog. Only the two of you know what the other can endure. Treat every day as if it is your last together and have no regrets. Hope for the best and prepare for the worst."

- Brad Burkholder, Galt, California

And finally, if you would like to see a full book on the subject of dog longevity, let me and my publisher know by taking a ten second survey at www.DogCancerVet.com/survey.

Appendix E:
Scientific & Medical References

There were many studies, articles and books used in writing this book. Here is a list of the most important, grouped alphabetically by subject matter. Please note that in vivo and clinical use citations were included whenever possible.

I frequently use the National Institute of Health's online library, PubMed. This site has citation information on more than nineteen million biomedical studies, articles, and books: www.ncbi.nlm.nih.gov/pubmed.

Acupuncture and acupressure

Acupuncture: role in comprehensive cancer care – a primer for the oncologist and review of the literature. Cohen AJ, Menter A, Hale L. *Integr Cancer Ther.* 2005 Jun;4(2):131–43. Review.

Efficacy of acupuncture in treatment of cancer pain: a systematic review. Peng H, et al. *Zhong Xi Yi Jie He Xue Bao.* 2010 Jun;8(6):501-9. Chinese.

Analgesic effect of auricular acupuncture for cancer pain: a randomized, blinded, controlled trial. Alimi D, et al. *J Clin Oncol.* 2003 Nov 15;21(22):4120–6.

Acupuncture as a treatment modality for the management of cancer pain: the state of the science. Hopkins Hollis AS. *Oncol Nurs Forum.* 2010 Sep 1;37(5):E344–8.

Acupuncture-point stimulation for chemotherapy-induced nausea or vomiting. Ezzo JM, et al. *Cochrane Database Syst Rev.* 2006 Apr 19;(2):CD002285. Review.

Acupressure for chemotherapy-induced nausea and vomiting: a randomized clinical trial. Dibble SL, Luce J, Cooper BA, Israel J, Cohen M, Nussey B, Rugo H. *Oncol Nurs Forum.* 2007 Jul;34(4):813-20.

Prolongation of the antiemetic action of P6 acupuncture by acupressure in patients having cancer chemotherapy. Dundee JW, Yang J. *J R Soc Med.* 1990 Jun;83(6):360-2.

Effect of acupressure on nausea and vomiting induced by chemotherapy in cancer patients. Gardani G, et al. *Minerva Med.* 2006 Oct;97(5):391-4.

A progress study of 100 cancer patients treated by acupressure for chemotherapy-induced vomiting after failure with the pharmacological approach. Gardani G, et al. *Minerva Med.* 2007 Dec;98(6):665-8.

Effect of acupressure on chemotherapy-induced nausea and vomiting in gynecologic cancer patients in Turkey. Taspinar A, Sirin A. *Eur J Oncol Nurs.* 2010 Feb;14(1):49-54. Epub 2009 Sep 11.

Antioxidants and Pro-Oxidants (also see maintenance multivitamin section)

Antioxidant supplements for preventing gastrointestinal cancers. Bjelakovic G, et al. *Cochrane Database Syst Rev.* 2008 Jul 16;(3):CD004183. Review.

Alpha-Tocopherol and beta-carotene supplements and lung cancer incidence in the alpha-tocopherol, beta-carotene cancer prevention study: effects of base-line characteristics and study compliance. Albanes D, et al. *J Natl Cancer Inst.* 1996 Nov 6;88(21):1560-70.

Incidence of cancer and mortality following alpha-tocopherol and beta-carotene supplementation: a postintervention follow-up. Virtamo J, et al. Taylor PR, Albert P; ATBC Study Group. *JAMA.* 2003 Jul 23;290(4):476-85.

Beta-carotene supplementation and cancer risk: a systematic review and metaanalysis of randomized controlled trials. Druesne-Pecollo N, et al. *Int J Cancer.* 2010 Jul 1;127(1):172-84. Review.

Antioxidant supplements for prevention of mortality in healthy participants and patients with various diseases. Bjelakovic G, et al. *Cochrane Database Syst Rev.* 2008 Apr 16;(2):CD007176. Review.

Mortality in randomized trials of antioxidant supplements for primary and secondary prevention: systematic review and meta-analysis. Bjelakovic G, et al. *JAMA.* 2007 Feb 28;297(8):842-57. Review. Erratum in: *JAMA.* 2008 Feb 20;299(7):765-6.

Anti- and pro-oxidative effects of flavonoids on metal-induced lipid hydroperoxide-dependent lipid peroxidation in cultured hepatocytes loaded with alpha-linolenic acid. Sugihara N, et al. *Free Radic Biol Med.* 1999 Dec;27(11-12):1313-23.

Free radicals, metals and antioxidants in oxidative stress-induced cancer. Valko M, et al. *Chem Biol Interact.* 2006 Mar 10;160(1):1-40. Epub 2006 Jan 23. Review.

Chemopreventive agents induce oxidative stress in cancer cells leading to COX-2 overexpression and COX-2-independent cell death. Sun Y, Chen J, Rigas B. *Carcinogenesis.* 2009 January;30(1): 93–100.

Breast cancer cell–targeted oxidative stress: enhancement of cancer cell uptake of conjugated linoleic acid, activation of p53, and inhibition of proliferation. Albright CD, et al. *Exp Mol Pathol.* 2005 Oct;79(2):118–25.

Targeting cancer cells by ROS-mediated mechanisms: a radical therapeutic approach? Trachootham D, Alexandre J, Huang P. *Nature Reviews Drug Discovery 8*, 579–591 (July 2009)

Apigenin

Antigenotoxic effect of apigenin against anti-cancerous drugs. Siddique YH, Beg T, Afzal M. *Toxicol In Vitro.* 2008 Apr;22(3):625–31.

5-Fluorouracil combined with apigenin enhances anticancer activity through induction of apoptosis in human breast cancer MDA-MB-453 cells. Choi EJ and Kim GH. *Oncol Rep.* 2009 Dec;22(6):1533–7.

The flavonoid apigenin potentiates the growth inhibitory effects of gemcitabine and abrogates gemcitabine resistance in human pancreatic cancer cells. Strouch MJ, et al. *Pancreas.* 2009 May;38(4):409–15.

Enhanced anti-tumor effect of combination therapy with gemcitabine and apigenin in pancreatic cancer. Lee SH, et al. *Cancer Lett.* 2008 Jan 18;259(1):39–49.

Flavonoids apigenin and quercetin inhibit melanoma growth and metastatic potential. Caltagirone S, et al. *Int J Cancer.* 2000 Aug 15;87(4):595–600.

Flavonoids Are Inhibitors of Breast Cancer Resistance Protein (ABCG2)-Mediated Transport. Zhang S, Yang X, Morris ME. *Molecular Pharmacology* May 2004 vol. 65 no. 5 1208–1216

The chemopreventive flavonoid apigenin confers radiosensitizing effect in human tumor cells grown as monolayers and spheroids. Watanabe N, Hirayama R, Kubota N. *J Radiat Res (Tokyo).* 2007 Jan;48(1):45–50.

Molecular targets for apigenin-induced cell cycle arrest and apoptosis in prostate cancer cell xenograft. Shukla S and Gupta S. *Mol Cancer Ther.* 2006 Apr;5(4):843–52.

Pharmacokinetics and metabolism of apigenin in female and male rats after a single oral administration. Gradolatto A, et al. *Drug Metab Dispos.* 2005 Jan;33(1):49–54.

Up-regulation of insulin-like growth factor binding protein-3 by apigenin leads to growth inhibition and apoptosis of 22Rv1 xenograft in athymic nude mice. Shukla S, et al. *FASEB J.* 2005 Dec;19(14):2042–4.

Dietary apigenin suppresses IgE and inflammatory cytokines production in C57BL/6N mice. Yano S, et al. *J Agric Food Chem.* 2006 Jul 12;54(14):5203–7.

Apigenin and luteolin modulate microglial activation via inhibition of STAT1-induced CD40 expression. Rezai-Zadeh K, et al. *J Neuroinflammation.* 2008; 5: 41.

Bioavailability of apigenin from apiin-rich parsley in humans. Meyer H, et al. *Ann Nutr Metab.* 2006;50(3):167–72.

Inhibition of proteasome activity by the dietary flavonoid apigenin is associated with growth inhibition in cultured breast cancer cells and xenografts. Chen D, et al. *Breast Cancer Res.* 2007; 9(6): R80.

Dietary flavonoids as proteasome inhibitors and apoptosis inducers in human leukemia cells. Chen D, et al. *Biochem Pharmacol.* 2005 May 15;69(10):1421–32.

Apigenin drives the production of reactive oxygen species and initiates a mitochondrial mediated cell death pathway in prostate epithelial cells. Morrissey C, et al. *Prostate.* 2005 May 1;63(2):131–42.

Apigenin-induced prostate cancer cell death is initiated by reactive oxygen species and p53 activation. Shukla S and Gupta S. *Free Radic Biol Med.* 2008 May 15;44(10):1833–45.

Induction of caspase-dependent, p53-mediated apoptosis by apigenin in human neuroblastoma. Torkin R, et al. *Mol Cancer Ther.* 2005 Jan;4(1):1–11.

Individual and interactive effects of apigenin analogs on G2/M cell-cycle arrest in human colon carcinoma cell lines. Wang W, et al. *Nutr Cancer.* 2004;48(1):106–14.

Induction of caspase-dependent, p53-mediated apoptosis by apigenin in human neuroblastoma. Torkin R, et al. *Mol Cancer Ther.* 2005 Jan;4(1):1–11.

Apigenin induced apoptosis through p53-dependent pathway in human cervical carcinoma cells. Zheng PW, Chiang LC, Lin CC. *Life Sci.* 2005 Feb 4;76(12):1367–79.

Suppression of constitutive and tumor necrosis factor alpha-induced nuclear factor (NF)-kappaB activation and induction of apoptosis by apigenin in human prostate carcinoma PC-3 cells: correlation with down-regulation of NF-kappaB-responsive genes. Shukla S and Gupta S. *Clin Cancer Res.* 2004 May 1;10(9):3169–78.

Cell-cycle arrest at G2/M and growth inhibition by apigenin in human colon carcinoma cell lines. Wang W, et al. *Mol Carcinog.* 2000 Jun;28(2):102–10.

Suppression of constitutive and tumor necrosis factor alpha-induced nuclear factor (NF)-kappaB activation and induction of apoptosis by apigenin in human prostate carcinoma PC-3 cells: correlation with down-regulation of NF-kappaB-responsive genes. Shukla S and Gupta S. *Clin Cancer Res.* 2004

May 1;10(9):3169-78.

Unbalanced activation of ERK1/2 and MEK1/2 in apigenin-induced HeLa cell death. Llorens F, et al. *Exp Cell Res.* 2004 Sep 10;299(1):15-26.

Flavonoids as DNA topoisomerase antagonists and poisons: structure-activity relationships. Constantinou A, et al. *J Nat Prod.* 1995 Feb;58(2):217-25.

Involvement of nuclear factor-kappa B, Bax and Bcl-2 in induction of cell cycle arrest and apoptosis by apigenin in human prostate carcinoma cells. Gupta S, Afaq F, Mukhtar H. *Oncogene.* 2002 May 23;21(23):3727-38.

Induction of cancer cell apoptosis by flavonoids is associated with their ability to inhibit fatty acid synthase activity. Brusselmans K, et al. *J Biol Chem.* 2005 Feb 18;280(7):5636-45.

Induction of apoptosis by apigenin and related flavonoids through cytochrome c release and activation of caspase-9 and caspase-3 in leukaemia HL-60 cells. Wang IK, Lin-Shiau SY, Lin JK. *Eur J Cancer.* 1999 Oct;35(10):1517-25.

Suppression of inducible cyclooxygenase and inducible nitric oxide synthase by apigenin and related flavonoids in mouse macrophages. Liang YC, et al. *Carcinogenesis.* 1999 Oct;20(10):1945-52.

Possible controversy over dietary polyphenols: benefits vs risks. Lambert JD, Sang S, Yang CS. *Chem Res Toxicol.* 2007 Apr;20(4):583-5.

Apoptosis

The hallmarks of cancer. Hanahan D, Weinberg RA. *Cell.* 2000 Jan 7;100(1):57-70. Review.

Apoptosis: A basic biological phenomenon with wide-ranging implications in tissue kinetics. Kerr JFR, Wyllie AH, Currie AR, *British Journal of Cancer* 1972, 26:239-257

Therapeutic targeting of death pathways in cancer: mechanisms for activating cell death in cancer cells. Tan TT and White E. *Adv Exp Med Biol.* 2008;615:81-104.

Targeting apoptosis pathways in cancer therapy. Fulda S and Debatin KM. *Curr Cancer Drug Targets.* 2004 Nov;4(7):569-76.

"Falling leaves": a survey of the history of apoptosis. Formigli L, Conti A, Lippi D. *Minerva Med.* 2004 Apr;95(2):159-64.

Apoptosis, oncosis, and necrosis. An overview of cell death. Majno G and Joris I. *Am J Pathol.* 1995 Jan;146(1):3-15.

Apoptosis signaling in tumor therapy. Fulda S and Debatin KM. *Ann NY Acad Sci.* 2004 Dec;1028:150-6.

Apoptosis in cancer. Lowe SW and Lin AW. Carcinogenesis.

2000 Mar;21(3):485-95. Review.

The molecular control of DNA damage-induced cell death. Coultas L and Strasser A. *Apoptosis.* 2000 Dec;5(6):491-507.

Role of alterations in the apoptotic machinery in sensitivity of cancer cells to treatment. Rodriguez-Nieto S, Zhivotovsky B. *Curr Pharm Des.* 2006;12(34):4411-25.

Artemisinin

Recent advances in artemisinin and its derivatives as antimalarial and antitumor agents. Jung M, et al. *Curr Med Chem.* 2004 May;11(10):1265-84. Review.

Artemisinin and its derivatives: a novel class of anti-malarial and anti-cancer agents. Chaturvedi D, et al. *Chem Soc Rev.* 2010 Feb;39(2):435-54. Epub 2009 Aug 24. Review.

Artesunate induces oncosis-like cell death in vitro and has antitumor activity against pancreatic cancer xenografts in vivo. Du, JH, et al. *Cancer Chemother Pharmacol.* 2010 April; 65(5): 895-902.

Artesunate in the treatment of metastatic uveal melanoma—first experiences. Berger TG, et al. *Oncol Rep.* 2005 Dec;14(6):1599-603.

Inhibition of angiogenesis in vivo and growth of Kaposi's sarcoma xenograft tumors by the anti-malarial artesunate. Dell'Eva R, et al. *Biochem Pharmacol.* 2004 Dec 15;68(12):2359-66.

The anti-malarial artesunate is also active against cancer. Efferth T, Dunstan H, Sauerbrey A, Miyachi H, Chitambar CR. *Int J Oncol.* 2001 Apr;18(4):767-73.

Oral artemisinin prevents and delays the development of 7,12-dimethylbenz[a]anthracene (DMBA)-induced breast cancer in the rat. Lai H, Singh NP. *Cancer Lett.* 2006 Jan 8;231(1):43-8.

Targeted treatment of cancer with artemisinin and artemisinin-tagged iron-carrying compounds. Lai H, Sasaki T, Singh NP. *Expert Opin Ther Targets.* 2005 Oct;9(5):995-1007. Review.

Inhibition of glutathione S-transferases by antimalarial drugs possible implications for circumventing anticancer drug resistance. Mukanganyama S, Widersten M, Naik YS, Mannervik B, Hasler JA. *Int J Cancer.* 2002 Feb 10;97(5):700-5.

Toxic brainstem encephalopathy after artemisinin treatment for breast cancer. Panossian LA, Garga NI, Pelletier D. *Ann Neurol.* 2005 Nov;58(5):812-3.

What made sesquiterpene lactones reach cancer clinical trials? Ghantous A, et al. *Drug Discov Today.* 2010 Aug;15(15-16):668-78. Epub 2010 Jun 9.

Berries

Anti-angiogenic property of edible berries. Roy S, et al. *Free Radic Res*. 2002 Sep;36(9):1023-31.

Anthocyanins in black raspberries prevent esophageal tumors in rats. Wang LS, et al. *Cancer Prev Res (Phila Pa)*. 2009 Jan;2(1):84-93.

Anthocyanidins induce apoptosis in human promyelocytic leukemia cells: structure-activity relationship and mechanisms involved. Hou DX, et al. *Int J Oncol*. 2003 Sep;23(3):705-12.

Do anthocyanins and anthocyanidins, cancer chemopreventive pigments in the diet, merit development as potential drugs? Thomasset S, et al. *Cancer Chemother Pharmacol*. 2009 Jun;64(1):201-11.

Effect of anthocyanin fractions from selected cultivars of Georgia-grown blueberries on apoptosis and phase II enzymes. Srivastava A, et al. *J Agric Food Chem*. 2007 Apr 18;55(8):3180-5

Beta Glucans

Oral administration of beta-1,3/1,6-glucan to dogs temporally changes total and antigen-specific IgA and IgM. Stuyven E, et al. *Clin Vaccine Immunol*. 2010 Feb;17(2):281-5.

Dietary modulation of immune function by beta-glucans. Volman JJ, Ramakers JD, Plat J. *Physiol Behav*. 2008 May 23;94(2):276-84.

[The biological activity of beta-glucans], Rondanelli M, Opizzi A, Monteferrario F. *Minerva Med*. 2009 Jun;100(3):237-45. Review. Italian.

Immunomodulatory activities of oat beta-glucan in vitro and in vivo. Estrada A, et al. *Microbiol Immunol*. 1997;41(12):991-8.

Effects of oat beta-glucan on innate immunity and infection after exercise stress. Davis JM, et al. *Med Sci Sports Exerc*. 2004 Aug;36(8):1321-7.

Oral delivery and gastrointestinal absorption of soluble glucans stimulate increased resistance to infectious challenge. Rice PJ, et al. *J Pharmacol Exp Ther*. 2005 Sep;314(3):1079-86

Immunomodulation by orally administered beta-glucan in mice. Suzuki I, et al. *Int J Immunopharmacol*. 1989;11(7):761-9.

Aggregating disparate epidemiological evidence: comparing two seminal EMF reviews. O'Carroll MJ, Henshaw DL. *Risk Anal*. 2008 Feb;28(1):225-34.

The effect of heated fat on the carcinogenic activity of 2-acetylaminofluorene. M. Sugai, et al. *Cancer Res* 22 (41): 510.

Formation of new heterocyclic amine mutagens by heating creatinine, alanine, threonine and glucose. Skog K, et al. *Mutat Res*. 1992 Aug;268(2):191-7.

Heterocyclic amines: Mutagens/carcinogens produced during cooking of meat and fish. Sugimura T, et al. *Cancer Sci*. 2004 Apr;95(4):290-9.

A new approach to risk estimation of food-borne carcinogens--heterocyclic amines--based on molecular information. Nagao M. *Mutat Res*. 1999 Dec 16;431(1):3-12. Review.

Verification of the findings of acrylamide in heated foods. Ahn JS, et al. *Food Addit Contam*. 2002 Dec;19(12):1116-24.

Analysis of acrylamide, a carcinogen formed in heated foodstuffs. Tareke E, et al. *J Agric Food Chem*. 2002 Aug 14;50(17):4998-5006.

A prospective study of dietary acrylamide intake and the risk of endometrial, ovarian, and breast cancer. Hogervorst JG, et al. *Cancer Epidemiol Biomarkers Prev*. 2007 Nov;16(11):2304-13.

The effects of beta-glucan on human immune and cancer cells. Chan GC, Chan WK, Sze DM. *J Hematol Oncol*. 2009 Jun 10;2:25.

[Biologically active compounds of edible mushrooms and their beneficial impact on health]. Rajewska J, Bałasińska B. *Postepy Hig Med Dosw* (Online). 2004;58:352-7.

Mushrooms, tumors, and immunity: an update. Borchers AT, Keen CL, Gershwin ME. *Exp Biol Med (Maywood)*. 2004 May;229(5):393-406.

Medicinal mushrooms as a source of antitumor and immunomodulating polysaccharides. Wasser SP. *Appl Microbiol Biotechnol*. 2002 Nov;60(3):258-74.

Phellinus Linteus Extract Sensitizes Advanced Prostate Cancer Cells to Apoptosis in Athymic Nude Mice. Takanori Tsuji, et al. *PLoS One*. 2010; 5(3): e9885.

Phellinus linteus sensitises apoptosis induced by doxorubicin in prostate cancer. Collins L, Zhu T, Guo J, Xiao ZJ, Chen CY. *Br J Cancer*. 2006 Aug 7;95(3):282-8.

Effect of Maitake (Grifola frondosa) D-Fraction on the activation of NK cells in cancer patients. Kodama N, Komuta K, Nanba H. *J Med Food*. 2003 Winter;6(4):371-7.

Maitake D-Fraction enhances antitumor effects and reduces immunosuppression by mitomycin-C in tumor-bearing mice. Kodama N, et al. *Nutrition*. 2005 May;21(5):624-9.

[Inhibitory effects of cordyceps extract on growth of colon cancer cells]. Huang H, Wang H, Luo RC. *Zhong Yao Cai*. 2007 Mar;30(3):310-3. Chinese.

Induction of apoptosis by aqueous extract of Cordyceps militaris through activation of caspases and inactivation of Akt in human breast cancer MDA-MB-231 Cells. Jin CY, Kim GY, Choi YH. *J Microbiol Biotechnol*. 2008 Dec;18(12):1997-2003.

Growth inhibition of U937 leukemia cells by aqueous extract of Cordyceps militaris through induction of apoptosis. Park C, et al. *Oncol Rep*. 2005 Jun;13(6):1211-6.

Inhibitory mechanisms of Agaricus blazei Murill on the growth of prostate cancer in vitro and in vivo. Yu CH, Kan SF, Shu CH, Lu TJ, Sun-Hwang L, Wang PS. *J Nutr Biochem*. 2009 Oct;20(10):753-64.

Suppressing effects of daily oral supplementation of beta-glucan extracted from Agaricus blazei Murill on spontaneous and peritoneal disseminated metastasis in mouse model. Kobayashi H, et al. *J Cancer Res Clin Oncol*. 2005 Aug;131(8):527-38.

Effects of the medicinal mushroom Agaricus blazei Murill on immunity, infection and cancer. Hetland G, et al. *Scand J Immunol*. 2008 Oct;68(4):363-70.

Induction of apoptosis in human prostatic cancer cells with beta-glucan (Maitake mushroom polysaccharide). Fullerton SA, Samadi AA, Tortorelis DG, Choudhury MS, Mallouh C, Tazaki H, Konno S. *Mol Urol*. 2000 Spring;4(1):7-13.

Can maitake MD-fraction aid cancer patients? Kodama N, Komuta K, Nanba H. *Altern Med Rev*. 2002 Jun;7(3):236-9.

Effects of mushroom-derived beta-glucan-rich polysaccharide extracts on nitric oxide production by bone marrow-derived macrophages and nuclear factor-kappaB transactivation in Caco-2 reporter cells: can effects be explained by structure? Volman JJ, Heet et al. *Mol Nutr Food Res*. 2010 Feb;54(2):268-76.

Beta-glucan functions as an adjuvant for monoclonal antibody immunotherapy by recruiting tumoricidal granulocytes as killer cells. Hong F, et al. *Cancer Res*. 2003 Dec 15;63(24):9023-31.

The polysaccharide, PGG-glucan, enhances human myelopoiesis by direct action independent of and additive to early-acting cytokines. Turnbull JL, Patchen ML, Scadden DT. *Acta Haematol*. 1999;102(2):66-71.

In vitro cytostatic and immunomodulatory properties of the medicinal mushroom Lentinula edodes. Israilides C, Kletsas D, Arapoglou D, Philippoussis A, Pratsinis H, Ebringerová A, Hríbalová V, Harding SE. *Phytomedicine*. 2008 Jun;15(6-7):512-9.

Inhibition of human colon carcinoma development by lentinan from shiitake mushrooms (Lentinus edodes). Ng ML, Yap AT. *J Altern Complement Med*. 2002 Oct;8(5):581-9.

Efficacy of orally administered superfine dispersed lentinan (beta-1,3-glucan) for the treatment of advanced colorectal cancer. Hazama S, et al. *Anticancer Res*. 2009 Jul;29(7):2611-7.

Improvement of QOL and prognosis by treatment of superfine dispersed lentinan in patients with advanced gastric cancer. Yoshino S, Watanabe S, Imano M, Suga T, Nakazawa S, Hazama S, Oka M. *Hepatogastroenterology*. 2010 Jan-Feb;57(97):172-7.

Differential anti-tumor activity of coriolus versicolor (Yunzhi) extract through p53- and/or Bcl-2-dependent apoptotic pathway in human breast cancer cells. Ho CY, et al. *Cancer Biol Ther*. 2005 Jun;4(6):638-44.

Coriolus versicolor (Yunzhi) extract attenuates growth of human leukemia xenografts and induces apoptosis through the mitochondrial pathway. Ho CY, et al. *Oncol Rep*. 2006 Sep;16(3):609-16.

Coriolus versicolor polysaccharide peptide slows progression of advanced non-small cell lung cancer. Tsang KW, Lam CL, Yan C, Mak JC, Ooi GC, Ho JC, Lam B, Man R, Sham JS, Lam WK. *Respir Med*. 2003 Jun;97(6):618-24.

Coriolus versicolor: a medicinal mushroom with promising immunotherapeutic values. Chu KK, Ho SS, Chow AH. *J Clin Pharmacol*. 2002 Sep;42(9):976-84.

Polysaccharide immunomodulators as therapeutic agents: structural aspects and biologic function. Tzianabos AO. *Clin Microbiol Rev*. 2000 Oct;13(4):523-33.

Mechanism by which orally administered beta-1,3-glucans enhance the tumoricidal activity of antitumor monoclonal antibodies in murine tumor models. Hong F, et al. *J Immunol*. 2004 Jul 15;173(2):797-806.

Oral delivery and gastrointestinal absorption of soluble glucans stimulate increased resistance to infectious challenge. Rice PJ, et al. *J Pharmacol Exp Ther*. 2005 Sep;314(3):1079-86.

Immunomodulation by orally administered beta-glucan in mice. Suzuki I, et al. *Int J Immunopharmacol*. 1989;11(7):761-9.

Effect of orally administered beta-glucan on macrophage function in mice. Suzuki I, et al. *Int J Immunopharmacol*. 1990;12(6):675-84.

Body Fat and Adiponectin

Adiponectin and cancer: a systematic review. Kelesidis I, Kelesidis T, Mantzoros CS. *Br J Cancer*. 2006 May 8;94(9):1221-5. Review.

Adiponectin in relation to malignancies: a review of existing basic research and clinical evidence. Barb D, et al. *Am J Clin Nutr*. 2007 Sep;86(3):s858-66. Review.

Adiponectin: a link between obesity and cancer. Barb D, Pazaitou-Panayiotou K, Mantzoros CS. *Expert Opin Investig Drugs*. 2006 Aug;15(8):917-31. Review.

Reducing the weight of cancer: mechanistic targets for breaking the obesity-carcinogenesis link. Hursting SD, et al. *Best Pract Res Clin Endocrinol Metab.* 2008 Aug;22(4):659-69. Review.

Prevalence of obese dogs in a population of dogs with cancer. Weeth LP, et al. *Am J Vet Res.* 2007 Apr;68(4):389-98.

Body conformation, diet, and risk of breast cancer in pet dogs: a case-control study. Sonnenschein EG, et al. *Am J Epidemiol.* 1991 Apr 1;133(7):694-703.

Relation between habitual diet and canine mammary tumors in a case-control study. Pérez Alenza D, et al. *J Vet Intern Med.* 1998 May-Jun;12(3):132-9.

Epidemiologic study of insecticide exposures, obesity, and risk of bladder cancer in household dogs. Glickman LT, et al. *J Toxicol Environ Health.* 1989;28(4):407-14.

Brain Cancer

Nervous System Neoplasia. Coates JR, Johnson GC, in Henry CJ, Higginbotham ML (ed): *Cancer Management in Small Animal Practice.* Missouri. Saunders Elsevier 2010, p 186-194.

Tumors of the Nervous System. LeCouteur RA, Withrow SJ, in Withrow SJ, Vail DM (eds): *Withrow & MacEwen's Small Animal Clinical Oncology.* St Louis Missouri, Saunders Elsevier, 2007, pp 659-685.

Treatment of Intracranial tumors. Narak J, Axlund TW, Smith AN, in Bonagura JD, Twedt DC (ed): *Kirk's Current Veterinary Therapy XIV.* Missouri. Saunders Elsevier 2009, p 1078-1083.

Brain Neoplasia. Troxel MT, in Cote E (2nd ed), *Clinical Veterinary Advisor: Dogs and Cats.* Missouri, Mosby Elsevier, 2011, p 153-155.

Meningioma. Troxel MT, in Cote E (2nd ed), *Clinical Veterinary Advisor: Dogs and Cats.* Missouri, Mosby Elsevier, 2011, p 715-716.

Analysis of survival in a retrospective study of 86 dogs with brain tumors. Heidner GL, Kornegay JN, Page RL, et al. *J Vet Intern Med.* 5(4):219-26. 1991

Influence of tumor cell proliferation and sex-hormone receptors on effectiveness of radiation therapy for dogs with incompletely resected meningiomas. Theon AP, LeCouteur RA, Carr EA, et al: *J Am Vet Med Assoc* 216:701, 2000.

Evaluation of progesterone and estrogen receptor expression in 15 meningiomas of dogs and cats. Adamo FP, Cantile C, Steinberg H: *Am J Vet Res* 64:1310, 2003.

Clinical signs associated with brain tumors in dogs: 97 cases (1992-1997). Bagley RS, Gavin PR, Moore MP, et al: *J Am Vet Med Assoc* 215:818, 1999.

Cyberknife radiosurgery for irradiation of brain tumors in dogs and cats. Charney SC, Witten MR, Berg JM et al. *Proc Annual ACVIM Forum* p. 326, 2010.

Characteristics of cisternal cerebrospinal fluid associated with primary brain tumors in the dog: a retrospective study. Bailey CS, Higgins RJ. *J Am Vet Med Assoc.* 188(4):414-7. 1986

Canine intracranial primary neoplasia: 173 cases (1986-2003), Snyder JM, Shofer FS, Van Winkle TJ, et al. *J Vet Intern Med* 20:669, 2006.

Intracranial meningioma with pulmonary metastasis in three dogs, Schulman FY, Ribas JL, Carpenter JL, et al. *Vet Pathol* 29:196, 1992.

Primary optic nerve meningioma and pulmonary metastasis in a dog. Dugan SJ, Schwarz PD, Roberts SM, et al. *J Am Anim Hosp Assoc* 29:11, 1993.

Current concepts in the diagnosis and treatments of brain tumours in dogs and cats. LeCouteur RA. *J Small Anim Pract* 40:411, 1999.

Radiosurgery using a stereotactic headframe system for irradiation of brain tumors in dogs. Lester NV, Hopkins AL, Bova FJ, et al. *J Am Vet Med Assoc* 219:1562, 2001.

Primary irradiation of canine intracranial masses. Spugnini EP, Thrall DE, Price GS, et al. *Vet Radiol Ultrasound* 41:377, 2000.

Surgery alone or in combination with radiation therapy for treatment of intracranial meningiomas in dogs: 31 cases (1989-2002). Axlund TW, McGlasson ML, Smith AN. *J Am Vet Med Assoc* 221:1597, 2002.

Calcium

Absorption of calcium as the carbonate and citrate salts, with some observations on method. Heaney RP, Dowell MS, Barger-Lux MJ. *Osteoporos Int.* 1999;9(1):19-23.

Calcium supplementation in clinical practice: a review of forms, doses, and indications. Straub DA. *Nutr Clin Pract.* 2007 Jun;22(3):286-96.

Cancer as a disease of civilization

The effect of diet on risk of cancer. Key TJ, et al. *Lancet.* 2002 Sep 14;360(9336):861-8. Review.

Evolution of the human diet: linking our ancestral diet to modern functional foods as a means of chronic disease prevention. Jew S, AbuMweis SS, Jones PJ. *J Med Food.* 2009 Oct;12(5):925-34. Review.

Population causes and consequences of leading chronic diseases: a comparative analysis of prevailing explanations. Stuckler D. *Milbank Q.* 2008 Jun;86(2):273-326. Review.

Disease without borders. Sener SF. *CA Cancer J Clin.* 2005 Jan-Feb;55(1):7-9.

Cancer risk diversity in non-western migrants to Europe: An overview of the literature. Arnold M, Razum O, Coebergh JW. *Eur J Cancer.* 2010 Sep;46(14):2647-59.

Testicular cancer risk in first- and second-generation immigrants to Denmark. Myrup C, et al. *J Natl Cancer Inst.* 2008 Jan 2;100(1):41-7. Epub 2007 Dec 25.

Migrant studies aid the search for factors linked to breast cancer risk. Nelson NJ. *J Natl Cancer Inst.* 2006 Apr 5;98(7):436-8.

[Mortality among non-western migrants in The Netherlands] Mackenbach JP, et al. *Ned Tijdschr Geneeskd.* 2005 Apr 23;149(17):917-23.

Origins and evolution of the Western diet: health implications for the 21st century. Cordain L, et al. *Am J Clin Nutr.* 2005 Feb;81(2):341-54. Review.

Between and within: international perspectives on cancer and health disparities. Jones LA, et al. *J Clin Oncol.* 2006 May 10;24(14):2204-8. Review.

The rising burden of cancer in the developing world. Kanavos P. *Ann Oncol.* 2006 Jun;17 Suppl 8:viii15-viii23. Review.

The exploding worldwide cancer burden: the impact of cancer on women. Wilson CM, Tobin S, Young RC. *Int J Gynecol Cancer.* 2004 Jan-Feb;14(1):1-11. Review.

Cancer Initiation, Promotion and Progression

Mutation-selection networks of cancer initiation: tumor suppressor genes and chromosomal instability. Komarova NL, et al., *J Theor Biol.* 2003 Aug 21;223(4):433-50.

Genome maintenance mechanisms for preventing cancer. Hoeijmakers JH. *Nature.* 2001 May 17;411(6835):366-74. Review.

Cancer initiation and progression: an unsimplifiable complexity. Grizzi F, et al. *Theor Biol Med Model.* 2006 Oct 17;3:37.

Cancer as a complex adaptive system. Schwab ED and Pienta KJ. *Med Hypotheses.* 1996 Sep;47(3):235-41.

"Blazing a genetic trial." Pines, M. *Howard Hughes Medical Institute.* http://www.hhmi.org/genetictrail/d100.html. Retrieved on 2010-6-25.

Cancer-related inflammation. Mantovani A, et al., *Nature.* 2008 Jul 24;454(7203):436-44. Review.

Molecular pathways and targets in cancer-related inflammation. Mantovani A, et al., *Ann Med.* 2010 Apr;42(3):161-70. Review.

The Yin-Yang of tumor-associated macrophages in neoplastic progression and immune surveillance. Allavena P, et al. *Immunol Rev.* 2008 Apr;222:155-61. Review.

Cancer-related inflammation, the seventh hallmark of cancer: links to genetic instability. Colotta F, et al., *Carcinogenesis.* 2009 Jul;30(7):1073-81.

Emergentism as a default: cancer as a problem of tissue organization. Soto AM and Sonnenschein C. *J Biosci.* 2005 Feb;30(1):103-18. Review.

A Malignant Flame, Stix, G., *Scientific American Special.* 2008; 18(3): 48-55.

Carbohydrates and sugars

Tumors show enhanced dependency on glucose and glycolytic pathway. Dwarakanath BS and Huilgol NG. *J Can Res Ther* [serial online] 2009 [cited 2010 Apr 2];5:1.

Why do cancers have high aerobic glycolysis? Gatenby RA and Gillies RJ. *Nat Rev Cancer.* 2004 Nov;4(11):891-9. Review.

Metabolic changes during carcinogenesis: potential impact on invasiveness. Smallbone K, et al. *J Theor Biol.* 2007 Feb 21;244(4):703-13.

The glycolytic phenotype in carcinogenesis and tumor invasion: insights through mathematical models. Gatenby RA and Gawlinski ET. *Cancer Res.* 2003 Jul 15;63(14):3847-54.

Cancer's sweet tooth: the Janus effect of glucose metabolism in tumorigenesis. Ashrafian H. *Lancet.* 2006 Feb 18;367(9510):618-21.

Diabetes and Cancer. Gatenby R, Masur, K. (Witten) (eds), *Front Diabetes.* Basel, Karger, 2008, vol 19, pp 59-70.

Carcinogens in the Air

An alternative approach for investigating the carcinogenicity of indoor air pollution: pets as sentinels of environmental cancer risk. J A Bukowski and D Wartenberg. *Environ Health Perspect.* 1997 December; 105(12): 1312–1319.

Environmental tobacco smoke and canine urinary cotinine level, Bertone-Johnson, E.R. et al. *Environ Res.* 2008 March; 106(3): 361–364.

Passive Smoking and Canine Lung Cancer Risk, John S. Reif, et al. *Am. J. Epidemiol.* (1992) 135 (3): 234–239.

Carcinogenicity studies of inhaled cigarette smoke in laboratory animals: old and new. Hecht SS. *Carcinogenesis.* 2005 Sep;26(9):1488-92. Epub 2005 Jun 1. Review. Erratum in: *Carcinogenesis.* 2005 Nov;26(11):2029.

The following is an article which concludes that cigarette smoke does not cause cancer in the animals studied, (by the way, it's funded by Lorillard Tobacco Company): A review of chronic inhalation studies with mainstream cigarette smoke, in hamsters, dogs, and nonhuman primates. Coggins CR. *Toxicol Pathol.* 2001 Sep-Oct;29(5):550-7. Review.

Metabolic activation of carcinogenic aromatic amines by dog bladder and kidney prostaglandin H synthase. Wise RW, et al. *Cancer Res.* 1984 May;44(5):1893-7.

Cancer risk assessment, indicators, and guidelines for polycyclic aromatic hydrocarbons in the ambient air. Boström CE, et al. *Environ Health Perspect.* 2002 Jun;110 Suppl 3:451-88. Review.

Role of radical cations in aromatic hydrocarbon carcinogenesis. Cavalieri, E and Rogan, E. *Environ Health Perspect.* 1985 December; 64: 69–84.

Nitrated polycyclic aromatic hydrocarbons: a risk assessment for the urban citizen. Möller L, Lax I, Eriksson LC. *Environ Health Perspect.* 1993 Oct;101 Suppl 3:309-15.

Indoor levels of polycyclic aromatic hydrocarbons in homes with or without wood burning for heating. Gustafson P, Ostman C, Sällsten G. *Environ Sci Technol.* 2008 Jul 15;42(14):5074-80.

Carcinogens and Synergy

Gene induction studies and toxicity of chemical mixtures. Mumtaz MM, et. al. *Environ Health Perspect.* 2002 Dec;110 Suppl 6:947-56.

Public health challenges posed by chemical mixtures. Hansen H, et. al. *Environ Health Perspect.* 1998 December; 106(Suppl 6): 1271–1280.

Mixtures and interactions. Groten JP. *Food Chem Toxicol.* 2000;38(1 Suppl):S65-71. Review.

Biochemical Reaction Network Modeling: Predicting Metabolism of Organic Chemical Mixtures. Mayeno AN, Yang RSH, Reisfeld B., *Environ. Sci. Technol.*, 2005, 39 (14), pp 5363–5371

Development of a research strategy for integrated technology-based toxicological and chemical evaluation of complex mixtures of drinking water disinfection byproducts. Simmons JE, et. al. *Environ Health Perspect.* 2002 December; 110(Suppl 6): 1013–1024.

Environmental causes of cancer: endocrine disruptors as carcinogens. Soto AM and Sonnenschein C. *Nat Rev Endocrinol.* 2010 Jul;6(7):363-70. Epub 2010 May 25. Review.

Endocrine-disrupting chemicals: an Endocrine Society scientific statement. Diamanti-Kandarakis E, et. al. *Endocr Rev.* 2009 Jun;30(4):293-342. Review.

Fifteen years after "Wingspread"--environmental endocrine disrupters and human and wildlife health: where we are today and where we need to go. Hotchkiss AK, et. al. *Toxicol Sci.* 2008 Oct;105(2):235-59. Epub 2008 Feb 16. Review.

Carcinogen Avoidance after a Cancer Diagnosis

A conundrum in molecular toxicology: molecular and biological changes during neoplastic transformation of human cells. Milo GE, et al. *Cell Biol Toxicol.* 1995 Dec;11(6):329-45. Review.

Diminished DNA repair and elevated mutagenesis in mammalian cells exposed to hypoxia and low pH. Yuan J, et al. *Cancer Res.* 2000 Aug 15;60(16):4372-6.

Genetic instability induced by the tumor microenvironment. Reynolds TY, Rockwell S, Glazer PM. *Cancer Res.* 1996 Dec 15;56(24):5754-7.

Mutagenesis induced by the tumor microenvironment. Yuan J, Glazer PM. *Mutat Res.* 1998 May 25;400(1-2):439-46. Review.

Chemotherapy

Chemotherapy. Rodriquez CO, Rankin WV, Henry CJ, et al, in Henry CJ, Higginbotham ML (ed): *Cancer Management in Small Animal Practice.* Missouri. Saunders Elsevier 2010, p 101-121.

Managing Oncologic Emergencies. Dhaliwal RS, Wiebe VJ, Simonson E, et al, in Henry CJ, Higginbotham ML (ed): *Cancer Management in Small Animal Practice.* Missouri. Saunders Elsevier 2010, p 122-135

Cancer chemotherapy. Chun R, Garrett LD, Vail DM, in Withrow SJ, Vail DM (eds): *Withrow & MacEwen's Small Animal Clinical Oncology.* Missouri, Saunders Elsevier, 2007, pp 163-192.

Impact of chemotherapeutic dose intensity and hematologic toxicity on first remission duration in dogs with lymphoma treated with a chemoradiotherapy protocol. Vaughan A, Johnson JL, Williams LE. *J Vet Intern Med* 21(6):1332-9, 2007.

Prophylactic trimethoprim-sulfadiazine during chemotherapy in dogs with lymphoma and osteosarcoma: a double-blind, placebo-controlled study. Chretin JD, Rassnick KM, Shaw NA, et al. *J Vet Intern Med* 21(1):141-8, 2007.

Risk factors for sterile hemorrhagic cystitis in dogs with lymphoma receiving cyclophosphamide with or without concurrent administration of furosemide: 216 cases (1990-1996). Charney SC, Bergman PJ, Hohenhaus AE, et al. *J Am Vet Med Assoc*.222(10):1388-93, 2003.

Metronomic therapy with cyclophosphamide and piroxicam effectively delays tumor recurrence in dogs with incompletely resected soft tissue sarcomas. Elmslie RE, Glawe P, Dow SW. *J Vet Intern Med*. 22(6):1373-9, 2008.

Safety of concurrent administration of dexrazoxane and doxorubicin in the canine cancer patient. FitzPatrick WM, Dervisis NG. Kitchell B. *Veterinary and Comparative Oncology*, 8: 273–282. 2010

Acute reactions in dogs treated with doxorubicin: increased frequency with the use of a generic formulation. Phillips BS, Kraegel SA, Simonson E, et al. *J Vet Intern Med*. 12(3):171-2, 1998.

Multi-center, placebo-controlled, double-blind, randomized study of oral toceranib phosphate (SU11654), a receptor tyrosine kinase inhibitor, for the treatment of dogs with recurrent (either local or distant) mast cell tumor following surgical excision. London CA, Malpas PB, Wood-Follis SL, et al. *Clin Cancer Res*. Jun 1;15(11):3856-65, 2009.

MOPP chemotherapy for treatment of resistant lymphoma in dogs: a retrospective study of 117 cases (1989-2000). Rassnick KM, Mauldin GE, Al-Sarraf R et al. *J Vet Intern Med*.16(5):576-8, 2002.

Efficacy of Maropitant in the Prevention of Delayed Vomiting Associated with Administration of Doxorubicin to Dogs. Rau S, Barber L, and Burgess K. *J Vet Intern Med*, 24: 1452–1457, 2010.

Tolerability of Metronomic Administration of Lomustine in Dogs with Cancer. Tripp C, Fidel J, Anderson C, et al. *J Vet Intern Med*, 25: 278–284, 2011.

Cimetidine

Cimetidine inhibits cancer cell adhesion to endothelial cells and prevents metastasis by blocking E-selectin expression. Kobayashi K, et al. *Cancer Res*. 2000 Jul 15;60(14):3978-84.

Effect of histamine on the growth of human gastrointestinal tumours: reversal by cimetidine. Watson SA, et al. *Gut*. 1993 Aug;34(8):1091-6.

Cimetidine inhibits in vivo growth of human colon cancer and reverses histamine stimulated in vitro and in vivo growth. Ad-

ams WJ, Lawson JA, Morris DL. *Gut*. 1994 Nov;35(11):1632-6.

Cimetidine increases survival of colorectal cancer patients with high levels of sialyl Lewis-X and sialyl Lewis-A epitope expression on tumour cells. Matsumoto, S. et al. *Br J Cancer*. 2002 January 21; 86(2): 161–167.

Cimetidine in colorectal cancer--are the effects immunological or adhesion-mediated? Eaton D, Hawkins RE. *Br J Cancer*. 2002 Jan 21;86(2):159-60.

Characterization and development of cimetidine as a histamine H2-receptor antagonist. Brimblecombe RW, Duncan WA, Durant GJ, Emmett JC, Ganellin CR, Leslie GB, Parsons ME. *Gastroenterology*. 1978 Feb;74(2 Pt 2):339-47.

Does cimetidine improve prospects for cancer patients? A reappraisal of the evidence to date. Siegers CP, Andresen S, Keogh JP. *Digestion* 1999 Sep-Oct;60(5):415-21.

Evaluation of Cimetidine Treatment for Melanomas in Seven Horses. Preliminary Report 16 Refs. *Lorin D. Warnick, DVM, PhD, Mary E. Graham, DVM, and Beth A. Valentine, DVM, PhD. *Equine Pract* 17[7]:16–22 Jul'95.

Cimetidine for the Treatment of Melanomas in Horses: Efficacy Determined by Client Questionnaire. *Equine Pract* 16[5]:18-21 May'94. Retrospective Study 12 Refs. *Jonathan E. Hare; Henry R. Staempfli. *Am J Clin Oncol* 1991 Oct;14(5):397-9.

Phase II trial of cimetidine in metastatic melanoma. A Hoosier Oncology Group trial. Mandanas R, Schultz S, Scullin D, Einhorn LH. *J Am Vet Med Assoc* 1990 Feb 1;196(3):449-52.

Cimetidine for treatment of melanomas in three horses. Goetz TE, Ogilvie GK, Keegan KG, Johnson PJ. *J Am Vet Med Assoc*. 1990 Feb 1;196(3):449-52.

Treatment of advanced malignant melanoma with coumarin and cimetidine: a pilot study. Marshall ME, Butler K, Cantrell J, Wiseman C, Mendelsohn L. *Cancer Chemother Pharmacol* 1989;24(1):65-6.

Regression of melanoma nodules in a patient treated with ranitidine. Smith T, Clark JW, Popp MB. *Arch Intern Med* 1987 Oct;147(10):1815-6.

Coenzyme Q10

Coenzyme q10 for prevention of anthracycline-induced cardiotoxicity. Conklin KA. *Integr Cancer Ther*. 2005 Jun;4(2):110-30.

Adriamycin cardiotoxicity: early detection by systolic time interval and possible prevention by coenzyme Q10. Cortes EP, et al. *Cancer Treat Rep*. 1978 Jun;62(6):887-91.

[Investigation of the preventive effect of CoQ10 against the side-effects of anthracycline antineoplastic agents] Tsubaki K, et al. *Gan To Kagaku Ryoho.* 1984 Jul;11(7):1420-7. [Article in Japanese]

[Chronic cardiotoxicity of anthracycline derivatives and possible prevention by coenzyme Q10] Tajima M. *Gan No Rinsho.* 1984 Jul;30(9 Suppl):1211-6. [Article in Japanese]

Cardioprotection against the toxic effects of anthracyclines given to children with cancer: a systematic review. Bryant J, et al. *Health Technol Assess.* 2007 Jul;11(27):iii, ix-x, 1-84. Review.

Effect of coenzyme Q10 on the disposition of doxorubicin in rats. Zhou Q, Chowbay B. *Eur J Drug Metab Pharmacokinet.* 2002 Jul-Sep;27(3):185-92.

Reduction by coenzyme Q10 of the acute toxicity of adriamycin in mice. Combs AB, et al. *Res Commun Chem Pathol Pharmacol.* 1977 Nov;18(3):565-8.

Effect of coenzyme Q10 on the survival time and lipid peroxidation of adriamycin (doxorubicin) treated mice. Shinozawa S, et al. *Acta Med Okayama.* 1984 Feb;38(1):57-63.

Protective effect of exogenous coenzyme Q against damage by adriamycin in perfused rat liver. Valls V, et al. *Biochem Mol Biol Int.* 1994 Jul;33(4):633-42.

Efficacy of coenzyme Q10 for improved tolerability of cancer treatments: a systematic review. Roffe L, Schmidt K, Ernst E. *J Clin Oncol.* 2004 Nov 1;22(21):4418-24. Review.

Comparative cancer medicine: Dogs and Humans

Naturally occurring cancer in pet dogs: important models for developing improved cancer therapy for humans. Knapp DW and Waters DJ. *Mol Med Today.* 1997 Jan;3(1):8-11.

Spontaneously occurring tumors of companion animals as models for human cancer. Vail DM and MacEwen EG. *Cancer Invest.* 2000;18(8):781-92.

Using the canine genome to cure cancer and other diseases. Olson PN. *Theriogenology.* 2007 Aug;68(3):378-81.

Leading the way: canine models of genomics and disease. Shearin AL and Ostrander EA. *Dis Model Mech.* 2010 Jan-Feb;3(1-2):27-34.

Translation of new cancer treatments from pet dogs to humans. Paoloni M, Khanna C. *Nat Rev Cancer.* 2008 Feb;8(2):147-56. Review.

Pet models in cancer research: general principles. Porrello A, Cardelli P, Spugnini EP. *J Exp Clin Cancer Res.* 2004 Jun;23(2):181-93.

Cordyceps sinensis (also see beta glucans for related citations)

Medicinal herbal extracts--renal friend or foe? Part two: herbal extracts with potential renal benefits. Wojcikowski K, Johnson DW, Gobé G. *Nephrology (Carlton).* 2004 Dec;9(6):400-5.

Effects of Cordyceps sinensis on dimethylnitrosamine-induced liver fibrosis in rats. Li FH, Liu P, Xiong WG, Xu GF. *Zhong Xi Yi Jie He Xue Bao.* 2006 Sep;4(5):514-7. Chinese.

Cordyceps mycelia extract decreases portal hypertension in rats with dimethylnitrosamine-induced liver cirrhosis: a study on its histological basis. Wang XB, Liu P, Tang ZP, Li FH, Liu CH, Hu YY, Xu LM. *Zhong Xi Yi Jie He Xue Bao.* 2008 Nov;6(11):1136-44. Chinese.

Effects of cordyceps sinensi on bleomycin-induced pulmonary fibrosis in mice. Wang SJ, et al. *Zhongguo Zhong Yao Za Zhi.* 2007 Dec;32(24):2623-7. Chinese.

Cordyceps sinensis extract suppresses hypoxia-induced proliferation of rat pulmonary artery smooth muscle cells. Gao BA, Yang J, Huang J, Cui XJ, Chen SX, Den HY, Xiang GM. *Saudi Med J.* 2010 Sep;31(9):974-9.

Protection against radiation-induced bone marrow and intestinal injuries by Cordyceps sinensis, a Chinese herbal medicine. Liu WC, et al. *Radiat Res.* 2006 Dec;166(6):900-7.

Effect of Cordyceps sinesis on T-lymphocyte subsets in chronic renal failure. Guan YJ, Hu Z, Hou M. *Zhongguo Zhong Xi Yi Jie He Za Zhi.* 1992 Jun;12(6):338-9, 323. Chinese.

Effects of Chinese medicinal fungus water extract on tumor metastasis and some parameters of immune function. Zhang W, Wang Y, Hou Y. *Int Immunopharmacol.* 2004 Mar;4(3):461-8.

Cordyceps sinensis health supplement enhances recovery from taxol-induced leukopenia. Liu WC, et al. *Exp Biol Med (Maywood).* 2008 Apr;233(4):447-55.

Curcumin

Chemosensitization to cisplatin by inhibitors of the Fanconi anemia/BRCA pathway. Chirnomas D, et al. *Mol Cancer Ther.* 2006 Apr;5(4):952-61.

Curcumin potentiates the apoptotic effects of chemotherapeutic agents and cytokines through down-regulation of nuclear factor-kappaB and nuclear factor-kappaB-regulated gene products in IFN-alpha-sensitive and IFN-alpha-resistant human bladder cancer cells. Kamat AM, Sethi G, Aggarwal BB. *Mol Cancer Ther.* 2007 Mar;6(3):1022-30.

Curcumin potentiates antitumor activity of gemcitabine in an orthotopic model of pancreatic cancer through suppression of proliferation, angiogenesis, and inhibition of nuclear factor-kappaB-regulated gene products. Kunnumakkara AB, et al. *Cancer Res.* 2007 Apr 15;67(8):3853-61.

Possible benefits of curcumin regimen in combination with taxane chemotherapy for hormone-refractory prostate cancer treatment. Cabrespine-Faugeras A, et al. *Nutr Cancer.* 2010;62(2):148-53.

Curcumin sensitizes human colorectal cancer to capecitabine by modulation of cyclin D1, COX-2, MMP-9, VEGF and CXCR4 expression in an orthotopic mouse model. Kunnumakkara AB, et al. *Int J Cancer.* 2009 Nov 1;125(9):2187-97.

Curcumin potentiates the apoptotic effects of chemotherapeutic agents and cytokines through down-regulation of nuclear factor-kappaB and nuclear factor-kappaB-regulated gene products in IFN-alpha-sensitive and IFN-alpha-resistant human bladder cancer cells. Kamat AM, Sethi G, Aggarwal BB. *Mol Cancer Ther.* 2007 Mar;6(3):1022-30.

Curcumin prevents adriamycin nephrotoxicity in rats. Venkatesan N, Punithavathi D, Arumugam V, *Br J Pharmacol.* 2000 January; 129(2): 231–234.

Modulation of human multidrug-resistance MDR-1 gene by natural curcuminoids. Limtrakul P, Anuchapreeda S, Buddhasukh D. *BMC Cancer.* 2004 Apr 17;4:13.

Thioredoxin reductase-1 mediates curcumin-induced radiosensitization of squamous carcinoma cells. Javvadi P, et al. *Cancer Res.* 2010 Mar 1;70(5):1941-50.

Curcumin confers radiosensitizing effect in prostate cancer cell line PC-3. Chendil D, et al. *Oncogene.* 2004 Feb 26;23(8):1599-607.

The chemopreventive agent curcumin is a potent radiosensitizer of human cervical tumor cells via increased reactive oxygen species production and overactivation of the mitogen-activated protein kinase pathway. Javvadi P, et al. *Mol Pharmacol.* 2008 May;73(5):1491-501.

Curcumin sensitizes human colorectal cancer xenografts in nude mice to gamma-radiation by targeting nuclear factor-kappaB-regulated gene products. Kunnumakkara AB, et al. *Clin Cancer Res.* 2008 Apr 1;14(7):2128-36.

Curcumin protects against radiation-induced acute and chronic cutaneous toxicity in mice and decreases mRNA expression of inflammatory and fibrogenic cytokines. Okunieff P, et al. *Int J Radiat Oncol Biol Phys.* 2006 Jul 1;65(3):890-8.

Phase I clinical trial of oral curcumin: biomarkers of systemic activity and compliance. Sharma RA, et al. *Clin Cancer Res.* 2004 Oct 15;10(20):6847-54.

Phase II trial of curcumin in patients with advanced pancreatic cancer. Dhillon N, et al. *Clin Cancer Res.* 2008 Jul 15;14(14):4491-9.

Curcumin acts as anti-tumorigenic and hormone-suppressive agent in murine and human pituitary tumour cells in vitro and in vivo. Schaaf C, et al. *Endocr Relat Cancer.* 2009 Dec;16(4):1339-50.

Curcumin inhibits tumor growth and angiogenesis in ovarian carcinoma by targeting the nuclear factor-kappaB pathway. Lin YG, et al. *Clin Cancer Res.* 2007 Jun 1;13(11):3423-30.

Therapeutic potential of curcumin in human prostate cancer. III. Curcumin inhibits proliferation, induces apoptosis, and inhibits angiogenesis of LNCaP prostate cancer cells in vivo. Dorai T, et al. *Prostate.* 2001 Jun 1;47(4):293-303.

Spleen tyrosine kinase (Syk), a novel target of curcumin, is required for B lymphoma growth. Gururajan M, et al. *J Immunol.* 2007 Jan 1;178(1):111-21.

Curcumin sensitizes TRAIL-resistant xenografts: molecular mechanisms of apoptosis, metastasis and angiogenesis. Shankar S, et al. *Mol Cancer.* 2008 Jan 29;7:16.

Curcumin: the story so far. Sharma RA, Gescher AJ, Steward WP. *Eur J Cancer.* 2005 Sep;41(13):1955-68.

Bioavailability of curcumin: problems and promises. Anand P, et al. *Mol Pharm.* 2007 Nov-Dec;4(6):807-18.

Induction of apoptosis by curcumin and its implications for cancer therapy. Karunagaran D, Rashmi R, Kumar TR. *Curr Cancer Drug Targets.* 2005 Mar;5(2):117-29.

Modulation of anti-apoptotic and survival pathways by curcumin as a strategy to induce apoptosis in cancer cells. Reuter S, et al. *Biochem Pharmacol.* 2008 Dec 1;76(11):1340-51.

Curcumin-induced antiproliferative and proapoptotic effects in melanoma cells are associated with suppression of IkappaB kinase and nuclear factor kappaB activity and are independent of the B-Raf/mitogen-activated/extracellular signal-regulated protein kinase pathway and the Akt pathway. Siwak DR, et al. *Cancer.* 2005 Aug 15;104(4):879-90.

Curcumin synergistically potentiates the growth-inhibitory and pro-apoptotic effects of celecoxib in osteoarthritis synovial adherent cells. Lev-Ari S, et al. *Rheumatology* (Oxford). 2006 Feb;45(2):171-7.

Celecoxib and curcumin synergistically inhibit the growth of colorectal cancer cells. Lev-Ari S, et al. *Clin Cancer Res.* 2005 Sep 15;11(18):6738-44.

Digestive enzymes as cancer treatments

Bromelain's activity and potential as an anti-cancer agent: Current evidence and perspectives. Chobotova K, Vernallis AB,

Majid FA. *Cancer Lett.* 2010 Apr 28;290(2):148–56. Epub 2009 Aug 22. Review.

Bromelain: biochemistry, pharmacology and medical use. Maurer HR. *Cell Mol Life Sci.* 2001 Aug;58(9):1234–45. Review.

Effects of oral bromelain administration on the impaired immunocytotoxicity of mononuclear cells from mammary tumor patients. Eckert K, et al. *Oncol Rep.* 1999 Nov–Dec;6(6):1191–9.

On the pharmacology of bromelain: an update with special regard to animal studies on dose-dependent effects. Lotz–Winter H. *Planta Med.* 1990 Jun;56(3):249–53. Review.

Bioavailability of 125I bromelain after oral administration to rats. White RR, et al. *Biopharm Drug Dispos.* 1988 Jul–Aug;9(4):397–403.

In vivo antitumoral activity of stem pineapple (Ananas comosus) bromelain. Báez R, et al. *Planta Med.* 2007 Oct;73(13):1377–83. Epub 2007 Sep 24.

Modulation of murine tumor growth and colonization by bromelaine, an extract of the pineapple plant (Ananas comosum L.). Beuth J, Braun JM. *In Vivo.* 2005 Mar–Apr;19(2):483–5.

Bromelain. Orsini RA; Plastic Surgery Educational Foundation Technology Assessment Committee. *Plast Reconstr Surg.* 2006 Dec;118(7):1640–4. Review.

Bromelain inhibits COX-2 expression by blocking the activation of MAPK regulated NF-kappa B against skin tumor-initiation triggering mitochondrial death pathway. Bhui K, et al. *Cancer Lett.* 2009 Sep 18;282(2):167–76. Epub 2009 Mar 31.

Bromelain reversibly inhibits invasive properties of glioma cells. Tysnes BB, et al. *Neoplasia.* 2001 Nov–Dec;3(6):469–79.

Doctor's literature reviews, Communication, and Patient Preferences

A focus group study of veterinarians' and pet owners' perceptions of veterinarian-client communication in companion animal practice. Coe JB, Adams CL, Bonnett BN., *J Am Vet Med Assoc.* 2008 Oct 1;233(7):1072–80

Evidence-based approach to the medical literature. Fletcher RH, Fletcher SW. *J Gen Intern Med.* 1997 Apr;12 Suppl 2:S5–14. Review.

Building on existing models from human medical education to develop a communication curriculum in veterinary medicine. Adams CL, Kurtz SM. *J Vet Med Educ.* 2006 Spring;33(1):28–37. Review.

Viewpoint: power and communication: why simulation training ought to be complemented by experiential and humanist learning. Hanna M, Fins JJ. *Acad Med.* 2006 Mar;81(3):265–70.

What veterinary clients really want, too? Milani M., *Can Vet J.* 2008 Oct;49(10):1021–4.

Patient preferences versus physician perceptions of treatment decisions in cancer care. Bruera E, et. al. *J Clin Oncol.* 2001 Jun 1;19(11):2883–5.

Doxycyline

Effect of doxycycline on bone turnover and tumor markers in breast cancer (BC) patients with skeletal metastases. Dhesy-Thind SK, et al. *Journal of Clinical Oncology,* 2005 ASCO Annual Meeting Proceedings. Vol 23, No 16S (June 1 Supplement), 2005: 3198

Doxycycline decreases tumor burden in a bone metastasis model of human breast cancer. Duivenvoorden WC, et al. *Cancer Res.* 2002 Mar 15;62(6):1588–91.

Doxycycline and other tetracyclines in the treatment of bone metastasis. Saikali Z and Singh G. *Anticancer Drugs.* 2003 Nov;14(10):773–8. Review.

Use of tetracycline as an inhibitor of matrix metalloproteinase activity secreted by human bone-metastasizing cancer cells. Duivenvoorden WC, Hirte HW, Singh G. *Invasion Metastasis.* 1997;17(6):312–22.

Does doxycycline work in synergy with cisplatin and oxaliplatin in colorectal cancer? Sagar J, et al. *World J Surg Oncol.* 2009 Jan 6;7:2.

Specificity of inhibition of matrix metalloproteinase activity by doxycycline: relationship to structure of the enzyme. Smith GN Jr, et al. *Arthritis Rheum.* 1999 Jun;42(6):1140–6.

Doxycycline inhibits neutrophil (PMN)-type matrix metalloproteinases in human adult periodontitis gingiva. Golub LM, et al. *J Clin Periodontol.* 1995 Feb;22(2):100–9.

Effects of tetracyclines on angiogenesis in vitro. Fife RS, et al. *Cancer Lett.* 2000 May 29;153(1–2):75–8.

Doxycycline Induces Expression of P Glycoprotein in MCF-7 Breast Carcinoma Cells. Mealey, KL, et al. *Antimicrob Agents Chemother.* 2002 March; 46(3): 755–761

Early Cancer Development and Detection

Biomarkers for the Early Detection of Cancer An Inflammatory Concept, Roy, H.K. et al., *Arch Intern Med.* 2007;167(17):1822-1824.

Detection of associations between diseases in animal carcinogenicity experiments. Mitchell TJ, Turnbull BW., *Biometrics.*

1990 Jun;46(2):359-74.

Multistep tumorigenesis and the microenvironment. Schedin P, Elias A., *Breast Cancer Res.* 2004;6(2):93-101. Epub 2004 Feb 12. Review.

Electromagnetic Fields

Residential exposure to magnetic fields and risk of canine lymphoma. Reif JS, Lower KS, Ogilvie GK. *Am J Epidemiol.* 1995 Feb 15;141(4):352-9.

Childhood cancer in relation to distance from high voltage power lines in England and Wales: a case-control study. Draper G, et al. *BMJ.* 2005 Jun 4;330(7503):1290.

Extremely low frequency electric fields and cancer: assessing the evidence. Kheifets L, et al. *Bioelectromagnetics.* 2010 Feb;31(2):89-101. Review.

Aggregating disparate epidemiological evidence: comparing two seminal EMF reviews. O'Carroll MJ, Henshaw DL. *Risk Anal.* 2008 Feb;28(1):225-34.

Emotional Self-Management and Oxygen Mask Exercises

A different perspective to approaching cancer symptoms in children. Woodgate RL, Degner LF, Yanofsky R., *J Pain Symptom Manage.* 2003 Sep;26(3):800-17.

The emotional harbinger effect: poor context memory for cues that previously predicted something arousing. Mather M and Knight M., *Emotion.* 2008 Dec;8(6):850-60.

Dispositional optimism predicts survival status 1 year after diagnosis in head and neck cancer patients. Allison PJ, et. al., *J Clin Oncol.* 2003 Feb 1;21(3):543-8.

Gratitude influences sleep through the mechanism of pre-sleep cognitions. Wood AM, Joseph S, Lloyd J, Atkins S., *J Psychosom Res.* 2009 Jan;66(1):43-8.

Gratitude and subjective well-being in early adolescence: examining gender differences. Froh JJ, Yurkewicz C, Kashdan TB., *J Adolesc.* 2009 Jun;32(3):633-50.

Dispositional anger and risk decision-making, Gambetti E and Giusberti F. *Mind & Society.* 2009 Jun; 8(1): 7-20

Immediate effect of high-frequency yoga breathing on attention, Telles, S. et al. *Indian Journal of Medical Sciences.* 2008; 62 (1): 20-22

Cognitive predictors of vigilance. Matthews G, Davies DR, Holley PJ., *Hum Factors.* 1993 Mar;35(1):3-24.

Intensive meditation training improves perceptual discrimination and sustained attention. MacLean KA, et al., *Psychol Sci.* 2010 Jun;21(6):829-39.

White Coat Hypertension: Relevance to Clinical and Emergency Medical Services Personnel, Khan TV, et al., *MedGenMed.* 2007; 9(1): 52.

Counting blessings versus burdens: an experimental investigation of gratitude and subjective well-being in daily life. Emmons RA and McCullough ME., *J Pers Soc Psychol.* 2003 Feb;84(2):377-89.

The effects of deep breathing training on pain management in the emergency department. Downey LV and Zun LS., *South Med J.* 2009 Jul;102(7):688-92.

Frames, Biases, and Rational Decision Making in the Human Brain, De Martino, B. et al., *Science.* 2006 August 4; 313(5787): 684-687.

Jumping to conclusions and delusion proneness: the impact of emotionally salient stimuli. Warman DM and Martin JM., *J Nerv Ment Dis.* 2006 Oct;194(10):760-5.

Acute stress modulates risk taking in financial decision making. Porcelli AJ and Delgado MR., *Psychol Sci.* 2009 Mar;20(3):278-83.

Ethoxyquin

The Antioxidant Ethoxyquin and its analogues: a review. Adrianus J. de Koning. *International Journal of Food Properties,* Volume 55, Issue 2 July 2002, pages 451-461

Ethoxyquin alone induces preneoplastic changes in rat kidney whilst preventing induction of such lesions in liver by aflatoxin B1. Manson MM, Green JA, Driver HE. *Carcinogenesis.* 1987 May;8(5):723-8.

Accumulation and depuration of the synthetic antioxidant ethoxyquin in the muscle of Atlantic salmon (Salmo salar L.). Bohne VJ, Lundebye AK, Hamre K. *Food Chem Toxicol.* 2008 May;46(5):1834-43. Epub 2008 Jan 26.

Petfood Insights: Ethoxyquin Redux. Dzanis D., *Petfood Industry,* December 2009

Ethoxyquin in fish meal, Spark A. *A. Journal of the American Oil Chemists' Society.* Volume 59, Number 4 / April, 1982

To see the federal regulations that mandate fishmeal be packed with ethoxyquin when shipped, see Code of Federal Regulations, Title 49, Volume 2, Revised as of October 1, 2004, CITE: 49CFR173.218.

Food and Cooking Carcinogens

Fluoride in canine diets: http://www.ewg.org/pets/fluorideindogfood

Formation of N–Nitrosopyrrolidine in a dog's stomach. Amiysliwny, TS, et al., *Br. J. Cancer* (1974) 30, 279

Acrylamide: a cooking carcinogen?, Tareke E, et. al., *Chem Res Toxicol*. 2000 Jun;13(6):517–22.

Analysis of acrylamide, a carcinogen formed in heated foodstuffs. Tareke E, et. al., *J Agric Food Chem*. 2002 Aug 14;50(17):4998–5006.

Verification of the findings of acrylamide in heated foods. Ahn JS et. al. *Food Addit Contam*. 2002 Dec;19(12):1116–24.

A review of mechanisms of acrylamide carcinogenicity. Besaratinia A and Pfeifer GP., *Carcinogenesis*. 2007 Mar;28(3):519–28. Epub 2007 Jan 18. Review.

Acrylamide carcinogenicity. Klaunig JE., *J Agric Food Chem*. 2008 Aug 13;56(15):5984–8. Epub 2008 Jul 15. Review.

A prospective study of dietary acrylamide intake and the risk of endometrial, ovarian, and breast cancer. Hogervorst JG et. al., *Cancer Epidemiol Biomarkers Prev*. 2007 Nov;16(11):2304–13.

Determination of acrylamide in processed foods by LC/MS using column switching. Takatsuki S, et al., *Shokuhin Eiseigaku Zasshi*. 2003 Apr;44(2):89–95.

Nitrate and human cancer: a review of the evidence. Fraser P, et al. *Int J Epidemiol*. 1980 Mar;9(1):3–11.

Renal carcinogenicity of concurrently administered fish meal and sodium nitrite in F344 rats. Furukawa F, et. al., *Jpn J Cancer Res*. 2000 Feb;91(2):139–47.

Volatile N-nitrosamine formation after intake of nitrate at the ADI level in combination with an amine-rich diet. Vermeer IT, et. al., *Environ Health Perspect*. 1998 Aug;106(8):459–63.

Endogenously formed N-nitroso compounds and nitrosating agents in human cancer etiology. Bartsch H, et. al., *Pharmacogenetics*. 1992 Dec;2(6):272–7. Review.

Animal Species in which N-nitroso compounds induce cancer. Bogovski P and Bogovski S., *Int J Cancer*. 1981;27(4):471–4.

N-nitroso compounds and human cancer: where do we stand? Bartsch H., *IARC Sci Publ*. 1991;(105):1–10. Review.

Inhibition of nitrosation. Bartsch H, et. al., *Basic Life Sci*. 1993;61:27–44. Review.

Role of N-nitroso compounds (NOC) and N-nitrosation in etiology of gastric, esophageal, nasopharyngeal and bladder cancer and contribution to cancer of known exposures to NOC. Mirvish SS., *Cancer Lett*. 1995 Jun 29;93(1):17–48. Review. Erratum in: *Cancer Lett* 1995 Nov 6;97(2):271.

Production of dog food from protein meal obtained from processed poultry slaughter by-products. Slavko, F et al. *Acta agriculturae Serbica* 2010, vol. 15, iss. 29, pp. 25–30

Genotoxic and carcinogenic risk to humans of drug-nitrite interaction products. Brambilla G and Martelli A. *Mutat Res*. 2007 Jan-Feb;635(1):17–52. Epub 2006 Dec 6. Review.

DNA adducts of heterocyclic amine food mutagens: implications for mutagenesis and carcinogenesis. Schut HA and Snyderwine EG. *Carcinogenesis*. 1999 Mar;20(3):353–68. Review.

Heterocyclic amines: Mutagens/carcinogens produced during cooking of meat and fish. Sugimura T, et. al. *Cancer Sci*. 2004 Apr;95(4):290–9. Review.

Comments on the history and importance of aromatic and heterocyclic amines in public health. Weisburger JH. *Mutat Res*. 2002 Sep 30;506–507:9–20.

Heterocyclic amines: Mutagens/carcinogens produced during cooking of meat and fish. Sugimura T, et. al. *Cancer Sci*. 2004 Apr;95(4):290–9.

A new approach to risk estimation of food-borne carcinogens--heterocyclic amines--based on molecular information. Nagao M. *Mutat Res*. 1999 Dec 16;431(1):3–12. Review.

Garlic

Possible mechanism by which allyl sulfides suppress neoplastic cell proliferation. Knowles LM, Milner JA. *J Nutr*. 2001 Mar;131(3s):1061S–6S.

Reversal of P-glycoprotein-mediated multidrug resistance by diallyl sulfide in K562 leukemic cells and in mouse liver. Arora A, Seth K and Shukla Y. *Carcinogenesis*. 2004 Jun;25(6):941–9. Epub 2004 Jan 16.

Antiproliferative effects of allium derivatives from garlic. Pinto JT and Rivlin RS. *J Nutr*. 001 Mar;131(3s):1058S–60S.

Garlic and cancer: a critical review of the epidemiologic literature. Fleischauer AT and Arab L. *J Nutr*. 2001 Mar;131(3s):1032S–40S.

Ginger

Zerumbone, a Southeast Asian ginger sesquiterpene, markedly suppresses free radical generation, proinflammatory protein production, and cancer cell proliferation accompanied by apoptosis: the alpha,beta-unsaturated carbonyl group is a prerequisite. Murakami A, et al. *Carcinogenesis*. 2002 May;23(5):795-802.

Cancer preventive properties of ginger: a brief review. Shukla Y and Singh M. *Food Chem Toxicol*. 2007 May;45(5):683-90.

Anti-tumor-promoting activities of selected pungent phenolic substances present in ginger. Surh YJ, et al. *J Environ Pathol Toxicol Oncol*. 1999;18(2):131-9.

Inhibitory effects of [6]-gingerol, a major pungent principle of ginger, on phorbol ester-induced inflammation, epidermal ornithine decarboxylase activity and skin tumor promotion in ICR mice. Park KK, et al. *Cancer Lett*. 1998 Jul 17;129(2):139-44. Erratum in: *Cancer Lett* 1998 Sep 25;131(2):231.

Efficacy of ginger for nausea and vomiting: a systematic review of randomized clinical trials. Ernst E and Pittler MH. *Br J Anaesth*. 2000 Mar;84(3):367-71.

Cancer preventive properties of ginger: a brief review. Shukla Y and Singh M. *Food Chem Toxicol*. 2007 May;45(5):683-90.

Ginger (Zingiber officinale) reduces muscle pain caused by eccentric exercise. Black CD, Herring MP, Hurley DJ, O'Connor PJ. *J Pain*. 2010 Sep;11(9):894-903.

Identification of serotonin 5-HT1A receptor partial agonists in ginger. Nievergelt A, Huonker P, Schoop R, Altmann KH, Gertsch J. *Bioorg Med Chem*. 2010 May 1;18(9):3345-51

Heartworm preventative and flea/tick control products

Spinosad insecticide: subchronic and chronic toxicity and lack of carcinogenicity in Fischer 344 rats. Yano BL, Bond DM, Novilla MN, McFadden LG, Reasor MJ. *Toxicol Sci*. 2002 Feb;65(2):288-98.

Fipronil: environmental fate, ecotoxicology, and human health concerns. Tingle CC, et al. *Rev Environ Contam Toxicol*. 2003;176:1-66. Review.

Permrethrin
http://toxnet.nlm.nih.gov/cgi-bin/sis/search/a?dbs+hsdb:@term+@DOCNO+6790

Imidacloprid
http://www.pesticideinfo.org/Detail_Chemical.jsp?Rec_Id=PC35730

Ivermectin
http://potency.berkeley.edu/chempages/IVERMECTIN.html

Selamectin
http://www.pesticideinfo.org/Detail_Chemical.jsp?Rec_Id=PC41305

Nitenpyram
http://www.pesticideinfo.org/Detail_Chemical.jsp?Rec_Id=PC43609

Hemangiosarcoma

Johnson KD Splenic Tumors, in Henry CJ, Higginbotham ML (ed): *Cancer Management in Small Animal Practice*. Missouri. Saunders Elsevier 2010, p 264-68.

Tumors of the Skin, Subcutis and other soft tissues. Northrup N, Geiger T, in Henry CJ, Higginbotham ML (ed): *Cancer Management in Small Animal Practice*. Missouri. Saunders Elsevier 2010, p 299.

Hemangiosarcoma. Chun R, in Cote E (2nd ed), *Clinical Veterinary Advisor: Dogs and Cats*. Missouri, Mosby Elsevier, 2011, p 482-486.

Hemangiosarcoma, Cardiac. Edwards NJ, in Cote E (ed), *Clinical Veterinary Advisor: Dogs and Cats*. Missouri, Mosby Elsevier, 2007, p 473-75.

Miscellaneous Tumors. Thamm DH, in Withrow SJ, Vail DM (eds): *Withrow & MacEwen's Small Animal Clinical Oncology*. Missouri, Saunders Elsevier, 2007, pp 785-823.

Hemangiosarcoma in dogs and cats. Smith A. *Vet Clin Small Anim* 33:533-552, 2003.

Prevalence, type, and importance of splenic diseases in dogs: 1,480 cases (1985-1989), Spangler WL, Culbertson MR. *J Am Vet Med Assoc* 200:829, 1992.

Treatment of canine hemangiosarcoma: 2000 and beyond. Clifford CA, Mackin AJ, Henry CJ. *J Vet Intern Med* 14:479, 2000.

Magnetic resonance imaging of focal splenic and hepatic lesions in the dog. Clifford CA, Pretorius ES, Weisse C et al. *J Vet Intern Med*. 18(3):330-8. 2004\

Vascular endothelial growth factor concentrations in body cavity effusions in dogs. Clifford CA, Hughes D, Beal MW, et al. *J Vet Intern Med*. 16(2):164-8. 2002

Ventricular arrhythmias in dogs with splenic masses. Keyes M, Rush J. *Vet Emerg Crit Care* 3:33-38. 1994

Liposome-encapsulated muramyl tripeptide phosphatidylethanolamine adjuvant immunotherapy for splenic hemangiosarcoma in the dog: a randomized multi-institutional clinical trial. Vail DM, MacEwen EG, Kurzman ID, et al. *Clin Cancer Res* 81:935, 1995.

Continuous low-dose oral chemotherapy for adjuvant therapy of splenic hemangiosarcoma in dogs. Lana S, U'ren L, Plaza S, et al. *J Vet Intern Med* 21:764, 2007.

Splenomegaly in dogs. Predictors of neoplasia and survival after splenectomy. Johnson KA, Powers BE, Withrow SJ, et al. *J Vet Intern Med* 3:160, 1989.

Pathologic factors affecting postsplenectomy survival in dogs. Spangler WL, Kass PH. *J Vet Intern Med* 11:166, 1997

Metastatic pattern in dogs with splenic hemangiosarcoma. Waters D, Hayden D, Walter P. *J Small Anim Pract* 3:222, 1988.

Efficacy and toxicity of a dose-intensified doxorubicin protocol in canine hemangiosarcoma. Sorenmo KU, Beaz JL, Clifford CA, et al. *J Vet Intern Med* 18:209-213, 2004

Canine hemangiosarcoma treated with standard chemotherapy and minocycline. Sorenmo K, Duda L, Barber L, et al. *J Vet Intern Med.* 14(4): 395-8. 2000

Evaluation of intracavitary mitoxantrone and carboplatin for treatment of carcinomatosis, sarcomatosis, and mesothelioma, with or without malignant effusions: a retrospective analysis of 12 cases (1997-2002). Charney SC, Bergman PJ, McKnight JA, et al. *Vet Comp Oncol* 3:171, 2005.

Hemangiosarcoma: Cardiac

Cardiac tumors in dogs: 1982-1995. Ware WA, Hopper DL. *J Vet Intern Med* 13:95, 1999.

Cardiac troponins I and T in dogs with pericardial effusion. Shaw SP, Rozanski EA, Rush JE. *J Vet Intern Med;* 18:322-324. 2004

Use of pericardial fluid pH to distinguish between idiopathic and neoplastic effusions. Fine DM, Tobias AH, Jacob KA. *J Vet Intern Med.* 17:525-9. 2003

The diagnostic value of pericardial fluid pH determination. Edwards NJ. *J Am Anim Hops Assoc Intern Med.* 32:63-67. 1996

Analysis of prognostic indicators for dogs with pericardial effusion: 46 cases (1985-1996). Dunning D, Monnet E, Orton EC, et al. *J Am Vet Med Assoc.* 212:1276-80. 1998

Cardiac hemangiosarcoma in the dog: a review of 38 cases. Aronsohn M. *J Am Vet Med Assoc* 187:922, 1985.

Survival times in dogs with right atrial hemangiosarcoma treated by means of surgical resection with or without adjuvant chemotherapy: 23 cases (1986-2000). Weisse C, Soares N, Beal MW, et al. *J Am Vet Med Assoc.* 226(4):575-9. 2005

Cardiac HSA risk associated with spay/neuter (Cardiac tumors in dogs: 1982-1995). Ware WA, Hopper DL. *J Vet Intern Med.* 1999 Mar-Apr;13(2):95-103.

Hemangiosarcoma: Skin, Subcutaneous and Intra-

muscular

Cutaneous hemangiosarcoma in 25 dogs: A retrospective study. Ward J, Fox LE, Calderwood-Mays MB, et al. *J Vet Intern Med* 8:345-48, 1994

A retrospective study of visceral and nonvisceral hemangiosarcoma and hemangiomas in domestic animals. Schultheiss PC. *J Vet Diagn Invest* 16(6):522, 2004.

Evaluation of outcome associated with subcutaneous and intramuscular hemangiosarcoma treated with adjuvant doxorubicin in dogs: 21 cases (2001-06). Bulakowski EJ, Philibert JC, Siegel S, et al. *J Am Vet Med Assoc* 233(1):122, 2008.

Effects of palliative radiation therapy for nonsplenic hemangiosarcoma in dogs. Hillers KR, Lana SE, Fuller CR, et al. *J Am Anim Hosp Assoc* 43(4):187, 2007

Herbicides, Pesticides, and Other Chemicals

Herbicide exposure and the risk of transitional cell carcinoma of the urinary bladder in Scottish Terriers. Glickman LT, et al. *J Am Vet Med Assoc.* 2004 Apr 15;224(8):1290-7.

Topical flea and tick pesticides and the risk of transitional cell carcinoma of the urinary bladder in Scottish Terriers. Raghavan M, et al. *J Am Vet Med Assoc.* 2004 Aug 1;225(3):389-94.

Epidemiologic study of insecticide exposures, obesity, and risk of bladder cancer in household dogs. Glickman LT, et al. *J Toxicol Environ Health.* 1989;28(4):407-14.

Canine exposure to herbicide-treated lawns and urinary excretion of 2,4-dichlorophenoxyacetic acid. Reynolds PM, et al. *Cancer Epidemiol Biomarkers Prev.* 1994 Apr–May;3(3):233-7.

On the association between canine malignant lymphoma and opportunity for exposure to 2,4-dichlorophenoxyacetic acid. Hayes HM, Tarone RE, Cantor KP. *Environ Res.* 1995 Aug;70(2):119-25.

Re-analysis of 2,4-D use and the occurrence of canine malignant lymphoma. Kaneene JB, Miller R. *Vet Hum Toxicol.* 1999 Jun;41(3):164-70.

Case-control study of canine malignant lymphoma: positive association with dog owner's use of 2,4-dichlorophenoxyacetic acid herbicides. Hayes HM, et al. *J Natl Cancer Inst.* 1991 Sep 4;83(17):1226-31.

Bladder cancer in pet dogs: a sentinel for environmental cancer? Hayes HM Jr, Hoover R, Tarone RE. *Am J Epidemiol.* 1981 Aug;114(2):229-33.

Disinfection byproducts and bladder cancer: a pooled analysis. Villanueva CM, et al. *Epidemiology.* 2004 May;15(3):357-67.

Association between canine malignant lymphoma, living in industrial areas, and use of chemicals by dog owners. Gavazza A, et al. *J Vet Intern Med.* 2001 May-Jun;15(3):190-5.

Homeopathy

Ruta 6 selectively induces cell death in brain cancer cells but proliferation in normal peripheral blood lymphocytes: A novel treatment for human brain cancer. Pathak S, et al. *Int J Oncol.* 2003 Oct;23(4):975-82.

Can homeopathic treatment slow prostate cancer growth? Jonas WB, et al. *Integr Cancer Ther.* 2006 Dec;5(4):343-9.

Homeopathy in cancer care. Frenkel M. *Altern Ther Health Med.* 2010 May-Jun;16(3):12-6. Review.

Efficacy of homeopathic therapy in cancer treatment. Milazzo S, Russell N, Ernst E. *Eur J Cancer.* 2006 Feb;42(3):282-9. Epub 2006 Jan 11. Review.

Homeopathic medicines for adverse effects of cancer treatments. Kassab S, et al. *Cochrane Database Syst Rev.* 2009 Apr 15;(2):CD004845. Review.

Hospice Care

Early palliative care for patients with metastatic non-small-cell lung cancer. Temel JS, Greer JA, Muzikansky A, Gallagher ER, Admane S, Jackson VA, Dahlin CM, Blinderman CD, Jacobsen J, Pirl WF, Billings JA, Lynch TJ. *N Engl J Med.* 2010 Aug 19;363(8):733-42.

Incredible Canine

Olfactory detection of human bladder cancer by dogs: proof of principle study. Willis CM, et. al. *BMJ.* 2004 Sep 25;329(7468):712.

Diagnostic accuracy of canine scent detection in early- and late-stage lung and breast cancers. McCulloch M, et al., *Integr Cancer Ther.* 2006 Mar;5(1):30-9.

"Seizure Alert Dogs", *Orlando Sentinel*, May 6, 1990

How Dogs Think. Coren, Stanley (2004) First Free Press. Simon and Schuster.

"Dog Sense of Hearing". seefido.com. http://www.seefido.com/html/dog_sense_of_hearing.htm. Retrieved on 2008-10-22.

"Smell". nhm.org. 6 May 2004. http://www.nhm.org/exhibitions/dogs/formfunction/smell.html. Retrieved on 2008-10-22.

Dogs: How to Take Care of Them and Understand Them. Wegler, M. New York: Barrons Educational Series, 1996.

Indole 3 carbinol

Prevention of chromosomal aberration in mouse bone marrow by indole-3-carbinol. Agrawal RC, Kumar S. *Toxicol Lett.* 1999 Jun 1;106(2-3):137-41.

Protective effects of indole-3-carbinol on cyclophosphamide-induced clastogenecity in mouse bone marrow cells. Shukla Y, Srivastava B, Arora A, Chauhan LK. *Hum Exp Toxicol.* 2004 May;23(5):245-50.

Prevention of cyclophosphamide-induced micronucleus formation in mouse bone marrow by indole-3-carbinol. Agrawal RC, Kumar S. *Food Chem Toxicol.* 1998 Nov;36(11):975-7.

Clinical development plan: indole-3-carbinol. [No authors listed]. *J Cell Biochem Suppl.* 1996; 26:127-36.

Krill Oil & Fish Oil

Fish oil and treatment of cancer cachexia. Giacosa A and Rondanelli M. *Genes Nutr.* 2008 Apr;3(1):25-8.

Eicosapentaenoic acid in treatment-resistant depression associated with symptom remission, structural brain changes and reduced neuronal phospholipid turnover. Puri BK, et al. *Int J Clin Pract.* 2001 Oct;55(8):560-3.

Omega-3 fatty acids and major depression: A primer for the mental health professional, Logan A. C. *Lipids in Health and Disease.* 2004, 3:25

The importance of the ratio of omega-6/omega-3 essential fatty acids. Simopoulos AP. *Biomed Pharmacother.* 2002 Oct;56(8):365-79.

Dietary omega-3 polyunsaturated fatty acids plus vi tamin E restore immunodeficiency and prolong survival for severely ill patients with generalized malignancy: a randomized control trial. Gogos CA, et al. *Cancer.* 1998 Jan 15;82(2):395-402.

Omega-3 fatty acids in major depressive disorder. A preliminary double-blind, placebo-controlled trial. Su KP, et al. *Eur Neuropsychopharmacol.* 2003 Aug;13(4):267-71. Erratum in: EurNeuropsychopharmacol. 2004 Mar;14(2):173.

Eicosapentaenoic acid in treatment-resistant depression associated with symptom remission, structural brain changes and reduced neuronal phospholipid turnover. Puri BK, et al. *Int J Clin Pract.* 2001 Oct;55(8):560-3.

Depression and cancer: mechanisms and disease progression. Spiegel D and Giese-Davis J. *Biol Psychiatry.* 2003 Aug

1;54(3):269–82. Review.

Depression as a predictor of disease progression and mortality in cancer patients: a meta-analysis. Satin JR, Linden W, Phillips MJ. *Cancer*. 2009 Nov 15;115(22):5349–61.

Psychological depression and 17-year risk of death from cancer. Shekelle RB, et al. *Psychosom Med*. 1981 Apr;43(2):117–25.

Psychological distress and cancer mortality. Hamer M, Chida Y, Molloy GJ. *J Psychosom Res*. 2009 Mar;66(3):255–8.

Luteolin

Phosphorylation and stabilization. Shi R, et al. *Mol Cancer Ther*. 2007 Apr;6(4):1338–47.

Anti-proliferative and chemosensitizing effects of luteolin on human gastric cancer AGS cell line. Wu B, et al. *Mol Cell Biochem* (2008) Jun;313(1–2):125–32. Epub 2008 Apr 9.

Luteolin as a glycolysis inhibitor offers superior efficacy and lesser toxicity of doxorubicin in breast cancer cells. Du GJ, et al. *Biochem Biophys Res Commun*. 2008 Aug 1;372(3):497–502

Radiosensitization effect of luteolin on human gastric cancer SGC-7901 cells. Zhang Q, et al. *J Biol Regul Homeost Agents*. 2009 Apr-Jun;23(2):71–8.

Intestinal absorption of luteolin and luteolin 7-O-beta-glucoside in rats and humans. Shimoi K, et al. *FEBS Lett*. 1998 Nov 6;438(3):220–4.

Distribution and biological activities of the flavonoid luteolin. López-Lázaro M. *Mini Rev Med Chem*. 2009 Jan;9(1):31–59. Review.

Absorption and excretion of luteolin and apigenin in rats after oral administration of Chrysanthemum morifolium extract. Chen T, et al. *J Agric Food Chem*. 2007 Jan 24;55(2):273–7.

Intestinal absorption of luteolin from peanut hull extract is more efficient than that from individual pure luteolin. Zhou P, et al. J Agric Food Chem. 2008 Jan 9;56(1):296–300.

Luteolin as an anti-inflammatory and anti-allergic constituent of Perilla frutescens. Ueda H, Yamazaki C, Yamazaki M. *Biol Pharm Bull*. 2002 Sep;25(9):1197–202.

Luteolin, a flavonoid with potentials for cancer prevention and therapy, Lin Y, et al. *Curr Cancer Drug Targets*. 2008 November; 8(7): 634–646.

Luteolin, an emerging anti-cancer flavonoid, poisons eukaryotic DNA topoisomerase I. Chowdhury AR, et al. *Biochem J*. 2002 Sep 1;366(Pt 2):653–61.

Design of new anti-cancer agents based on topoisomerase poisons targeted to specific DNA sequences. Arimondo PB and Hélène C. *Curr Med Chem Anticancer Agents*. 2001 Nov;1(3):219–35. Review.

Luteolin induces apoptosis via death receptor 5 upregulation in human malignant tumor cells. Horinaka M, et al. *Oncogene*. 2005 Nov 3;24(48):7180–9.

Luteolin induces apoptosis in oral squamous cancer cells. Yang SF, et al. *J Dent Res*. 2008 Apr;87(4):401–6.

Sensitizing HER2-overexpressing cancer cells to luteolin-induced apoptosis through suppressing p21(WAF1/CIP1) expression with rapamycin. Chiang CT, Way TD, Lin JK. *Mol Cancer Ther*. 2007 Jul;6(7):2127–38.

Luteolin and luteolin-7-O-glucoside from dandelion flower suppress iNOS and COX-2 in RAW264.7 cells. Hu C and Kitts DD. *Mol Cell Biochem*. 2004 Oct;265(1–2):107–13.

Luteolin inhibits insulin-like growth factor 1 receptor signaling in prostate cancer cells. Fang J, et al. *Carcinogenesis*. 2007 Mar;28(3):713–23. Epub 2006 Oct 25.

Luteolin suppresses inflammation-associated gene expression by blocking NF-kappaB and AP-1 activation pathway in mouse alveolar macrophages. Chen CY, et al. *Life Sci*. 2007 Nov 30;81(23–24):1602–14.

Luteolin inhibits invasion of prostate cancer PC3 cells through E-cadherin. Zhou Q, et al. *Mol Cancer Ther*. 2009 Jun;8(6):1684–91.

Pro-apoptotic effects of the flavonoid luteolin in rat H4IIE cells. Michels G, et al. *Toxicology*. 2005 Jan 31;206(3):337–48.

Lymphoma General References

Lymphoma. Bryan JN, in Henry CJ, Higginbotham ML (ed): *Cancer Management in Small Animal Practice*. Missouri. Saunders Elsevier 2010, p 343–350.

Principles of treatment for canine lymphoma. Ettinger SN. *Clin Tech Small Anim Pract* 18:92–97, 2003.

Canine lymphoma and lymphoid leukemias. Vail DM, Young KM, in Withrow SJ, Vail DM (eds): *Withrow & MacEwen's Small Animal Clinical Oncology*. Missouri, Saunders Elsevier, 2007, pp 699–733.

Lymphoma, Dog (Multicentric). Williams LE, in Cote E (2nd ed), *Clinical Veterinary Advisor: Dogs and Cats*. Missouri, Mosby Elsevier, 2011, p 675–678.

Proteomic identification and profiling of canine lymphoma patients. Ratcliffe L, Mian S, Slater K, et al. *Vet Comp Oncol*. 7(2):92–105. 2009

Lymphoma Risks

Association between canine malignant lymphoma, living in industrial areas, and use of chemicals by dog owners. Gavazza A, Presciuttini S, Barale R, et al. *J Vet Intern Med* 15:190, 2001.

On the association between canine malignant lymphoma and opportunity for exposure to 2,4-dichlorophenoxyacetic acid. Hayes HM, Tarone RE, Cantor KP. *Environ Res* 70:119, 1995.

Re-analysis of 2,4-D use and the occurrence of canine malignant lymphoma. Kaneene JB, Miller R. *Vet Hum Toxicol* 41:164, 1999.

Distinct B-cell and T-cell lymphoproliferative disease prevalence among dog breeds indicates heritable risk. Modiano JF, Breen M, Burnett RC, et al. *Cancer Res* 65:5654, 2005

The occurrence of tumors in domestic animals. Preister WA, McKay FW, in Zeigler JL (ed): *National Cancer Institute Monographs,* Bethesda, 1980, U.S. Dept of Health and Human Services.

Canine exposure to herbicide-treated lawns and urinary excretion of 2,4-dichlorophenoxyacetic acid. Reynolds PM, Reif JS, Ramsdell HS, et al. *Cancer Epidemiol Biomarkers Prev* 3:233, 1994.

Lymphoma Diagnostics, Staging, and Prognosis

Radiographic abnormalities in canine multicentric lymphoma: a review of 84 cases. Blackwood L, Sullivan M, Lawson H. *J Small Anim Pract* 38:62-9, 1997

Canine lymphoma: immunocytochemical analysis of fine-needle aspiration biopsy. Caniatti M, Roccabianca P, Scanziani E, et al. *Vet Pathol* 33:204-12, 1996

Gastrointestinal lymphoma in 20 dogs. A retrospective study. Couto CG, Rutgers HC, Sherding RG, et al. *J Vet Intern Med* 3:73-8, 1989

Central nervous system lymphosarcoma in the dog. Couto CG, Cullen J, Pedroia V, et al. *J Am Vet Med Assoc.* 184:809-13, 1984

Updates on the management of canine epitheliotropic cutaneous T-cell lymphoma. de Lorimier LP. *Vet Clin North Am Small Anim Pract* 36:213, 2006.

Flow cytometric immunophenotype of canine lymph node aspirates. Gibson D, Aubert I, Woods JP, et al. *J Vet Intern Med* 18:710, 2004.

Hematologic and bone marrow cytological abnormalities in 75 dogs with malignant lymphoma. Madewell BR. *J An Anim Hosp Assoc* 22:235-240, 1986

Canine cutaneous epitheliotropic lymphoma (mycosis fungoides) is a proliferative disorder of CD8+ T cells. Moore PF, Olivry T, Naydan D. *Am J Pathol.* 144:421-9, 1994

Prevalence of leukemic blood and bone marrow in dogs with multicentric lymphoma. Raskin RE, Krehbiel JD. *J Am Vet Med Assoc* 194:1427-9, 1989

Prognostic factors in dogs with lymphoma and associated hypercalcemia. Rosenberg MP, Matus RE, Patnaik AK. *J Vet Intern Med* 5:268-71, 1991

Parathyroid hormone (PTH)-related protein, PTH, and 1,25-dihydroxyvitamin D in dogs with cancer-associated hypercalcemia. Rosol TJ, Nagode LA, Couto CG, et al. *Endocrinology* 131:1157-64, 1992

Immunophenotypic characterization of canine lymphoproliferative disorders. Ruslander DA, Gebhard DH, Tompkins MB, et al. *In Vivo* 11:169-72, 1997

Utility of polymerase chain reaction for analysis of antigen receptor rearrangement in staging and predicting prognosis in dogs with lymphoma. Lana SE, Jackson TL, Burnett RC, et al. *J Vet Intern Med* 20:329, 2006.

Use of fine needle aspirates and flow cytometry for the diagnosis, classification, and immunophenotyping of canine lymphomas. Sozmen M, Tasca S, Carli E, et al. *J Vet Diagn Invest* 17:323, 2005.

Correlation between thoracic radiographic changes and remission/survival duration in 270 dogs with lymphosarcoma. Starrak GS, Berry CR, Page RL, et al. *Vet Radiol Ultrasound.* 38:411-8, 1997

Humoral hypercalcemia of malignancy in canine lymphosarcoma. Weir EC, Norrdin RW, Matus RE, et al. *Endocrinology* 122:602-8, 1988

Lymphoma Chemotherapy

Systemic therapy of cutaneous T-cell lymphoma (Mycosis fungoides and the Sezary Syndrome). Bunn PA, Hoffman SJ, Norris D, et al. *Ann Intern Med* 121:592-602, 1994.

Monoclonal antibody C219 immunohistochemistry against P-glycoprotein: sequential analysis and predictive ability in dogs with lymphoma. Bergman PJ, Ogilvie GK, Powers BE. *J Vet Intern Med* 10:354, 1996.

Chemotherapy of canine lymphoma with histopathological correlation: doxorubicin alone compared to COP as first treatment regimen. Carter RF, Harris CK, Withrow SJ. *J Am Anim Hosp Assoc* 23:221, 1987.

Treatment of lymphoma and leukemia with cyclophosphamide, vincristine, and prednisone. Cotter SM, Goldstein MA. *J Am Anim Hosp Assoc* 19:159, 1983.

Evaluation of a 6-month chemotherapy protocol with no maintenance therapy for dogs with lymphoma. Garrett LD, Thamm DH, Chun R, et al. *J Vet Intern Med* 16:704, 2002.

Influence of asparaginase on a combination chemotherapy protocol for canine multicentric lymphoma. Jeffreys AB, Knapp DW, Carlton WW, et al. *J Am Anim Hosp Assoc* 41:221, 2005.

Does L-asparaginase influence efficacy or toxicity when added to a standard CHOP protocol for dogs with lymphoma? MacDonald VS, Thamm DH, Kurzman ID, et al. *J Vet Intern Med* 19:732, 2005

Evaluation of a discontinuous treatment protocol (VELCAP-S) for canine lymphoma. Moore AS, Cotter SM, Rand WM, et al. *J Vet Intern Med* 15:348, 2001.

Comparison of the effects of asparaginase administered subcutaneously versus intramuscularly for treatment of multicentric lymphoma in dogs receiving doxorubicin. Valerius KD, Ogilvie GK, Fettman MJ, et al. *J Am Vet Med Assoc* 214:353, 1999.

The expression of P-glycoprotein in canine lymphoma and its association with multidrug resistance. Moore AS, Leveille CR, Reimann KA, et al. *Cancer Invest* 13:475, 1995.

Increased toxicity of P-glycoprotein-substrate chemotherapeutic agents in a dog with the MDR1 deletion mutation associated with ivermectin sensitivity. Mealey KL, Northrup NC, Bentjen SA. *J Am Vet Med Assoc* 223:1453, 1434, 2003.

Impact of Chemotherapeutic Dose Intensity and Hematologic Toxicity on First Remission Duration in Dogs with Lymphoma Treated with a Chemoradiotherapy Protocol. Vaughan A, Johnson JL, Williams, LE. *J Vet Intern Med*, 21: 1332–1339, 2007.

CCNU in the treatment of canine epitheliotropic lymphoma. Williams LE, Rassnick KM, Power HT, et al. *J Vet Intern Med* 20:136, 2006.

Lymphoma Rescue Protocols

Doxorubicin for treatment of canine lymphosarcoma after development of resistance to combination chemotherapy. Calvert CA, Leifer CE. *J Am Vet Med Assoc* 179:1011, 1981.

Treatment of tumor-bearing dogs with actinomycin D. Hammer AS, Couto CG, Ayl RD, et al. *J Vet Intern Med* 8:236, 1994.

Efficacy and toxicity of BOPP and LOPP chemotherapy for the treatment of relapsed canine lymphoma. LeBlanc AK, Mauldin GE, Milner RJ, et al. *Vet Comp Oncol* 4:21, 2006.

Lomustine (CCNU) for the treatment of resistant lymphoma in dogs. Moore AS, London CA, Wood CA, et al. *J Vet Intern Med* 13:395, 1999.

Evaluation of mitoxantrone for the treatment of lymphoma in dogs. Moore AS, London CA, Wood CA, et al. *J Am Vet Med Assoc* 204:1903-5, 1994

Actinomycin D for reinduction of remission in dogs with resistant lymphoma. Moore AS, Ogilvie GK, Vail DM. *J Vet Intern Med* 8:343, 1994.

MOPP chemotherapy for treatment of resistant lymphoma in dogs: a retrospective study of 117 cases (1989-2000). Rassnick KM, Mauldin GE, Al-Sarraf R, et al. *J Vet Intern Med* 16:576, 2002.

Treatment of relapsed canine lymphoma with doxorubicin and dacarbazine. Van Vechten M, Helfand SC, Jeglum KA. *J Vet Intern Med* 4:187, 1990

Lymphoma: Other Treatment Options

A feasibility study of low-dose total body irradiation for relapsed canine lymphoma. Brown EM, Ruslander DM, Azuma C, et al. *Vet Comp Oncol* 4:75, 2006.

A combination chemotherapy protocol with dose intensification and autologous bone marrow transplant (VELCAP-HDC) for canine lymphoma. Frimberger AE, Moore AS, Rassnick KM, et al. *J Vet Intern Med* 20:355, 2006.

Half-body radiotherapy in the treatment of canine lymphoma. Laing EJ, Fitzpatrick PJ, Binnington AG, et al. *J Vet Intern Med* 3:102-8, 1989

Use of multigeneration-family molecular dog leukocyte antigen typing to select a hematopoietic cell transplant donor for a dog with T-cell lymphoma. Lupu M, Sullivan EW, Westfall TE, et al. *J Am Vet Med Assoc* 228:728, 2006.

The role of radiotherapy in the treatment of lymphoma and thymoma. Meleo KA. *Vet Clin North Am Small Anim Pract* 27:115-29, 1997

Effect of fish oil, arginine, and doxorubicin chemotherapy on remission and survival time for dogs with lymphoma: a double-blind, randomized placebo-controlled study. Ogilvie GK, Fettman MJ, Mallinckrodt CH, et al. *Cancer* 88:1916, 2000.

Total skin electron beam irradiation for generalized cutaneous lymphoma. Prescott D.M., Gordon J. *Vet Comp Oncol* 3:32, 2005.

Evaluation of the effects of dietary n-3 fatty acid supplementation on the pharmacokinetics of doxorubicin in dogs with lymphoma. Selting KA, Ogilvie GK, Gustafson DL, et al. *Am J*

Vet Res 67:145, 2006.

Chemotherapy followed by half-body radiation therapy for canine lymphoma. Williams LE, Johnson JL, Hauck ML, et al. *J Vet Intern Med* 18:703, 2004.

Maintenance multivitamins (also see antioxidants and pro-oxidants for related citations)

Antioxidants and cancer therapy: a systematic review. Ladas EJ, et al. *J Clin Oncol.* 2004 Feb 1;22(3):517-28. Review.

Should patients undergoing chemotherapy and radiotherapy be prescribed antioxidants? Moss RW. *Integr Cancer Ther.* 2006 Mar;5(1):63-82. Review.

Antioxidant Supplementation in Cancer: Potential Interactions with Conventional Chemotherapy and Radiation Therapy. [No author listed.] Thomas Jefferson University Hospital, Myrna Brind Center of Integrative Medicine. July, 2006. Available at: http://jdc.jefferson.edu/cgi/viewcontent.cgi?article=1009&context=jmbcim

Antioxidants and other nutrients do not interfere with chemotherapy or radiation therapy and can increase kill and increase survival, part 1. Simone CB 2nd, et al. *Altern Ther Health Med.* 2007 Jan-Feb;13(1):22-8. Review.

Antioxidants and other nutrients do not interfere with chemotherapy or radiation therapy and can increase kill and increase survival, Part 2. Simone CB 2nd, et al. *Altern Ther Health Med.* 2007 Mar-Apr;13(2):40-7. Review.

Dietary antioxidants during cancer chemotherapy: impact on chemotherapeutic effectiveness and development of side effects. Conklin KA. *Nutr Cancer.* 2000;37(1):1-18. Review.

The antioxidant conundrum in cancer. Seifried HE, et al. *Cancer Res.* 2003 Aug 1;63(15):4295-8. Review.

Antioxidant vitamins and minerals in prevention of cancers: lessons from the SU.VI.MAX study. Hercberg S, Czernichow S, Galan P. *Br J Nutr.* 2006 Aug;96 Suppl 1:S28-30.

A review of the interaction among dietary antioxidants and reactive oxygen species. Seifried HE, et al. *J Nutr Biochem.* 2007 Sep;18(9):567-79. Epub 2007 Mar 23. Review.

Antioxidant effects of natural bioactive compounds. Balsano C and Alisi A. *Curr Pharm Des.* 2009;15(26):3063-73. Review.

Free radicals and antioxidants in normal physiological functions and human disease. Valko M, et al. *Int J Biochem Cell Biol.* 2007;39(1):44-84. Epub 2006 Aug 4. Review.

Clinical and experimental experiences with intravenous vitamin C. Riordan NH, Riordan HD, Casciari JP. *J Orthomol Med.* 2000;15:201-213. Available at: http://orthomolecular. org/library/jom/2000/pdf/2000-v15n04-p201.pdf. Accessed February 12, 2007.

Mammary Tumors

Canine Mammary Gland Tumors. Henry CJ, in Henry CJ, Higginbotham ML (ed): *Cancer Management in Small Animal Practice.* Missouri. Saunders Elsevier 2010, p 275-280.

Tumors of the mammary gland, in. Lana SE, Rutteman GR, Withrow SJ. Withrow SJ, Vail DM (eds): *Withrow & MacEwen's Small Animal Clinical Oncology.* Missouri, Saunders Elsevier, 2007, pp 619-628

Mammary Gland Neoplasia, Dog. Balkman C, in Cote E (2nd ed), *Clinical Veterinary Advisor: Dogs and Cats.* Missouri, Mosby Elsevier, 2011, p 692-694.

Canine Mammary Gland Tumors. Sorenmo K. *Vet Clin Small Anim* 33: 573-596, 2003.

Mammary Cancer. Henry CJ, in Bonagura JD, Twedt DC (ed): *Kirk's Current Veterinary Therapy XIV.* Missouri. Saunders Elsevier 2009, p 363-368.

A population-based case-control study of canine mammary tumours and clinical use of medroxyprogesterone acetate. Stovring M, Moe L, Glattre E. *APMIS* 105:590, 1997.

Mammary gland tumors in male dogs. Saba CF, Rogers KS, Newman SJ, et al. *J Vet Intern Med* 21:1056, 2007.

Factors influencing canine mammary cancer development and postsurgical survival. Schneider R, Dorn CR, Taylor DON. *J Natl Cancer Inst* 43(6):1249, 1969.

Body confirmation, diet and risk of breast cancer in pet dogs: a case-control study. Sonnenschein EG, Glickman LT, Goldschmidt MH, et al. *Am J Epidemiol* 133:694, 1991.

Cyclooxygenase-2 expression is associated with histologic tumor type in canine mammary carcinoma. Heller DA, Clifford CA, Goldschmidt MH, et al. *Vet Pathol.* 42(6):776-80. 2005

Meta-analysis: dietary fat intake, serum estrogen levels, and the risk of breast cancer. Wu AH, Pike MC, Stram DO. *J Natl Cancer Inst.* 17;91(6):529-34. 1999

Relation between habitual diet and canine mammary tumors in a case-control study. Perez Alenza MD, Rutteman GR, Pena L, et al. *J Vet Intern Med* 12:132, 1998.

Factors influencing the incidence and prognosis of canine mammary tumours. Perez Alenza MD, Pena L, del Castillo N, Nieto AI. *J Small Anim Pract* 41:287, 2000.

Prognostic factors in canine mammary tumours: a multivariate study of 202 consecutive cases. Hellmen E, Bergstrom R,

Holmberg L, et al. *Vet Pathol* 30:20, 1993

Histopathologic and dietary prognostic factors for canine mammary carcinoma. Shofer FS, Sonnenschein EG, Goldschmidt MH, et al. *Breast Cancer Res Treat*.13(1):49-60. 1989

The lymph drainage of the neoplastic mammary glands in the bitch: a lymphographic study. Patsikas MN, Karayannopoulou M, Kaldrymidoy E, et al. *Anat Histol Embryol*. 2006 Aug;35(4):228-34.

Effect of spaying and timing of spaying on survival of dogs with mammary carcinoma. Sorenmo KU, Shofer FS, Goldschmidt MH. *J Vet Intern Med* 14:266, 2000.

Clinicopathological survey of 101 canine mammary gland tumors: differences between small-breed dogs and others. Itoh T, Uchida K, Ishikawa K, et al. *J Vet Med Sci* 67:345, 2005.

Adjuvant post-operative chemotherapy in bitches with mammary cancer. Karayannopoulou M, Kaldrymidou E, Constantinidis TC, et al. *J Vet Med A Physiol Pathol Clin Med*. 48(2):85-96. 2001

Evaluation of the effect of levamisole and surgery on canine mammary cancer. MacEwen EG, Harvey HJ, Patnaik AK, et al. *J Biol Resp Mod* 25:540, 1985.

Mammary tumor recurrence in bitches after regional mastectomy. Stratmann N, Failing K, Richter A, et al. *Vet Surg* 37(1):82, 2008.

Prognostic factors associated with survival two years after surgery in dogs with malignant mammary tumors: 79 cases (1998-2002). Chang S, Chang C, Chang T, Wong M. *J Am Vet Med Assoc* 227:1625, 2005.

Massage and Touch Therapies

Safety and efficacy of massage therapy for patients with cancer. Corbin L. *Cancer Control*. 2005 Jul;12(3):158-64. Review.

Massage Therapy vs. Simple Touch to Improve Pain and Mood in Patients with Advanced Cancer: A Randomized Trial, Kutner, JS et al. *Ann Intern Med*. 2008 September 16; 149(6): 369-379.

Massage therapy for symptom control: outcome study at a major cancer center. Cassileth BR and Vickers AJ. *J Pain Symptom Manage*. 2004 Sep;28(3):244-9.

WITHDRAWN: Aromatherapy and massage for symptom relief in patients with cancer. Fellowes D, Barnes K, Wilkinson SS. *Cochrane Database Syst Rev*. 2008 Oct 8;(4)

The effect of massage on immune function and stress in women with breast cancer--a randomized controlled trial. Billhult A, et al. *Auton Neurosci*. 2009 Oct 5;150(1-2):111-5.

Role of massage therapy in cancer care. Russell NC, et al. *J Altern Complement Med*. 2008 Mar;14(2):209-14.

Impact of massage therapy on anxiety levels in patients undergoing radiation therapy: randomized controlled trial. Campeau MP, et al. *J Soc Integr Oncol*. 2007 Fall;5(4):133-8.

The use of therapeutic massage as a nursing intervention to modify anxiety and the perception of cancer pain. Ferrell-Torry AT, Glick OJ. *Cancer Nurs*. 1993 Apr;16(2):93-101.

Efficacy of complementary and alternative medicine therapies in relieving cancer pain: a systematic review. Bardia A, et al. *J Clin Oncol*. 2006 Dec 1;24(34):5457-64.

Safety and efficacy of massage therapy for patients with cancer. Corbin L. *Cancer Control*. 2005 Jul;12(3):158-64.

Mast Cell Tumors

Mast Cell Tumors. McCaw DL, in Henry CJ, Higginbotham ML (ed): *Cancer Management in Small Animal Practice*. Missouri. Saunders Elsevier 2010, p 317-321.

Mast cell tumors. Thamm DH, Vail DM, in Withrow SJ, Vail DM (eds): *Withrow & MacEwen's Small Animal Clinical Oncology*. Missouri, Saunders Elsevier, 2007, pp 402-424.

Mast cell tumors, Dog, Geiger T, in Cote E (2nd ed), *Clinical Veterinary Advisor: Dogs and Cats*. Missouri, Mosby Elsevier, 2011, p 701-703.

Canine cutaneous mast cell tumor: morphologic grading and survival time in 83 dogs. Patnaik AK, Ehler WJ, MacEwen EG. *Vet Pathol*. 21:469-74. 1984

Biologic behavior and prognostic factors for mast cell tumors of the canine muzzle: 24 cases (1990-2001). Gieger TL, Théon AP, Werner JA, et al. *J Vet Intern Med*. 17:687. 2003

Mitotic index is predictive for survival for canine cutaneous mast cell tumors. Romansik EM, Reilly DM, Moore PF, et al. *Vet Pathol* 44:355, 2007.

Evaluation of prognostic factors associated with outcome in dogs with multiple cutaneous mast cell tumors treated with surgery with and without adjuvant treatment: 54 cases (1998-2004). Mullins MN, Dernell WS, Withrow SJ, et al. *J Am Vet Med Assoc* 228:91, 2000.

Canine mastocytoma: excess risk as related to ancestry. Peters JA. *J Natl Cancer Inst* 42:435, 1969.

Proposal of a 2-Tier Histologic Grading System for Canine Cutaneous Mast Cell Tumors to More Accurately Predict Biological Behavior. Kiupel M, Webster JD, Bailey KL, et al. *Vet Pathol* 48:147-155, 2011.

Mast Cell Treatment

Evaluation of a two-centimeter lateral surgical margin for excision of grade I and grade II cutaneous mast cell tumors in dogs. Fulcher RP, Ludwig LL, Bergman PJ, et al. *J Am Vet Med Assoc.* 228:210. 2006.

Radiotherapy of incompletely resected, moderately differentiated mast cell tumors in the dog: 37 cases (1989-1993). Frimberger AE, Moore AS, LaRue SM, et al. *J Am Anim Hosp Assoc.* 33(4):320. 1997

A prospective study of radiation therapy for the treatment of grade 2 mast cell tumors in 32 dogs. al-Sarraf R, Mauldin GN, Patnaik AK et al. *J Vet Intern Med.* 10:376. 1996

Treatment of canine mast cell tumours with prednisolone and radiotherapy. Dobson J, Cohen S, Gould S. *Vet Comp Oncol.* 2:132. 2004

Efficacy of radiation therapy for incompletely resected grade III MCT in dogs: 31 cases. Hahn KA, King GK, Carrera JK. *J Am Vet Med Assoc.* 224:79, 2004.

Melanoma

Oral and Salivary Gland Tumors. Henry CJ, Higginbotham ML, in Henry CJ, Higginbotham ML (ed): *Cancer Management in Small Animal Practice.* Missouri. Saunders Elsevier 2010, p 195-203.

Tumors of the Skin, Subcutis and other soft tissues. Northrup N, Geiger T, in Henry CJ, Higginbotham ML (ed): *Cancer Management in Small Animal Practice.* Missouri. Saunders Elsevier 2010, p 299-311.

Oral Tumors. Liptak JM, Withrow SJ. Withrow SJ, Vail DM (eds): *Withrow & MacEwen's Small Animal Clinical Oncology.* Missouri, Saunders Elsevier, 2007, pp 455-475

Melanomain. Proulx DR. Cote E (2nd ed), *Clinical Veterinary Advisor: Dogs and Cats.* Missouri, Mosby Elsevier, 2011, p 711-713.

Multimodality therapy for head and neck cancer. Klein MK. *Vet Clin Small Anim* 33: 615-628, 2003.

Tumors of the Skin and Subcutaneous tissues. Vail DM, Withrow SJ. Withrow SJ, Vail DM (eds): *Withrow & MacEwen's Small Animal Clinical Oncology.* Missouri, Saunders Elsevier, 2007, pp 375-401

Tumors of the Nasal Cavity and Paranasal Sinuses, Nasopharynx, Oral Cavity, and Oropharynx. Schantz SP, Harrison LB, Forastiere AA, in Devita VT, Hellman A, Rosenberg SA (ed.): *Cancer Principles & Practice of Oncology.* NY. Lippincott Williams & Wilkens, 2001. p 797-860

Oral cavity risk factors: experts' opinions and literature sup-

port. Stucken E, Weissman J, Spiegel JH. *J Otolaryngol Head Neck Surg.* 39(1):76-89. 2010

Body Mass Index, Cigarette Smoking, and Alcohol Consumption and Cancers of the Oral Cavity, Pharynx, and Larynx: Modeling Odds Ratios in Pooled Case-Control Data. Lubin JH, Gaudet MM, Olshan AF, et al. *Am J Epidemiol.* 2010 May 21. [Epub ahead of print]

Association between lymph node size and metastasis in dogs with oral malignant melanoma: 100 cases (1987-2001). Williams LE, Packer RA. *J Am Vet Med Assoc* 222:1234, 2003.

Sensitivity and specificity of methods of assessing the regional lymph nodes for evidence of metastasis in dogs and cats with solid tumors. Lagenbach A, McManus PM, Hendrick MJ, et al. *J Am Vet Med Assoc* 218:1424, 2001.

The molecular basis of canine melanoma: pathogenesis and trends in diagnosis and therapy. Modiano JF, Ritt MG, Wojcieszyn J. *J Vet Intern Med* 13:163, 1999.

Histologic features and clinical outcomes of melanomas of lip, haired skin, and nail bed location of dogs. Schultheiss PC. *J Vet Diagn Invest* 18(4):422, 2006.

Retrospective study of 338 canine oral melanomas with clinical, histologic, and immunohistochemical review of 129 cases. Ramos-Vara, JA, Miller MA, Beissenherz ME, et al. *Vet Pathol* 37:597, 2000

Histologic features and clinical outcomes of melanomas of lip, haired skin, and nail bed location of dogs. Schultheiss PC. *J Vet Diagn Invest* 18(4):422, 2006.

Oral Melanoma Treatment

Prognosis after surgical excision of canine melanomas. Bostock DE. *Vet Pathol* 16:32, 1979

Owner satisfaction with partial mandibulectomy or maxillectomy for treatment of oral tumors in 27 dogs. Fox LE, Geoghegan SL, Davis LH, et al. *J Am Anim Hosp Assoc* 33:25, 1997

A retrospective analysis of 140 dogs with oral melanoma treated with external beam radiation. Proulx DR, Ruslander DM, Dodge RK, et al. *Vet Radiol Ultrasound.* 44(3):352-9. 2003

Radiotherapy of oral malignant melanomas in dogs. Blackwood L, Dobson JM. *J Am Vet Med Assoc* 209:98, 1996

Treatment of dogs with oral melanoma by hypofractionated radiation therapy and platinum-based chemotherapy (1987-1997). Freeman KP, Hahn KA, Harris FD, et al. *J Vet Int Med* 17:96, 2003.

Use of carboplatin for treatment of dogs with malignant melanoma: 27 cases (1989-2000). Rassnick KM, Ruslander DM, Cotter SM et al. *J Am Vet Med Assoc.* 218(9):1444-8. 2001

Development of a xenogeneic DNA vaccine program for canine malignant melanoma at the Animal Medical Center. Bergman PJ, et al. *Vaccine* 24:4582-4585. 2006

Long-Term Survival of Dogs with Advanced Malignant Melanoma after DNA Vaccination with Xenogeneic Human Tyrosinase: A Phase I Trial. Bergman PJ, et al. *Clinical Cancer Research* 9:1284-1290. 2003

Vaccination with human tyrosinase DNA induces antibody responses in dogs with advanced melanoma. Liao JCF, et al. *Cancer Immunity* 6:8-17. 2006

Retrospective evaluation of lingual tumors in 42 dogs: 1999-2005. Syrcle JA, Bonczynski JJ, Monette S, et al. *J Am Anim Hosp Assoc* 44:308, 2008.

Digit Melanoma Treatment

Xenogeneic Murine Tyrosinase DNA Vaccine for Malignant Melanoma of the Digit is Dogs. Manley CA, Leibman NF, Wolchok JD, et al. *J Vet Int Med* 25:94, 2011.

Evaluation of dogs with digit masses: 117 cases (1981-1991). Marino DJ, Matthiesen DT, Stefanacci JD, et al. *J Am Vet Med Assoc.* 207(6):726-8. 1995

Canine digital tumors: a veterinary cooperative oncology group retrospective study of 64 dogs. Henry CJ, Brewer WG, Whitley EM, et al. *J Vet Intern Med* 19:720, 2005

Skin Melanoma Treatment

Muller and Kirk's small animal dermatology, ed 5. Scott DW, Miller WH, Griffin CE. Philadelphia, 1995, WB Saunders.

A comparative review of melanocytic neoplasms. Smith SH, Goldschmidt MH, McManus PM. *Vet Pathol* 39:651, 2002.

Characteristics of canine melanomas and comparison of histology and DNA ploidy to their biologic behavior. Bolon B, Calderwood Mays MB, Hall BJ. *Vet Pathol.* 27(2):96-102. 1990

PCNA and Ki67 proliferation markers as criteria for prediction of clinical behaviour of melanocytic tumours in cats and dogs. Roels S, Tilmant K, Ducatelle R. *J Comp Pathol.* 121(1):13-24. 1999

Modified Citrus Pectin

Modified citrus pectin anti-metastatic properties: one bullet, multiple targets. Glinsky VV, Raz A. *Carbohydr Res.* 2009 Sep 28;344(14):1788-91. Epub 2008 Sep 26. Review.

Inhibition of human cancer cell growth and metastasis in nude mice by oral intake of modified citrus pectin. Nangia-Makker P, et al. *J Natl Cancer Inst.* 2002 Dec 18;94(24):1854-62.

Inhibition of spontaneous metastasis in a rat prostate cancer model by oral administration of modified citrus pectin. Pienta KJ, et al. *J Natl Cancer Inst.* 1995 Mar 1;87(5):348-53.

Inhibitory effect of modified citrus pectin on liver metastases in a mouse colon cancer model. Liu HY, Huang ZL, Yang GH, Lu WQ, Yu NR. *World J Gastroenterol.* 2008 Dec 28;14(48):7386-91.

Modified citrus pectin (MCP) increases the prostate-specific antigen doubling time in men with prostate cancer: a phase II pilot study. Guess BW, Scholz MC, Strum SB, Lam RY, Johnson HJ, Jennrich RI. *Prostate Cancer Prostatic Dis.* 2003;6(4):301-4.

Galectin-3 is an important mediator of VEGF- and bFGF-mediated angiogenic response. Markowska AI, Liu FT, Panjwani N. *J Exp Med.* 2010 Aug 30;207(9):1981-93.

PectaSol-C modified citrus pectin induces apoptosis and inhibition of proliferation in human and mouse androgen-dependent and- independent prostate cancer cells. Yan J, Katz A. *Integr Cancer Ther.* 2010 Jun;9(2):197-203.

Pectin induces apoptosis in human prostate cancer cells: correlation of apoptotic function with pectin structure. Jackson CL, et al. *Glycobiology.* 2007 Aug;17(8):805-19.

The role of modified citrus pectin as an effective chelator of lead in children hospitalized with toxic lead levels. Zhao ZY, et al. *Altern Ther Health Med.* 2008 Jul-Aug;14(4):34-8. Erratum in: Altern Ther Health Med. 2008 Nov-Dec;14(6):18.

Integrative medicine and the role of modified citrus pectin/alginates in heavy metal chelation and detoxification—five case reports. Eliaz I, Weil E, Wilk B. *Forsch Komplementmed.* 2007 Dec;14(6):358-64.

The effect of modified citrus pectin on urinary excretion of toxic elements. Eliaz I, et al. *Phytother Res.* 2006 Oct;20(10):859-64.

Nasal Tumors

Nasal Tumors. Higginbotham ML, Henry CJ, in Henry CJ, Higginbotham ML (ed): *Cancer Management in Small Animal Practice.* Missouri. Saunders Elsevier 2010, p 203-210.

Nasosinal Tumors. Turek MM, Lana SE. Withrow SJ, Vail DM (eds): *Withrow & MacEwen's Small Animal Clinical Oncology.* Missouri, Saunders Elsevier, 2007, pp 525-539

Nasal Neoplasia. Fidel JL. in Cote E (2nd ed), *Clinical Veterinary Advisor: Dogs and Cats.* Missouri, Mosby Elsevier, 2011, p 749-751.

Squamous cell carcinomas, Oral (Mucosal, Tonsillar). Garrett LD, in Cote E (ed), *Clinical Veterinary Advisor: Dogs and Cats.* Missouri, Mosby Elsevier, 2007, p 1034-1035.

Multimodality therapy for head and neck cancer. Klein MK. *Vet Clin Small Anim* 33: 615-628, 2003.

Environmental causes for sinonasal cancers in pet dogs, and their usefulness as sentinels of indoor cancer risk. Bukowski JA, Wartenberg D. *J Toxicol Environ Health* 54:579, 1998.

Cancer of the nasal cavity and paranasal sinuses and exposure to environmental tobacco smoke in pet dogs. Reif JS, Bruns C, Lower KS. *Am J Epidemiol* 147:488, 1998.

Nasal tumors in the dog: retrospective evaluation of diagnosis, prognosis, and treatment. MacEwen EG, Withrow SJ, Patnaik AK. *J Am Vet Med Assoc* 170:45, 1977.

Comparison of computed tomography and radiography for detecting changes induced by malignant nasal neoplasia in dogs. Park RD, Beck ER, LeCouteur RA. *J Am Vet Med Assoc* 201:1720, 1992.

Megavoltage irradiation of neoplasms of the nasal and paranasal cavities in 77 dogs. Théon AP, Madewell BR, Harb MF, et al. *J Am Vet Med Assoc* 202:1469, 1993.

Surgical therapy of canine nasal tumors: a retrospective study (1982-1986). Laing EJ, Binnington AG. *Can Vet J* 29:809, 1988

Outcome of accelerated radiotherapy alone or accelerated radiotherapy followed by exenteration of the nasal cavity in dogs with intranasal neoplasia: 53 cases (1990-2002). Adams WM, Bjorling DE, McAnulty JF, et al. *J Am Vet Med Assoc* 227:936, 2005.

Failure patterns following cobalt irradiation in dogs with nasal carcinoma. Thrall DE, Heidner GL, Novotney CA, et al. *Vet Radiol Ultrasound* 34:295-300, 1993.

Factors influencing survival after radiotherapy of nasal tumors in 130 dogs. Ladue TA, Dodge R, Page RL, et al. *Vet Radiol Ultrasound* 40:312-317, 1999.

Use of radiation and a slow-release cisplatin formulation for treatment of canine nasal tumors. Lana SE, Dernell WS, Lafferty MH, et al. *Vet Radiol Ultrasound* 45:577, 2004.

Treatment of eight dogs with nasal tumours with alternating doses of doxorubicin and carboplatin in conjunction with oral piroxicam. Langova V, Mustsaers AJ, Phillips B, et al. *Aust Vet J* 82:676, 2004.

Evaluation of factors associated with survival in dogs with untreated nasal carcinomas: 139 cases (1993-2003). Rassnick KM, Goldkamp CE, Erb HN, et al. *J Am Vet Med Assoc* 229:401, 2006.

Long-term outcome of 56 dogs with nasal tumours treated with four doses of radiation at intervals of seven days. Mellanby RJ, Stevenson RK, Herrtage ME, et al. *Vet Rec* 151:253, 2002.

Oral Cancer

Oral and Salivary Gland Tumors. Henry CJ, Higginbotham ML, in Henry CJ, Higginbotham ML (ed): *Cancer Management in Small Animal Practice.* Missouri. Saunders Elsevier 2010, p 195-203.

Oral Tumors. Liptak JM, Withrown SJ. Withrow SJ, Vail DM (eds): *Withrow & MacEwen's Small Animal Clinical Oncology.* Missouri, Saunders Elsevier, 2007, pp 455-475

Oral Tumors, Malignant. Lewis JR in Cote E (2nd ed), *Clinical Veterinary Advisor: Dogs and Cats.* Missouri, Mosby Elsevier, 2011, p788-790.

Squamous cell carcinomas, Oral (Mucosal, Tonsillar). Garrett LD in Cote E (ed), *Clinical Veterinary Advisor: Dogs and Cats.* Missouri, Mosby Elsevier, 2007, p 1034-1035.

Epulides. Ettinger SN in Cote E (2nd ed), *Clinical Veterinary Advisor: Dogs and Cats.* Missouri, Mosby Elsevier, 2011, p 359-361.

Multimodality therapy for head and neck cancer. Klein MK. *Vet Clin Small Anim* 33: 615-628, 2003.

Malignant tumor formation in dogs previously irradiated for acanthomatous epulis. McEntee MC, Page RL, Theon A, et al. *Vet Radiol Ultrasound* 45:357, 2004.

Orthovoltage radiotherapy of acanthomatous epulides in 39 dogs. Thrall D. *J Am Vet Med Assoc* 184:826, 1984.

Tumors of the Nasal Cavity and Paranasal Sinuses, Nasopharynx, Oral Cavity, and Oropharynx. Schantz SP, Harrison LB, Forastiere AA in Devita VT, Hellman A, Rosenberg SA (ed.): *Cancer Principles & Practice of Oncology.* NY. Lippincott Williams & Wilkens, 2001. p 797-860

Oral cavity risk factors: experts' opinions and literature support. Stucken E, Weissman J, Spiegel JH. *J Otolaryngol Head Neck Surg.* 39(1):76-89. 2010

Body Mass Index, Cigarette Smoking, and Alcohol Consumption and Cancers of the Oral Cavity, Pharynx, and Larynx: Modeling Odds Ratios in Pooled Case-Control Data. Lubin JH, Gaudet MM, Olshan AF, et al. *Am J Epidemiol.* 2010 May 21. [Epub ahead of print]

Association between lymph node size and metastasis in dogs with oral malignant melanoma: 100 cases (1987-2001). Williams LE, Packer RA. *J Am Vet Med Assoc* 222:1234, 2003.

Sensitivity and specificity of methods of assessing the regional lymph nodes for evidence of metastasis in dogs and cats with solid tumors. Lagenbach A, McManus PM, Hendrick MJ, et al. *J Am Vet Med Assoc* 218:1424, 2001.

Owner satisfaction with partial mandibulectomy or maxillectomy for treatment of oral tumors in 27 dogs. Fox LE, Geoghegan SL, Davis LH, et al. *J Am Anim Hosp Assoc* 33:25, 1997

Analysis of prognostic factors and patterns of failure in dogs with malignant oral tumors treated with megavoltage irradiation. Theon AP, Rodriquez C, Madewell BR. *J Am Vet Med Assoc* 210:778, 1997.

Piroxicam and carboplatin as a combination treatment of canine oral non-tonsillar squamous cell carcinoma: a pilot study and a literature review of a canine model of human head and neck squamous cell carcinoma. de Vos JP, Burm AGD, Focker AP, et al. *J Vet Comp Oncol* 3:16, 2005.

Evaluation of piroxicam for the treatment of oral squamous cell carcinoma in dogs. Schmidt BR, Glickman NW, DeNicola DB, et al. *J Am Vet Med Assoc* 218:1783, 2001

Analysis of prognostic factor and patterns of failure in dogs with periodontal tumors treated with megavoltage irradiation. Théon AP, et al. *J Am Vet Med Assoc* 210:785, 1997.

The effect of intralesional bleomycin on canine acanthomatous epulis. Yoshida K, et al. *J Am Anim Hosp Assoc* 34:457, 1998.

Clinicopathological study of canine oral epulides. Yoshida K, et al. *J Vet Med Sci* 61:897, 1999.

Epulides in the dog: A review. Gardner DG. *J Oral Pathol Med* 25:32, 1996.

Postoperative radiotherapy for canine soft tissue sarcoma. Forrest LJ, Chun R, Adams WM, et al. *J Vet Intern Med.* 14(6):578-82. 2000

Lymph node staging of oral and maxillofacial neoplasms in 31 dogs and cats. Herring ES, Smith MM, Robertson JL. *J Vet Dentistry* 19:122, 2002

Osteosarcoma

Tumors of the Musculoskeletal System. Ruslander D, in Henry CJ, Higginbotham ML (ed): *Cancer Management in Small Animal Practice.* Missouri. Saunders Elsevier 2010, p 333-342.

Tumors of the Skeletal System. Dernell WS, Ehrhart NP, Straw RC, et al. in Withrow SJ, Vail DM (eds): *Withrow & MacEwen's Small Animal Clinical Oncology.* Missouri, Saunders Elsevier, 2007, pp 540-582

Osteosarcoma. Bailey DB in Cote E (2nd ed), *Clinical Veterinary Advisor: Dogs and Cats.* Missouri, Mosby Elsevier, 2011, p 801-

803.

Host related risk factors for canine osteosarcoma. Ru G, Terracini B, Glickman LT. *Vet J.* 156(1):31-9. 1998

Osteosarcoma Treatment

Prognosis for dogs with appendicular osteosarcoma treated by amputation alone: 162 cases (1978-1988). Spodnick GJ, Berg J, Rand WM, et al. *J Am Vet Med Assoc.* 200(7):995-9. 1992

Alternating carboplatin and doxorubicin as adjunctive chemotherapy to amputation or limb-sparing surgery in the treatment of appendicular osteosarcoma in dogs. Kent MC, Strom A, London CA, et al. *J Vet Intern Med.* 2004 Jul-Aug;18(4):540-4.

Carboplatin and doxorubicin combination chemotherapy for the treatment of appendicular osteosarcoma in the dog. Bailey D, Erb H, Williams L, et al. *J Vet Intern Med.* 17(2):199-205, 2003

Stereotactic radiosurgery for treatment of osteosarcomas involving the distal portions of the limbs in dogs. Farese JP, Milner R, Thompson MS, et al. *J Am Vet Med Assoc.* 225(10):1567-72, 1548. 2004

Four fraction palliative radiotherapy for osteosarcoma in 24 dogs. Green EM, Adams WM, Forrest LJ. *J Am Anim Hosp Assoc* 38(5):445, 2002.

Palliative radiotherapy for canine appendicular osteosarcoma. McEntee MC, Page RL, Novotney CA, et al. *Vet Radiol Ultrasound* 34:367, 1993.

Palliative radiotherapy of appendicular osteosarcoma in 95 dogs. Ramirez O 3rd, Dodge RK, Page RL, et al. *Vet Radiol Ultrasound* 40:517, 1999.

Interleukin-2 liposome inhalation therapy is safe and effective for dogs with spontaneous pulmonary metastases. Khanna C, Anderson PM, Hasz DE, et al. *Cancer* 79(7):1409-21. 1997

Overfeeding

Effects of home-based diet and exercise on functional outcomes among older, overweight long-term cancer survivors: RENEW: a randomized controlled trial. Morey MC, et al. *JAMA.* 2009 May 13;301(18):1883-91.

Effects of diet restriction on life span and age-related changes in dogs. Kealy RD, et al. *J Am Vet Med Assoc.* 2002 May 1;220(9):1315-20.

Adiponectin and cancer: a systematic review. Kelesidis I, Kelesidis T, Mantzoros CS. *Br J Cancer.* 2006 May 8;94(9):1221-5.

Adiponectin in relation to malignancies: a review of existing basic research and clinical evidence. Barb D, Williams CJ, Neuwirth AK, Mantzoros CS. *Am J Clin Nutr.* 2007 Sep;86(3):s858-66. Review.

Diet and cancer. Divisi D, et al. *Acta Biomed.* 2006 Aug;77(2):118-23. Review.

Perianal and Anal Sac Tumors

Perianal and Anal sac tumors. Higginbotham ML, in Henry CJ, Higginbotham ML (ed): *Cancer Management in Small Animal Practice.* Missouri. Saunders Elsevier 2010, p 330-332.

Perianal Tumors. Turek MM, Withrow SJ. Withrow SJ, Vail DM (eds): *Withrow & MacEwen's Small Animal Clinical Oncology.* St Louis Missouri, Saunders Elsevier, 2007, pp 503-510.

Anal sac tumors. Chun R, in Bonagura JD, Twedt DC (ed): *Kirk's Current Veterinary Therapy XIV.* Missouri. Saunders Elsevier 2009, p 382-384.

Adenocarcinoma, Anal Sac. McNeil EA, in Cote E (2nd ed), *Clinical Veterinary Advisor: Dogs and Cats.* Missouri, Mosby Elsevier, 2011, p 36-37.

Adenoma/Adenocarcinoma, Perianal. McNeil EA, in Cote E (2nd ed), *Clinical Veterinary Advisor: Dogs and Cats.* Missouri, Mosby Elsevier, 2011, p 39-40.

Perianal adenocarcinoma in the canine male: a retrospective study of 41 cases. Vail DM, Withrow SJ, Schwarz PD, Powers BE. *J Am Anim Hosp Assoc* 26:329, 1990.

Hormone-dependent neoplasms of the canine perianal gland. Hayes HM, Wilson GP. *Cancer Res* 37:2068, 1977.

Adenocarcinoma of the apocrine glands of the anal sac in dogs: a review of 32 cases. Ross JT, Scavelli TD, Matthiesen DT, Patnaik AK. *J Am Anim Hosp Assoc* 27:349, 1991.

Canine anal sac adenocarcinomas: clinical presentation and response to therapy. Bennett PF, DeNicola DB, Bonney P, et al. *J Vet Intern Med* 16:100, 2002.

Carcinoma of the apocrine glands of the anal sac in dogs: 113 cases (1985-1995). Williams LE, Gliatto JM, Dodge RK, et al. *J Am Vet Med Assoc* 223:825, 2003

Late complications of pelvic irradiation in 16 dogs. Anderson CR, McNiel EA, Gillette EL, et al. *Vet Radiol Ultrasound* 43:187, 2002.

Clinical stage, therapy and prognosis in canine anal sac gland carcinoma. Polton GA, Brearley MJ. *Vet Intern Med* 21:274, 2007.

Identification of parathyroid hormone-related protein in canine apocrine adenocarcinoma of the anal sac. Rosol TJ, Capen CC, Danks JA, et al. *Vet Pathol* 27:89, 1990.

Parathyroid hormone (PTH)-related protein, PTH, and 1,25-dihydroxyvitamin D in dogs with cancer-associated hypercalcemia. Rosol TJ, Nagode LA, Couto CG, et al. *Endocrinology* 131:1157, 1992.

Cryosurgical treatment of perianal gland adenomas in the dog. Liska WD, Withrow SJ. *J Am Anim Hosp Assoc* 14:457, 1978.

X-irradiation of perianal gland neoplasms in the dog. Morgan JP, Carlson WD. *J Am Vet Med Assoc* 143:1227, 1963.

Surgery of metastatic anal sac adenocarcinoma in five dogs. Hobson HP, Brown MR, Rogers KS. *Vet Surg* 35:267, 2006.

Postoperative radiotherapy and mitoxantrone for anal sac adenocarcinoma in the dog: 15 cases (1991-2001). Turek MM, Forrest LJ, Adams WM, et al. *Veterinary and Comparative Oncology.* 1:94-104. 2003

Prayer

Effects of remote, retroactive intercessory prayer on outcomes in patients with bloodstream infection: randomised controlled trial. Leibovici L. *BMJ.* 2001 Dec 22-29;323(7327):1450-1.

Science, medicine, and intercessory prayer. Sloan RP, Ramakrishnan R. *Perspect Biol Med.* 2006 Autumn;49(4):504-14.

Does religious activity improve health outcomes? A critical review of the recent literature. Coruh B, Ayele H, Pugh M, Mulligan T. *Explore* (NY). 2005 May;1(3):186-91.

Intercessory prayer for the alleviation of ill health. Roberts L, Ahmed I, Hall S, Davison A. *Cochrane Database Syst Rev.* 2009 Apr 15;(2)

Radiation

Radiation therapy. Lattimer JC, Bommarito, et al, in Henry CJ, Higginbotham ML (ed): *Cancer Management in Small Animal Practice.* Missouri. Saunders Elsevier 2010, p 146-56.

Radiation therapy. LaRue SM, Gillette EL, in Withrow SJ, Vail DM (eds): *Withrow & MacEwen's Small Animal Clinical Oncology.* Missouri, Saunders Elsevier, 2007, pp 193-210.

Four fraction palliative radiotherapy for osteosarcoma in 24 dogs. Green EM, Adams WM, Forrest LJ. *J Am Anim Hosp Assoc* 38(5):445, 2002.

Palliative radiotherapy for canine appendicular osteosarcoma. McEntee MC, Page RL, Novotney CA, et al. *Vet Radiol Ultrasound* 34:367, 1993.

Palliative radiotherapy of appendicular osteosarcoma in 95

dogs. Ramirez O 3rd, Dodge RK, Page RL, et al. *Vet Radiol Ultrasound* 40:517, 1999.

Salt

Enhancing effects of dietary salt on both initiation and promotion stages of rat gastric carcinogenesis. Takahashi M and Hasegawa R. *Princess Takamatsu Symp*. 1985;16:169–82.

Dietary sodium chloride intake independently predicts the degree of hyperchloremic metabolic acidosis in healthy humans consuming a net acid-producing diet. Frassetto LA, Morris RC Jr, Sebastian A. *Am J Physiol Renal Physiol*. 2007 Aug;293(2):F521–5.

Silymarin/Silybinin

Effects of the flavonoids biochanin A, morin, phloretin, and silymarin on P-glycoprotein-mediated transport. Zhang S and Morris ME. *J Pharmacol Exp Ther*. 2003 Mar;304(3):1258–67.

Antiproliferative effect of silybin on gynaecological malignancies: synergism with cisplatin and doxorubicin. Scambia G, et al. *Eur J Cancer*. 1996 May;32A(5):877–82.

Silibinin synergizes with mitoxantrone to inhibit cell growth and induce apoptosis in human prostate cancer cells. Flaig TW, et al. *Int J Cancer*. 2007 May 1;120(9):2028–33.

The emerging pharmacotherapeutic significance of the breast cancer resistance protein (ABCG2) Hardwick LJA, Velamakanni S, van Veen HW, *Br J Pharmacol*. 2007 May; 151(2): 163–174.

Dietary feeding of silibinin inhibits prostate tumor growth and progression in transgenic adenocarcinoma of the mouse prostate model. Raina K, et al. *Cancer Res*. 2007 Nov 15;67(22):11083–91.

Oral silibinin inhibits in vivo human bladder tumor xenograft growth involving down-regulation of survivin. Singh RP, et al. *Clin Cancer Res*. 2008 Jan 1;14(1):300–8.

Stage-specific inhibitory effects and associated mechanisms of silibinin on tumor progression and metastasis in transgenic adenocarcinoma of the mouse prostate model. Raina K, et al. *Cancer Res*. 2008 Aug 15;68(16):6822–30.

Silibinin inhibits constitutive and TNFalpha-induced activation of NF-kappaB and sensitizes human prostate carcinoma DU145 cells to TNFalpha-induced apoptosis. Dhanalakshmi S, et al. *Oncogene*. 2002 Mar 7;21(11):1759–67.

Silymarin induces apoptosis primarily through a p53-dependent pathway involving Bcl-2/Bax, cytochrome c release, and caspase activation. Katiyar SK, Roy AM, Baliga MS. *Mol Cancer Ther*. 2005 Feb;4(2):207–16.

Multitargeted therapy of cancer by silymarin. Ramasamy K and Agarwal R. *Cancer Lett*. 2008 Oct 8;269(2):352–62. Epub 2008 May 9.

Comparative bioavailability of silibinin in healthy male volunteers. Kim YC, et al. *Int J Clin Pharmacol Ther*. 2003 Dec;41(12):593–6.

Silibinin activates p53-caspase 2 pathway and causes caspase-mediated cleavage of Cip1/p21 in apoptosis induction in bladder transitional-cell papilloma RT4 cells: evidence for a regulatory loop between p53 and caspase 2. Tyagi A, et al. *Carcinogenesis*. 2006 Nov;27(11):2269–80.

Silymarin causes caspases activation and apoptosis in K562 leukemia cells through inactivation of Akt pathway. Zhong X, et al. *Toxicology*. 2006 Oct 29;227(3):211–6.

Inhibition of P-glycoprotein by natural products in human breast cancer cells. Chung SY, et al. *Arch Pharm Res*. 2005 Jul;28(7):823–8.

Influence of silymarin and its flavonolignans on doxorubicin-iron induced lipid peroxidation in rat heart microsomes and mitochondria in comparison with quercetin. Psotová J, et al. *Phytother Res*. 2002 Mar;16 Suppl 1:S63–7.

Toward the definition of the mechanism of action of silymarin: activities related to cellular protection from toxic damage induced by chemotherapy. Comelli MC, et al. *Integr Cancer Ther*. 2007 Jun;6(2):120–9.

Effect of silibinin on the growth and progression of primary lung tumors in mice. Singh RP, et al. *J Natl Cancer Inst*. 2006 Jun 21;98(12):846–55.

Silibinin inhibits established prostate tumor growth, progression, invasion, and metastasis and suppresses tumor angiogenesis and epithelial-mesenchymal transition in transgenic adenocarcinoma of the mouse prostate model mice. Singh RP, et al. *Clin Cancer Res*. 2008 Dec 1;14(23):7773–80.

Sleep, Melatonin, and Cancer

Melatonin as a chronobiotic/anticancer agent: cellular, biochemical, and molecular mechanisms of action and their implications for circadian-based cancer therapy. Blask DE, Sauer LA, Dauchy RT. *Curr Top Med Chem*. 2002 Feb;2(2):113–32. Review.

Melatonin inhibition of cancer growth in vivo involves suppression of tumor fatty acid metabolism via melatonin receptor-mediated signal transduction events. Blask DE, et al. *Cancer Res*. 1999 Sep 15;59(18):4693–701.

New actions of melatonin on tumor metabolism and growth.

Blask DE, et al. *Biol Signals Recept.* 1999 Jan–Apr;8(1–2):49–55. Review.

Putting cancer to sleep at night: the neuroendocrine/circadian melatonin signal. Blask DE, Dauchy RT, Sauer LA. *Endocrine.* 2005 Jul;27(2):179–88. Review.

Melatonin as a chronobiotic/anticancer agent: cellular, biochemical, and molecular mechanisms of action and their implications for circadian-based cancer therapy. Blask DE, Sauer LA, Dauchy RT. *Curr Top Med Chem.* 2002 Feb;2(2):113–32. Review.

Therapeutic actions of melatonin in cancer: possible mechanisms. Srinivasan V, et al. *Integr Cancer Ther.* 2008 Sep;7(3):189–203. Review.

Circadian stage-dependent inhibition of human breast cancer metabolism and growth by the nocturnal melatonin signal: consequences of its disruption by light at night in rats and women. Blask DE et al. *Integr Cancer Ther.* 2009 Dec;8(4):347–53.

A randomized study of chemotherapy with cisplatin plus etoposide versus chemoendocrine therapy with cisplatin, etoposide and the pineal hormone melatonin as a first-line treatment of advanced non-small cell lung cancer patients in a poor clinical state. Lissoni P, et al. *J Pineal Res.* 1997 Aug;23(1):15–9.

Melatonin in cancer management: progress and promise. Jung B and Ahmad N. *Cancer Res.* 2006 Oct 15;66(20):9789–93.

Melatonin in the treatment of cancer: a systematic review of randomized controlled trials and meta-analysis. Mills E, Wu P, Seely D, Guyatt G. *J Pineal Res.* 2005 Nov;39(4):360–6.

Light at night, chronodisruption, melatonin suppression, and cancer risk: a review. Reiter RJ, et al. *Crit Rev Oncog.* 2007 Dec;13(4):303–28.

Lighting for the human circadian clock: recent research indicates that lighting has become a public health issue. Pauley SM. *Med Hypotheses.* 2004;63(4):588–96.

The modulatory role of melatonin on immune responsiveness. Carrillo-Vico A, et al. *Curr Opin Investig Drugs.* 2006 May;7(5):423–31.

Melatonin, immune function and aging. V Srinivasan, et al. *Immun Ageing.* 2005; 2: 17.

Melatonin for refractory idiopathic thrombocytopenic purpura: a report of 3 cases. Todisco M, Rossi N. *Am J Ther.* 2002 Nov–Dec;9(6):524–6.

Melatonin makes splenectomy unnecessary in two patients with idiopathic thrombocytopenic purpura refractory to corticosteroids. Todisco M. *J Pineal Res.* 2007 Sep;43(2):214.

Soft Tissue Sarcomas

Soft Tissue Sarcomas. Selting KA, in Henry CJ, Higginbotham ML (ed): *Cancer Management in Small Animal Practice.* Missouri. Saunders Elsevier 2010, p 321-325.

Soft Tissue Sarcomas. Liptak JM, Forrest LJ. Withrow SJ, Vail DM (eds): *Withrow & MacEwen's Small Animal Clinical Oncology.* St Louis Missouri, Saunders Elsevier, 2007, pp 425-454.

Soft-Tissue Sarcomas. Farrelly J, in Cote E (2nd ed), *Clinical Veterinary Advisor: Dogs and Cats.* Missouri, Mosby Elsevier, 2011, p 1064-1035.

Management of Soft Tissue Sarcomas. Rassnick KM. *Vet Clin Small Anim* 33: 517-531, 2003.

Principles of treatment for Soft-Tissue Sarcomas in the dog. Ettinger SN. *Clin Tech Small Anim Pract* 18:118-122, 2003.

Prognostic significance of intratumoral microvessel density in canine soft-tissue sarcomas. Luong RH, Baer KE, Craft DM, Ettinger SN, et al. *Vet Pathol.* 43(5):622-31. 2006

Association of argyrophilic nucleolar organizing regions, Ki-67, and proliferating cell nuclear antigen scores with histologic grade and survival in dogs with soft tissue sarcomas: 60 cases (1996-2002). Ettinger SN, Scase TJ, Oberthaler KT, et al. *J Am Vet Med Assoc.* 228(7):1053-62. 2006

Prognostic factors for surgical treatment of soft-tissue sarcomas in dogs: 75 cases (1986-1996). Kuntz CA, Dernell WS, Powers BE, et al. *J Am Vet Med Assoc* 211: 1147-1151, 1997

Radiation treatment for incompletely resected soft-tissue sarcomas in dogs. McKnight JA, Mauldin GN, McEntee MC, et al. *J Am Vet Med Assoc* 217:205-10, 2000

Prognosis after surgical excision of canine fibrous connective tissue sarcomas. Bostock DE, Dye MT. *Vet Pathol* 17:581-8, 1980

Radiotherapy of soft tissue sarcomas in dogs. McChesney SL, Withrow SJ, Gillette EL, et al. *J Am Vet Med Assoc* 194:60-3, 1989

Postoperative radiotherapy for canine soft tissue sarcoma. Forrest LJ, Chun R, Adams WM, et al. *J Vet Intern Med* 14:578-82, 2000

Efficacy of mitoxantrone against various neoplasms in dogs. Ogilvie GK, Obradovich JE, Elmslie RE, et al. *J Am Vet Med Assoc* 198:1618-21, 1991

Phase II evaluation of doxorubicin for treatment of various canine neoplasms. Ogilvie GK, Reynolds HA, Richardson RC, et al. *J Am Vet Med Assoc* 195:1580-3, 1989

Soft tissue sarcomas and mast cell tumours in dogs; clinical behaviour and response to surgery. Baker-Gabb M, Hunt GB,

France MP. *Aust Vet J* 81:732, 2003.

Immunohistochemical and histopathologic features of 14 malignant fibrous histiocytomas from Flat-Coated Retrievers. Morris JS, McInnes EF, Bostock DE, et al. *Vet Pathol* 39:473, 2002

Histopathological survey of neoplasms in flat-coated retrievers, 1990 to 1998. Morris JS, Bostock DE, McInnes EF, et al. *Vet Rec* 147:291, 2000

Outcome of dogs with high-grade soft tissue sarcomas treated with and without adjuvant doxorubicin chemotherapy: 39 cases (1996-2004). Selting KA, Powers BE, Thompson LJ, et al. *J Am Vet Med Assoc* 227:1442, 2005.

Metronomic therapy with cyclophosphamide and piroxicam effectively delays tumor recurrence in dogs with incompletely resected soft tissue sarcomas. Elmslie RE, Glawe P, Dow SW. *J Vet Intern Med.* 22(6):1373-9. 2008

Spaying and neutering

For a provocative look at the health considerations of spaying and neutering, see: Long-Term Health Risks and Benefits Associated with Spay / Neuter in Dogs http://www.naiaonline.org/pdfs/LongTermHealthEffectsOfSpayNeuterInDogs.pdf

Factors influencing canine mammary cancer development and postsurgical survival. Schneider R, Dorn CR, Taylor DO. *J Natl Cancer Inst.* 1969 Dec;43(6):1249-61.

Hormonal and Sex Impact on the Epidemiology of Canine Lymphoma. Villamil, JA, et al. *J Cancer Epidemiol.* 2009; 2009: 591753.

Endogenous gonadal hormone exposure and bone sarcoma risk. Cooley DM, et al. *Cancer Epidemiol Biomarkers Prev.* 2002 Nov;11(11):1434-40.

A population study of neutering status as a risk factor for canine prostate cancer. Bryan JN, et al. *Prostate.* 2007 Aug 1;67(11):1174-81.

Castration for treatment of perianal gland neoplasms in the dog. Wilson GP, Hayes HM Jr. *J Am Vet Med Assoc.* 1979 Jun 15;174(12):1301-3.

Effect of spaying and timing of spaying on survival of dogs with mammary carcinoma. Sorenmo KU, Shofer FS, Goldschmidt MH. *J Vet Intern Med.* 2000 May-Jun;14(3):266-70.

Long -term risks and benefits of pediatric gonadectomy in dogs. Spain CV, Scarlett JM, Houpt KA, *JAVMA.* 2004. 224(3):380-387.

Canine prostate carcinoma: epidemiological evidence of an increased risk in castrated dogs. Teske E, et al. *Mol Cell Endocrinol.*

2002 Nov 29;197(1-2):251-5.

Hormonal and Sex Impact on the Epidemiology of Canine Lymphoma, Villamil JA, et al. *J Cancer Epidemiol.* 2009; 2009: 591753.

Specific Cancer Tests (excluding cytology and biopsy)

Evaluation of a bladder tumor antigen test as a screening test for transitional cell carcinoma of the lower urinary tract in dogs. Henry CJ, et al., *Am J Vet Res.* 2003 Aug;64(8):1017-20.

Information about Pet Screen can be found on their website at www.pet-screen.com

Information about Oncopet can be found on their website at www.oncopetdiagnostics.com/

Stress, Depression and Psychoneuroimmunology

Chronic stress promotes tumor growth and angiogenesis in a mouse model of ovarian carcinoma. Thaker PH, et al. *Nat Med.* 2006 Aug;12(8):939-44. Epub 2006 Jul 23.

The neuroendocrine impact of chronic stress on cancer. Thaker PH, Lutgendorf SK, Sood AK. *Cell Cycle.* 2007 Feb 15;6(4):430-3. Epub 2007 Feb 9. Review.

Neuroendocrine influences on cancer biology. Thaker PH, Sood AK. *Semin Cancer Biol.* 2008 Jun;18(3):164-70. Epub 2007 Dec 8. Review.

Neuroendocrine modulation of cancer progression. Armaiz-Pena GN, et al. *Brain Behav Immun.* 2009 Jan;23(1):10-5. Epub 2008 Jun 27. Review.

Does the pineal gland have a role in the psychological mechanisms involved in the progression of cancer? Callaghan BD. *Med Hypotheses.* 2002 Sep;59(3):302-11.

Stress, cancer and circadian rhythm of melatonin, Kwiatkowski F, et al. *Pathol Biol (Paris).* 2005 Jun;53(5):269-72. Epub 2005 Jan 20. Review. French.

Major depression and cancer: the 13-year follow-up of the Baltimore epidemiologic catchment area sample (United States). Gallo JJ, et al. *Cancer Causes Control.* 2000 Sep;11(8):751-8.

Depression and cancer risk: 24 years of follow-up of the Baltimore Epidemiologic Catchment Area sample. Gross AL, Gallo JJ, Eaton WW. *Cancer Causes Control.* 2010 Feb;21(2):191-9. Epub 2009 Nov 3.

How chronic stress exacerbates cancer, Wells, WA. *J Cell Biol.* 2006 August 14; 174(4): 476.

Depression and cancer: recent data on clinical issues, research challenges and treatment approaches. Reich M. *Curr Opin Oncol.* 2008 Jul;20(4):353-9. Review.

The social-psychological precursors to cancer. Cooper CL. *J Human Stress.* 1984 Spring;10(1):4-11.

Incidence and perception of psychosocial stress: the relationship with breast cancer. Cooper CL, Cooper R, Faragher EB. *Psychol Med.* 1989 May;19(2):415-22.

Stress, cancer and immunity. New developments in biopsychosocial and psychoneuroimmunologic research. Baltrusch HJ, Stangel W, Titze I. *Acta Neurol (Napoli).* 1991 Aug;13(4):315-27. Review.

Personality Predictors of the Time Course for Lung Cancer Onset, Augustine AA, et al. *J Res Pers.* 2008 December; 42(6): 1448–1455.

Type A stress prone behaviour and breast cancer. Faragher EB, Cooper CL. *Psychol Med.* 1990 Aug;20(3):663-70.

Psychosocial stress and breast cancer: the inter-relationship between stress events, coping strategies and personality. Cooper CL, Faragher EB. *Psychol Med.* 1993 Aug;23(3):653-62.

Surgery

Surgical Interventions is Cancer. Pope ER, in Henry CJ, Higginbotham ML (ed): *Cancer Management in Small Animal Practice.* Missouri. Saunders Elsevier 2010, p 136-145.

Biopsy Principle. Ehrhart NP, Withrow SJ, in Withrow SJ, Vail DM (eds): *Withrow & MacEwen's Small Animal Clinical Oncology.* Missouri, Saunders Elsevier, 2007, pp 147-153.

Surgical Oncology. Withrow SJ In Withrow SJ, Vail DM (eds): *Withrow & MacEwen's Small Animal Clinical Oncology.* Missouri, Saunders Elsevier, 2007, pp 157-162.

Suppression of natural killer cell activity and promotion of tumor metastasis by ketamine, thiopental, and halothane, but not by propofol: mediating mechanisms and prophylactic measures. Melamed R, Bar-Yosef S, Shakhar G, Shakhar K, Ben-Eliyahu S. *Anesth Analg.* 2003 Nov;97(5):1331-9.

Transitional Cell Carcinoma

Bladder and Urethral Tumors. Henry CJ, in Henry
CJ, Higginbotham ML (ed): *Cancer Management in Small Animal Practice.* Missouri. Saunders Elsevier 2010, p 290-296.

Tumors of the urinary system. Knapp DW. Withrow SJ, Vail DM (eds): *Withrow & MacEwen's Small Animal Clinical Oncology.* St Louis Missouri, Saunders Elsevier, 2007, pp 649-658

Transitional Cell Carcinoma. Bryan JN, in Cote E (2nd ed), *Clinical Veterinary Advisor: Dogs and Cats.* Missouri, Mosby Elsevier, 2011, p 1112-1114.

Management of Transitional Cell Carcinoma. Henry CJ. *Vet Clin Small Anim* 33: 597-614, 2003.

Evaluation of a bladder tumor antigen test as a screening test for transitional cell carcinoma of the lower urinary tract in dogs. Henry CJ, Tyler JW, McEntee MC, et al. *Am J Vet Res* 64:1017, 2003.

Epidemiologic study of insecticide exposures, obesity, and risk of bladder cancer in household dogs. Glickman LT, Schofer FS, McKee LF, et al. *J Tox Environ Health* 28(4):407, 1989.

Herbicide exposure and the risk of transitional cell carcinoma of the urinary bladder in Scottish terrier dogs. Glickman LT, Raghyavan M, Knapp DW et al. *J Am Vet Med Assoc* 224:1290-1297, 2004.

Evaluation of the effect of dietary vegetable consumption on reducing risk of transitional cell carcinoma of the urinary bladder in Scottish Terriers. Raghavan M, Knapp DW, Bonney PL, et al. *J Am Vet Med Assoc.* 227(1):94-100. 2005

Clinical evaluation of mitoxantrone and piroxicam in a canine model of human invasive urinary bladder carcinoma. Henry CJ, McCaw DL, Turnquist SE, et al. *Clin Cancer Res* 9:906, 2003.

Piroxicam therapy in 34 dogs with transitional cell carcinoma of the urinary bladder. Knapp DW, Richardson RC, Chan TC, et al. *J Vet Int Med* 8:273, 1994.

Canine bladder and urethral tumors: a retrospective study of 115 cases (1980-1985). Norris AM, Laing EJ, Valli VEO, et al. *J Vet Intern Med* 6(3):145, 1992.

Surgically induced tumor-seeding in eight dogs and two cats. Gilson SD, Stone EA. *J Am Vet Med Assoc* 196(11):1811, 1990.

Piroxicam, mitoxantrone, and course fraction radiotherapy for the treatment of transitional cell carcinoma of the bladder in 10 dogs: a pilot study. Poirier VJ, Forrest LJ, Adams WM, et al. *J Am Anim Hosp Assoc* 40:131, 2004.

Surgically induced tumor-seeding in eight dogs and two cats. Gilson SD, Stone EA. *J Am Vet Med Assoc* 196(11):1811, 1990.

Needle-tract implantation following US-guided fine-needle aspiration biopsy of transitional cell carcinoma of the bladder, urethra, and prostate. Nyland TG, Wallack ST, Wisner ER. *Vet Radiol Ultrasound* 43(1):50, 2002.

Evaluation of a bladder tumor antigen test as a screening test for transitional cell carcinoma of the lower urinary tract in dogs. Henry CJ, Tyler JW, McEntee MC, et al. *Am J Vet Res* 64:1017, 2003.

Radiographic appearance of pulmonary metastases from transitional cell carcinoma of the bladder and urethra of the dog. Walter PA, Haynes JS, Feeney DA, et al. *J Am Vet Med Assoc* 185(4):411, 1984.

Evaluation of carbon dioxide laser ablation combined with mitoxantrone and piroxicam treatment in dogs with transitional cell carcinoma. Upton ML, Tangner CH, Payton ME. *J Am Vet Med Assoc* 228:549, 2006.

Prognostic factors in dogs with urinary bladder carcinoma. Rocha TA, Mauldin GN, Patnaik AK, et al. *J Vet Intern Med* 14(5): 486-90

Canine transitional cell carcinoma. Mutsaers AJ, Widmer WR, Knapp DW. *J Vet Intern Med* 17:136, 2003

Vaccination (infant) and TH2 shift with potential cancer impact

Optimization of vaccine responses in early life: the role of delivery systems and immunomodulators. Kovarik J, Siegrist CA. *Immunol Cell Biol*. 1998 Jun;76(3):222-36. Review.

The generation of Th memory in neonates versus adults: prolonged primary Th2 effector function and impaired development of Th1 memory effector function in murine neonates. Adkins B, Bu Y, Guevara P. *J Immunol*. 2001 Jan 15;166(2):918-25.

Molecular immunological approaches to biotherapy of human cancers--a review, hypothesis and implications. Becker Y. *Anticancer Res*. 2006 Mar-Apr;26(2A):1113-34. Review.

Development of neonatal Th1/Th2 function. Adkins B. *Int Rev Immunol*. 2000;19(2-3):157-71. Review.

The role of activation-induced cell death in the differentiation of T-helper-cell subsets. Roberts AI, Devadas S, Zhang X, Zhang L, Keegan A, Greeneltch K, Solomon J, Wei L, Das J, Sun E, Liu C, Yuan Z, Zhou JN, Shi Y. *Immunol Res*. 2003;28(3):285-93. Review.

Disease-associated Bias in T Helper Type 1 (Th1)/Th2 CD4+ T Cell Responses Against MAGE-6 in HLA-DRB1*0401+ Patients With Renal Cell Carcinoma or Melanoma, Tatsumi, T et al. *J Exp Med*. 2002 September 2; 196(5): 619–628.

Tumor antigen–specific T helper cells in cancer immunity and immunotherapy. Knutson KL, Disis ML. *Cancer Immunol Immunother*. 2005 Aug;54(8):721-8. Epub 2005 Jan 27. Review.

Vegetables

Allyl isothiocyanate, a constituent of cruciferous vegetables, inhibits growth of PC-3 human prostate cancer xenografts in vivo. Srivastava SK, et al. *Carcinogenesis*. 2003 Oct;24(10):1665-70.

Phytochemicals from cruciferous plants protect against cancer by modulating carcinogen metabolism. Talalay P, Fahey JW. *J Nutr*. 2001 Nov;131(11 Suppl):3027S-33S. Review.

Effects of cruciferous vegetables and their constituents on drug metabolizing enzymes involved in the bioactivation of DNA-reactive dietary carcinogens. Steinkellner H, et al. *Mutat Res*. 2001 Sep 1;480-481:285-97.

Human metabolism and excretion of cancer chemoprotective glucosinolates and isothiocyanates of cruciferous vegetables. Shapiro TA, et al. *Cancer Epidemiol Biomarkers Prev*. 1998 Dec;7(12):1091-100.

Phytochemicals from cruciferous plants protect against cancer by modulating carcinogen metabolism. Talalay P and Fahey JW. *J Nutr*. 2001 Nov;131(11 Suppl):3027S-33S.

Phytochemicals from cruciferous plants protect against cancer by modulating carcinogen metabolism. Talalay P and Fahey JW. *J Nutr*. 2001 Nov;131(11 Suppl):3027S-33S.

Evaluation of the effect of dietary vegetable consumption on reducing risk of transitional cell carcinoma of the urinary bladder in Scottish Terriers. Raghavan M, et al. *J Am Vet Med Assoc*. 2005 Jul 1;227(1):94-100.

Vitamin D and Sunlight

Ecologic studies of solar UV-B radiation and cancer mortality rates. Grant WB. *Recent Results Cancer Res*. 2003;164:371-7. Review.

Ecological studies of ultraviolet B, vitamin D and cancer since 2000. Grant WB, Mohr SB. *Ann Epidemiol*. 2009 Jul;19(7):446-54. Epub 2009 Mar 9. Review.

Current impediments to acceptance of the ultraviolet-B-vitamin D-cancer hypothesis. Grant WB, Boucher BJ. *Anticancer Res*. 2009 Sep;29(9):3597-604. Review.

How strong is the evidence that solar ultraviolet B and vitamin D reduce the risk of cancer?: An examination using Hill's criteria for causality. Grant WB. *Dermatoendocrinol*. 2009 Jan;1(1):17-24.

Lower vitamin-D production from solar ultraviolet-B irradiance may explain some differences in cancer survival rates. Grant WB. *J Natl Med Assoc*. 2006 Mar;98(3):357-64.

The association of solar ultraviolet B (UVB) with reducing risk of cancer: multifactorial ecologic analysis of geographic variation in age-adjusted cancer mortality rates. Grant WB and Garland CF. *Anticancer Res*. 2006 Jul-Aug;26(4A):2687-99.

Sunlight, vitamin D, and ovarian cancer mortality rates in US women. Lefkowitz ES and Garland CF. *Int J Epidemiol.* 1994 Dec;23(6):1133-6.

Sunlight-skin cancer association in the dog: a report of three cases. Madewell BR, Conroy JD, Hodgkins EM. *J Cutan Pathol.* 1981 Dec;8(6):434–43.

Canine conjunctival hemangioma and hemangiosarcoma: a retrospective evaluation of 108 cases (1989-2004). Pirie CG, et al. *Vet Ophthalmol.* 2006 Jul-Aug;9(4):215-26.

The role of vitamin D in cancer prevention. Garland CF, et al. *Am J Public Health.* 2006 Feb;96(2):252-61.

Vitamin D and intervention trials in prostate cancer: from theory to therapy. Schwartz GG. *Ann Epidemiol.* 2009 Feb;19(2):96-102. Epub 2008 Jul 10.

Commonly recommended daily intake of vitamin D is not sufficient if sunlight exposure is limited. Glerup H, et al. *J Intern Med.* 2000 Feb;247(2):260-8.

Impact of oral vitamin D supplementation on serum 25-hydroxyvitamin D levels in oncology. Vashi, PG, et al. *Nutr J.* 2010; 9: 60.

Estimates of beneficial and harmful sun exposure times during the year for major Australian population centres. Samanek AJ, Croager EJ, Gies P, Milne E, Prince R, McMichael AJ, Lucas RM, Slevin T; *Skin Cancer Prevention. Med J* Aust. 2006 Apr 3;184(7):338-41.

UK Food Standards Agency Workshop Report: an investigation of the relative contributions of diet and sunlight to vitamin D status. Ashwell M, Stone EM, Stolte H, Cashman KD, Macdonald H, Lanham-New S, Hiom S, Webb A, Fraser D. *Br J Nutr.* 2010 Aug;104(4):603-11.

Low vitamin D status: definition, prevalence, consequences, and correction. Binkley N, Ramamurthy R, Krueger D. *Endocrinol Metab Clin North Am.* 2010 Jun;39(2):287-301

Water

Center for Disease Control Statement on water fluoridation and osteosarcoma: http://www.cdc.gov/fluoridation/fact_sheets/osteosarcoma.htm

Occurrence, genotoxicity, and carcinogenicity of regulated and emerging disinfection by-products in drinking water: a review and roadmap for research. Richardson SD, et al. *Mutat Res.* 2007 Nov-Dec;636(1-3):178-242. Epub 2007 Sep 12. Review.

Age-specific fluoride exposure in drinking water and osteosarcoma (United States). Bassin EB, et al. *Cancer Causes Control.* 2006 May;17(4):421-8.

Municipal drinking water nitrate level and cancer risk in older women: the Iowa Women's Health Study. Weyer PJ, et al. *Epidemiology.* 2001 May;12(3):327-38.

Drinking water and cancer. Cantor KP. *Cancer Causes Control.* 1997 May;8(3):292-308. Review.

Effects and interactions in an environmentally relevant mixture of pharmaceuticals. Pomati F, Orlandi C, Clerici M, Luciani F, Zuccato E. *Toxicol Sci.* 2008 Mar;102(1):129-37. Epub 2007 Nov 28.

Ultra-trace analysis of multiple endocrine-disrupting chemicals in municipal and bleached kraft mill effluents using gas chromatography-high-resolution mass spectrometry. Ikonomou MG, et. al. *Environ Toxicol Chem.* 2008 Feb;27(2):243-51.

The asbestos cancer epidemic. LaDou J. *Environ Health Perspect.* 2004 Mar;112(3):285-90.

Asbestos is still with us: repeat call for a universal ban. Collegium Ramazzini. *Int J Occup Environ Health.* 2010 Jul-Sep;16(3):351-5.

Cancer incidence and asbestos in drinking water, Town of Woodstock, New York, 1980-1998. Browne ML, Varadarajulu D, Lewis-Michl EL, Fitzgerald EF. *Environ Res.* 2005 Jun;98(2):224-32.

Cancer incidence in relation to asbestos in drinking water in the Puget Sound region. Polissar L, Severson RK, Boatman ES, Thomas DB. *Am J Epidemiol.* 1982 Aug;116(2):314-28.

2008 Associated Press Investigative Series on Water Quality Professor at Harvard Is Being Investigated; Fluoride-Cancer Link May Have Been Hidden, Eilperin, J. *The Washington Post.* Washington, DC. The Washington Post Company; [updated 13 Jul 2005; cited 2 Jan 2009]

Nitrate in public water supplies and the risk of renal cell carcinoma. Ward MH, Rusiecki JA, Lynch CF, Cantor KP. *Cancer Causes Control.* 2007 Dec;18(10):1141-51. Epub 2007 Aug 24. Drinking water and cancer. Cantor KP. *Cancer Causes Control.* 1997 May;8(3):292-308.

Removal of pharmaceuticals during drinking water treatment. Ternes TA, et al. *Environ Sci Technol.* 2002 Sep 1;36(17):3855-63.

Fate and removal of pharmaceuticals and illicit drugs in conventional and membrane bioreactor wastewater treatment plants and by riverbank filtration. Petrovic M, et al. *Philos Transact A Math Phys Eng Sci.* 2009 Oct 13;367(1904):3979-4003.

From municipal sewage to drinking water: fate and removal of pharmaceutical residues in the aquatic environment in urban areas. Heberer T, Reddersen K, Mechlinski A. *Water Sci Technol.*

2002;46(3):81–8.

Ozonation and advanced oxidation technologies to remove endocrine disrupting chemicals (EDCs) and pharmaceuticals and personal care products (PPCPs) in water effluents. Esplugas S, et al. *J Hazard Mater.* 2007 Nov 19;149(3):631-42. Epub 2007 Jul 28.

Index

Symbols

3-D conformal radiation 364
5-FU 140, 146, 325

A

AAHA Helping Pets Fund 272, 426

abscess 381

acai 417

acanthomatous ameloblastoma 83, 353–354, 358

acetaminophen 335

acid 61, 81, 100, 145, 174, 208, 311, 458

acrylamide 75, 76, 434, 444

actinomycin-D 307

acupressure 223, 431

acupuncture 46, 258–259, 280, 425, 431

acute reactions 125, 439

acute tumor lysis syndrome 300

adaptive immune system 88

Addison's disease 143, 208, 382

adenocarcinomas 320, 322, 360, 379, 380, 381, 383, 402, 457–458

adenoma 82, 84, 122, 320, 379–381, 383, 457

adiponectin 198, 435, 456

adrenal glands 407

adrenal tumor 380

Adriamycin 139, 140, 385, 400–401, 439–441

aerosol chemotherapy 334

Afghan Hound 236

aggression, dog 84, 231, 268, 373

aggression, tumor 50, 72, 84, 97, 98, 100, 112, 160, 297, 309, 315–316, 320, 322, 326, 327, 331, 337–338, 354, 360, 366, 368, 370, 380, 382, 383, 387

AgNOR 314, 368

Agus, Dr. David 59

air quality 47, 72, 78–80, 113, 215, 217, 280, 286, 360, 437–438

Airedale Terrier 236, 298, 347, 361

Alaskan Malamutes 380

alcohol 354, 387, 453, 455

algae 139, 170, 417

alkaline phosphatase 329, 330, 332

alkylating agent 395–398

allergic reaction 116, 118, 179, 204, 213, 309, 401, 403

allergies 51, 107, 206, 244, 310, 314, 401, 422

aloe 125, 417

Aloha Medicinals 182, 186

alopecia 138–139

alternative medicine 5, 7, 63, 107, 111, 161, 452

Alzheimer's 64

amantadine 178, 233, 335

ameloblastomas 353, 354

American Academy of Veterinary Acupuncture 259, 425

American College of Veterinary Internal Medicine 53, 258, 425

American Holistic Veterinary Medical Association 258, 259, 425

amifostine 364

amino acid 146, 202, 402

amitriptyline 233

amputation 2, 121, 235, 244, 246, 272, 327, 328, 330–334, 335, 336, 370, 391, 409, 426, 456

anal gland tumors 379–386

anal sac 379, 380

anal sac adenocarcinoma 82, 379–383, 402, 457

anal sac carcinoma 82, 138, 406

analysis 54, 56, 239

analysis paralysis 252–253

anaphylaxis 310, 401, 403

anaplastic tumors 322

anemia 138, 140, 209, 298, 301, 314, 338, 339, 342, 400, 419, 440

anesthesia 113, 115, 118–119, 120, 125

Angels for Animals 271, 426

anger 4, 16, 28, 41, 54, 284, 340, 443

angiogenesis 46, 52, 61, 137, 163, 165, 167, 173, 181, 185, 191, 192, 214, 318, 334, 335, 341, 344, 358, 368, 406, 433, 440, 441, 442, 458, 460

angiosarcoma 337

Animal Cancer Therapy Subsidization Society 272, 426

Animal Specialty Center 10, 124

antacid 145, 193, 318

anthracyclines 400–402, 439, 440

antibiotic 113, 116–117, 120, 125, 126, 130, 131, 135, 137, 192, 205, 303, 332, 348, 351, 361, 364, 396, 397, 402, 405

antibody/antibodies 88, 435, 449, 454

anti-convulsant 375, 377

anti-estrogen therapy 326

antihistamine 146, 401, 403

anti-inflammatory 64, 74, 93, 125, 166, 169, 176, 179, 189, 190, 207, 232, 305, 335, 351, 358, 365, 407, 408, 417, 418, 419, 421, 448

antimetabolites 398

antioxidant/antioxidants 72, 91–94, 149, 150, 151, 165, 170–171, 175, 186–190, 401, 402, 413, 416, 417, 418, 419, 421, 422, 423, 431, 443, 451

antitumor metabolites 400

anus 379, 380, 384

anxiety 29, 144, 222, 223, 233, 256, 452

apathy 231

apigenin 92, 155, 156, 157, 162, 167–168, 172, 173, 432, 433, 448

Apocaps 53, 60, 105, 154, 155–172, 175, 176, 177, 178, 182, 232, 280, 407, 408, 414, 416, 425

apocrine adenocarcinoma 380, 457

apocrine gland adenocarcinoma 379

apocrine gland anal sac adenocarcinomas 380

apoptogen 8–9, 46, 70, 152–179, 189

apoptosis 8, 46–47, 54, 60, 61, 62, 64, 69–71, 152, 156, 163, 164, 165, 167, 176, 181, 192, 400, 432, 433, 434, 435, 441, 445, 448, 454, 458

apoptosis and stress 90–91,

apoptosis and free radicals 91–94

appendicular bones 327

appetite, loss of 22, 140–148. 162, 279–280

apples 190

appointment, preparing for 131, 134, 256–257, 281–283, 292

arctic breeds 82, 380

Armstrong, Lance 109

arrhythmias 300, 339, 342, 401, 445

artemether 171, 173, 174

artemisinin 164, 170–172, 172–176, 178, 187, 212, 409, 433

About the Authors

Demian Dressler, DVM

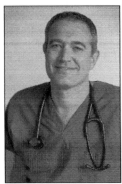

Photo Credit: Michelle Brady

Dr. Demian Dressler is internationally recognized as "the dog cancer vet" because of his innovations in the field of dog cancer management, and the popularity of his blog, www.DogCancerBlog.com. The owner of South Shore Veterinary Care, a full-service veterinary hospital in Maui, Hawaii, Dr. Dressler studied Animal Physiology and received a Bachelor of Science degree from the University of California at Davis before earning his Doctorate in Veterinary Medicine from Cornell University. After practicing at Killewald Animal Hospital in Amherst, New York, he returned to his home state, Hawaii, to practice at the East Honolulu Pet Hospital before heading home to Maui to open his own hospital. Dr. Dressler consults both dog lovers and veterinary professionals, and is sought after as a speaker on topics ranging from the links between lifestyle choices and disease, nutrition and cancer, and animal ethics. His television appearances include "Ask the Vet" segments on local news programs. Dr. Dressler is the cofounder of Functional Nutriments, LLC, a nutraceutical company, and is the inventor of Apocaps, the first clinical apoptogen formula. Dr. Dressler is a member of the American Veterinary Medical Association, the Hawaii Veterinary Medical Association, the American Association of Avian Veterinarians, the National Animal Supplement Council and CORE (Comparative Orthopedic Research Evaluation). He is also an advisory board member for Pacific Primate Sanctuary. He and his wife, Allison, live on Maui, Hawaii, with their dog, Bjorn, and their cat, Ginsu.

Susan Ettinger, DVM, Dip. ACVIM (Oncology)

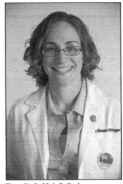

Photo Credit: Michelle Brady

Dr. Susan Ettinger is a staff medical oncologist at Animal Specialty Center in Yonkers, New York, and board-certified by the American College of Veterinary Internal Medicine (Oncology). After earning a B.S. in biology at Tufts University, she received a Doctorate in Veterinary Medicine from Cornell University. She completed her small animal medicine and surgery internship before joining the Department of Radiation Oncology at Duke University Medical Center in Durham, North Carolina, as a research associate and investigator in a five-year NIH program project grant. Dr. Ettinger was also an instructor in the Department of Molecular Medicine and an oncology associate with the Comparative Cancer Program at Cornell. During her residency in medical oncology at The Animal Medical Center in New York City she conducted research in soft tissue sarcomas in dogs. Dr. Ettinger served as a staff oncologist at South Bay Veterinary Associates in San Jose, California, and affiliated with the Veterinary Tumor Institute, a radiation oncology facility in Santa Cruz. After relocating to New York, she became a staff oncologist at Long Island Veterinary Specialists before rejoining Animal Specialty Center. She is well-known for compassionate, comprehensive cancer management with a focus on quality of life and palliative care. She and her husband, Kerry, who is also a veterinarian, live with their two sons, their dog, Matilda, and two cats, Jeter and Raziel, in New York.

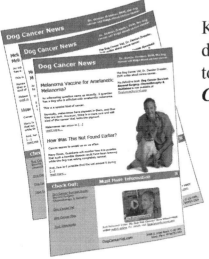
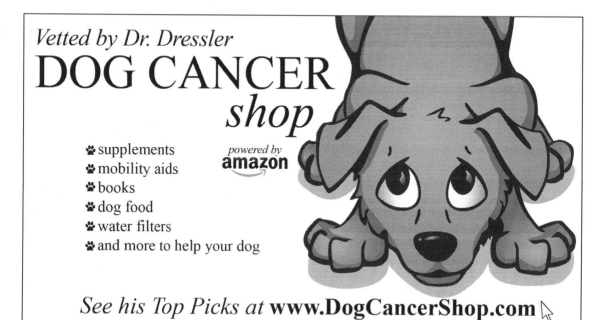

Made in the USA
Lexington, KY
21 September 2011